Promoting Health
Through Risk Reduction

Promoting Health Through Risk Reduction

Edited by

Marilyn M. Faber
Wellness Activities Director
Children's Hospital, Santa Rosa Medical Center

Clinical Instructor
University of Texas Health Science Center
San Antonio, Texas

Adina M. Reinhardt
Consultant, Community Care
University of Utah

Quality Assurance Specialist
Utah State Department of Health
Salt Lake City, Utah

Foreword by Anne R. Somers

Macmillan Publishing Co., Inc.
New York

COLLIER MACMILLAN PUBLISHERS
London

Macmillan Publishing Co., Inc.
866 Third Avenue, New York, New York 10022

Collier Macmillan Canada, Inc.

Library of Congress Cataloging in Publication Data

Main entry under title:

Promoting health through risk reduction.

  Bibliography: p.
  Includes index.
  1. Medicine, Preventive. 2. Preventive health
services. I. Faber, Marilyn M. II. Reinhardt,
Adina M., (Date)
RA425.P77   614.4'4   81-8245
ISBN 0-02-334850-X   AACR2

Printing:1 2 3 4 5 6 7 8   Year: 2 3 4 5 6 7 8 9

To Dotty and Hy

Contributors

Charles Althafer
Director
Professional Services and Consultation Division
Bureau of Health Education
Centers for Disease Control
Atlanta, Georgia

Katharine G. Bauer
Senior Professional Associate
Institute of Medicine
National Academy of Sciences
Washington, D.C.

William Beardslee, M.D.
Assistant Chief of Consultation-Liaison Service
Children's Hospital Medical Center
Instructor of Psychiatry
Harvard Medical School
Boston, Massachusetts

Jules R. Bemporad, M.D.
Associate Professor of Psychiatry
Harvard Medical School
Director of Children's Services
Massachusetts Mental Health Center
Boston, Massachusetts

William Blockstein, Ph.D.
Statewide Program Chairman, Health Sciences Unit
Professor of Pharmacy; Clinical Professor of Preventive Medicine
University of Wisconsin
Madison, Wisconsin

Henrik L. Blum, M.D., M.P.H.
Professor of Health Planning
School of Public Health
University of California, Berkeley
Berkeley, California

Tommie G. Cayton, Ph.D.
Chief, Stress Management Service
Chairman, Behavior Committee
Mental Health Director, Cardiac Rehab Unit
Department of Mental Health
USAF Medical Center, Lackland Air Force Base, Texas

Sabina Dunton, M.P.H.
Director
Well Aware About Health
University of Arizona Health Sciences Center
Tucson, Arizona

Felton Earls, M.D.
Director, Division of Child Psychiatry
Associate Professor of Child Psychiatry
Washington University School of Medicine
St. Louis, Missouri

Susan Evans
Staff Specialist, HSA II
Well Aware About Health
University of Arizona Health Sciences Center

Marilyn M. Faber, M.A., M.H.A.
Wellness Activities Director
Children's Hospital, Santa Rosa Medical Center
Clinical Instructor
University of Texas Health Science Center
San Antonio, Texas

Raymond A. Faber, M.D.
Assistant Professor of Clinical Psychiatry
University of Texas Health Science Center
Audie Murphy Veterans Administration Hospital
San Antonio, Texas

Jonathan E. Fielding, M.D., M.P.H.
Professor of Pediatrics and Public Health
Co-Director
Center for Health Enhancement Education and Research
University of California, Los Angeles
Los Angeles, California

Turkan K. Gardenier, Ph.D.
Health Statistician
U.S. Environmental Protection Agency
Washington, D.C.

Janet Brown Hall
Project Director
Stevens Point Area Wellness Commission
Stevens Point, Wisconsin

Bill Hettler, M.D.
Director
University Health Service
University of Wisconsin
Stevens Point, Wisconsin

Christopher Hitt, M.S.
American Farm Foundation
Formerly Professional Staff
Senate Agriculture, Nutrition, and Forestry Committee
Washington, D.C.

Harold Leppink, M.D.
Executive Officer
St. Louis County Board of Health
Duluth, Minnesota

Paul C. Mohl, M.D.
Assistant Professor of Psychiatry
University of Texas Health Science Center
Chief, Psychosomatic Consultation-Liaison Service
Audie Murphy Veterans Administration Hospital
San Antonio, Texas

Naomi Morris, M.D., M.P.H.
Professor and Director
Community Health Sciences, School of Public Health
University of Illinois
Chicago, Illinois

K. Michael Peddecord, Dr. P.H.
Assistant Professor
Graduate School of Public Health
San Diego State University
San Diego, California

Kenneth L. Rentmeester, M.P.H.
Director
Portage County Community Human Services Department
Stevens Point, Wisconsin

Ernest Schloss,
Director Health Systems Agency of Southeastern Arizona
Tucson, Arizona

Anne R. Somers, Ph.D.
Professor, Department of Environmental and Community Medicine and Department of
    Family Medicine
College of Medicine and Dentistry
New Jersey-Rutgers Medical School
Piscataway, New Jersey

R. G. Troxler, M.D.
Chief, Clinical Pathology
USAF School of Aerospace Medicine
Brooks Air Force Base, Texas

Christine Williams, M.D., M.P.H.
Associate Director of Research
Lederle Laboratories
Assistant Professor of Community Health and Preventive Medicine
New York Medical College
Pearl River, New York

Foreword

Anne R. Somers

"I would like to be remembered as the Secretary who put preventive health care and preventive medicine at the very top of the Federal medical agenda." Thus spoke Secretary of Health and Human Services Richard Schweiker at his Senate confirmation hearings in January 1981. This would include, he continued, emphasizing prevention in terms of reimbursement and research.

Secretary Schweiker was not the first to laud prevention. Secretary Joseph Califano had already done so and had demonstrated real commitment in one politically difficult area, cigarette smoking. There is no question but that we have witnessed a crescendo of interest and at least rhetorical commitment to health promotion and disease prevention over the past decade.

Evidence of the growing interest is everywhere—from the top reaches of government to the columns of the daily press and TV shows. The symbols of success are easy to identify: Looking first at the federal level, one thinks immediately of the establishment of OHIHP, the Office of Health Information and Health Promotion (now Office of Health Information, Health Promotion, Physical Fitness, and Sports Medicine) in the Office of the Assistant Secretary for Health, and the Bureau of Health Education (now Center for Health Promotion and Education) in the Centers for Disease Control; publication of *Healthy People: The Surgeon General's Report on Health Promotion and Disease Prevention* and the follow-up *Promoting Health/Preventing Disease: Objectives for the Nation*; the health promotion activities of the National Heart, Lung, and Blood Institute including the Multiple Risk-Factor Intervention Trials (MRFIT), the High Blood Pressure Education Program, and the Stanford Heart Disease Prevention programs; and the work and publications of the Senate Select Committee on Nutrition and Human Needs.

The private sector has also been active through the San Francisco-based National Center for Health Education; the Washington-based Advisory Committee on Education for Health (supported by the life and health insurance industries); the American Hospital Association's Center for Health Promotion; the Pittsburgh Center for Health Education—a model for community-based activities; the Office of Consumer Health Education in the College of Medicine and Dentistry of New Jersey, marking the first serious entry of a medical school into this field; and numerous programs sponsored by business and industry.

One of the most significant developments for the long-run was the establishment of the Division and Board of Health Promotion and Disease Prevention in the National Academy of Sciences-Institute of Medicine, a quasi-public institution bridging the sometimes considerable gap between public and private sectors and assuring attention to research and evaluation.

This list could be expanded to include literally thousands of smaller or more localized initiatives. Several are described in this volume. Indeed, the fact that so much is going on at the state or local level is perhaps the most encouraging part of the whole picture.

As it is, health promotion and its frequent synonym, health education, is sometimes praised as the answer to virtually all our national ills from teen-age pregnancies, to premature cardiovascular death, to the American "culture of violence," to excessive national expenditures for health care. Some enthusiasts have labelled health promotion "the second public health revolution", comparable in significance to the first public health revolution of the 19th century—the discovery of the germ theory of disease and the great sanitary reforms that led to near eradication of infectious diseases in the United States and most other advanced nations.

Naturally, there is no lack of critics who find as much to criticize in the new movement as its advocates do to praise. There are charges of faddism; unproved claims bordering on quackary; impractical or unethical approaches to human behavior; undermining the First Amendment of the Constitution; "blaming the victim" for circumstances, including poor health, beyond his or her control; even undermining existing health insurance programs as well as the now-stalled drive for national health insurance.

The debate is of more than casual significance. Unfortunately, the substance has not, thus far, matched the symbols. Most of the new health promotion and health education offices, agencies, and programs are seriously underfinanced, understaffed, and inadequately integrated with the mainstream of health care financing. Medicare, the nation's pattern-setting health care program, specifically prohibits reimbursement for preventive services, and no Administration has made any serious effort to repeal this ban. The same is true of most private health insurance, with the exception of health maintenance organizations (HMOs). Health promotion still receives very short shrift in medical schools and many other schools of the health professions.

As a result of these and numerous other obstacles, including a great deal of continuing consumer/patient apathy, the performance of some programs has fallen short of the promise; many are having trouble holding their own; and some new "initiatives" have turned out to be one-time events rather than significant break-throughs. Efforts to measure cost-effectiveness have been particularly difficult and in some cases inconclusive. How could it be otherwise, when most such evaluations have had to juxtapose additional short-term costs against presumed long-term economies?

Ironically, financial restrictions are becoming increasingly stringent at precisely the same time that the rhetoric of support is growing. The same Administration that claims to put prevention "at the very top of the Federal medical agenda" has also sharply cut the already minimal budgets of OHIHP and the Center for Health Promotion and Education. At the present writing, it is uncertain if the latter can survive. The same Administration that came up with the positive concept of a Federal–State Prevention Block Grant proposes to accompany such an innovation with a 25 percent cut in the programs that would be consolidated into the grant. The Senate Select Committee on Nutrition and Human Needs was abolished under the previous Administration.

In short, despite the widespread verbal support and considerable progress of the past decade, the future of health promotion in the U.S. is still far from assured. In an era of increasingly limited resources and emphasis on cost-benefit calculations and projections, future funds, personnel, and other essential resources—indeed the viability of the entire health promotion movement—will depend, in good part, on public and professional perceptions not only of the need for, but the effectiveness and practicality of, this approach to our major health problems.

Herein lies the importance of this volume. The editors and authors have moved beyond the traditional rhetoric, the pleas for support, and public exhortations, to detailed discussion of problems of risk reduction in specific situations—for different age groups and in different settings and with case studies of existing programs. They have not hesitated to engage in some generalizations and crystal-gazing of their own, especially in Part IV, but for the most part this is a useful "how to do it" guide for health care professionals and public policy-makers who are tired of clichés and determined to get on with the business of translating the high-level rhetoric of health promotion into practical grass roots programs, and reduced morbidity for the American people. Editors Faber and Reinhardt are also to be congratulated for assembling a group of down-to-earth authors with first-hand experience in the programs they describe and discuss.

In conclusion, it is my view that we are still far from the alleged health promotion "revolution." On the contrary, we still live in a hedonistic society, where jobs, incomes, and pleasures are generally given far higher priority than health. Within the health field, our resources remain overwhelmingly committed to the cure, rather than the prevention, of disease. Nevertheless there is reason for optimism. With the concept of limited resources comes more emphasis on social responsibility to balance our current great emphasis on individual rights, more on prevention as opposed to cure. Just as the individual—who has had a heart attack and for the first time in his life understands his vulnerability—reaches the "teachable moment" with respect to behavior change, so a society that suddenly discovers its economic vulnerability may also reach the "teachable moment" with respect to dominant social values and lifestyle.

The obstacles remain many and formidable. Persistence and patience are essential. Altering lifestyle is a long-term pursuit. Individual moderation and self-control in the presence of affluence will always be difficult to achieve, but there is evidence that gradual change can be effected.

Despite the new federal initiatives, the task is still primarily in the hands of health professionals, business and community leaders, and others in the private sector. It is likely to remain there for some time to come. That is probably inevitable. As in many other public issues, the signs are that the general public is already ahead of its officials in its thinking and response to the problem. If this continues, officialdom will follow, in a manner that will probably be more forceful, less equivocal, and better informed than if it had initially been in the forefront. It will then have the assurance of the public support that is required in a democratic society. In this quiet, grass roots evolution, this book should play an important contributory role.

Anne R. Somers

Preface

We have come to take the cures of modern medicine almost for granted, forgetting that our improved health has come more from disease prevention than from therapeutic intervention in the disease process. Preventive and health promoting measures such as improved sanitation, better nutrition and the control of infectious disease through immunizations are reasons why we are healthier than ever before in our history.

The existing medical model is largely therapeutic intervention in the disease process, the effectiveness of which is frequently limited. Health care providers and the public at large are increasingly cognizant of the potential personal benefits of including disease prevention, health maintenance and health promotion concepts in the accepted medical model. Individual health is very much linked to factors such as lifestyle, nutritional habits and physical fitness. Such factors are controlled by the individual, and health status is in large measure the responsibility of the individual.

The public at large needs to be alerted to health risks which all of us face. Some risks such as environment, heredity and quality of health care are usually beyond individual control. However, those risks that involve our personal habits—our lifestyle— are not only controllable but are often the key to dramatic improvements in health. Of the ten leading causes of death in the United States, at least seven could be substantially reduced by changes in dietary habits, cessation of smoking, adequate exercise, control of alcohol abuse and therapeutic intervention in so called "borderline" hypertension.

This book brings together a broad range of readings dealing with issues and topics that are relevant to the rapidly emerging field of health promotion.

The editors' primary goal in assembling these chapters is to provide under one cover source material on application of health promotion strategies and techniques from which both health care professionals and students can develop and expand their knowledge of this emerging field.

This text has also been prepared for the informed lay consumers who are interested in suggestions for improving and promoting their own health status and in keeping abreast of the current state of the art in health promotion.

Promoting Health through Risk Reduction is divided into four parts:

 I. Overview and Definition of Health Risk Estimation and Risk Reduction.
 II. Risk Reduction Methods.
 III. Present Programs for Risk Reduction and Health Promotion.
 IV. Future Directions for Risk Reduction.

These titles and their constituent chapters reflect the broad range of issues that should be the concern of physicians, community health nurses, family nurse practitioners, physician's assistants, public health administrators, private voluntary agency administrators and professionals employed by HMOs . . . a vast scope of health care providers can benefit from utilizing this information. A look to the immediate future and the issues addressed by the contributors should stimulate the reader to move beyond present practices.

Contributors to this volume have devoted many valuable hours seeking out and describing the latest techniques, questioning their value and finally presenting an accumulation of essential knowledge of health care providers of all disciplines. For sharing this knowledge with us, we are most grateful.

In addition, we extend our thanks to Carmela Rodriguez and Deborah Woitaske for helping with the preparation of this manuscript. And finally, we wish to thank our husbands for their contributions and support during the long hours devoted to the preparation of this manuscript.

Marilyn M. Faber
Adina M. Reinhardt

Contents

PART IV

PART I
Overview and Definition of Health Risk Estimation and Risk Reduction

In this introductory part, three chapters that provide a unifying overall framework for the text are presented. These chapters have a common and unifying theme: (1) health risk reduction and health from an individual and a social perspective, and (2) health risk estimation. Risk reduction is discussed and focused upon from several points of view. For example, in one Chapter interventions that might be formulated for each of a number of specific periods of life, each with its own health goal, are the focus; and in a second article risk reduction is focused upon from a broad social perspective.

Health risk estimation becomes the focus of the third chapter by Leppink who discusses in detail the Robbins and Hall health risk estimation instrument, Health Hazard Appraisal.

The introductory chapter by Jonathon Fielding, M.D., presents a wealth of insights contributed by a physician with wide experience in the field of health promotion and risk reduction. As Dr. Fielding notes, when physicians are requested to list the medical advances that have contributed substantial and objective improvements in indicators of health status, they usually cite improvements in mechanistic medicine such as improved diagnostic techniques, the advent of antibiotics, and a broader range of therapeutic weapons against disease. Dr. Fielding cautions that a more careful look at history is humbling. He notes that available evidence strongly suggests that the greatest improvements in health are derived from better housing, improved sanitation, water purification and sewage disposal, enhanced techniques of food preservation, and changes in reproductive behavior.

The author notes that when evaluating risk reduction activities in the 1980s, we must take a broad view of the determinants of health and illness. Recently the causes of the major killers were summarized by the Surgeon General in the following sentences:

> We are killing ourselves by our careless habits.
> We are killing ourselves by carelessly polluting the environment.
> We are killing ourselves by permitting harmful social conditions to persist—conditions like poverty, hunger and ignorance—which destroy health, especially for infants and children.*

Fielding describes the Breslow and Somers's "Lifetime Health Monitoring" Program that divided the life span into ten periods based on changing life-styles, health needs, and problems. Fielding believes that risk reduction requires looking not only at what medicine can do but what public health and public policy can contribute to health.

In each of the ten periods of the Lifetime Health Monitoring Program, the authors formulated brief general goals and professional services requirements related to these goals. For each period to which specific goals can be assigned, there are a number of types of interventions which may reduce health risks.

*Healthy People, the Surgeon General's Report on Health Promotion and Disease Prevention, Department of Health

One set of interventions deals with economic issues such as providing education and meaningful jobs, reduction of poverty, and so forth. Another set of interventions relates to environmental controls such as controls on air and water pollution. A third set of interventions focuses on human behavioral patterns such as smoking, alcohol and drug consumption, and poor nutritional habits that confer large increases in risk to the growing fetus. Yet another set of interventions involves the increasing availability of effective risk reduction services such as amniocentesis, increasing immunization levels among children, and increased screening for sensory defects in infants.

Finally, Fielding discusses the difficult question concerning the degree to which risk identification and reduction can and should be integrated into the clinical practice of medicine. The reader will find the author's discussion enlightened by his rich experience.

An eminent physician and health planner has contributed the second chapter, "Social Perspective on Risk Reduction." Dr. Blum looks at risk reduction (considers, evaluates, and discusses) from both micro and macro approaches and shows how these two approaches are interrelated. He noted that micro risk reduction efforts are made by individuals to minimize their exposure to health hazards. In contrast, macro risk reduction efforts are those made by a society to minimize the possibility of its members being exposed to health hazards. Blum accurately points out that meaningful macro efforts are required as enablers or inducers for most good micro behaviors. For example, he states that "On the job and community sponsorship and leadership—for periods for exercise and nutritious low cost meals at work, good public transportation, safe sidewalks and streets, and opportunities for nominal cost adult education and recreation—are examples of micro-based, micro-enabling efforts that far transcend macro-based exhortation in utility." Creative leadership will be needed in the coming decade to sponsor such on-the-job exercise programs. Escalating costs may hamper the development of good public transportation.

Numerous thought-provoking issues are discussed in this chapter. However, one that appears to be a key point is Blum's thoughtful observation that at present there are few tangible rewards for all but a few categories of health professionals to carry out risk reduction efforts. As a result, the medical community may even look with grave misgivings when someone else offers to undertake only the simplest and least socially threatening micro-promoting and enabling programs. Not until professionals are perhaps preferentially paid and applauded for performing risk minimizing tasks will risk reduction efforts be undertaken by a growing number in the medical community.

"Health Risk Estimation" is the subject of the third chapter by Harold B. Leppink, M.D. This chapter competently and comprehensively addresses health risk estimation as a technique of prospective medicine. Leppink suggests that health education may be the best method we have for implementing the primary prevention of noncommunicable diseases—with these diseases, prevention and control have become a matter of individual or societal choice. Therefore, the ultimate question is: How do health professionals go about helping individuals and society (or groupings in society, such as associations, communities, and so on) assuming they want to? How do we go about helping them to make such informed choices about healthful life-style behaviors and elimination of harmful environmental impacts (such as air and water pollution)?

Leppink answers his question by pointing out that the first step is informing people of the problems, that is, creating awareness. The second step is identifying those people with high risk, and the third is offering those so identified the benefits of what we know about motivating and supporting behavioral change.

In this outstanding and informative chapter, Leppink first discusses the rationale for the shift of emphasis to health education. Second, he describes the health risk estimation instrument (the Robbins and Hall Health Appraisal Instrument), and finally discusses some of the barriers to finding the persons at risk and offering them educational experiences which may affect their choices.

This is the dawning of the age of individual responsibility for health. Prospective medicine involves detecting precursors and operative risk factors in the patient's life and attempts to reduce these risks by some type of intervention which has behavioral change as the expected outcome.

In summary (p. 42) the steps in prospective preventive medicine are these:

1. Screening for risk factors, agents of disease, or precursors rather than for symptoms and signs of overt disease;
2. Quantification and appraisal of the degree of risk, systematic risk reduction planning, risk-specific health education aimed at permanent behavioral change; and
3. Societal support to sustain change.

Thus, what was required was an efficient, dignified, creditable screening instrument capable of identifying, quantifying, and appraising risks to continued wellness or health.

It was through the efforts of Dr. Lewis Robbins and Dr. Jack Hall at Indiana Methodist Hospital that a risk estimation instrument, which they called Health Hazard Appraisal (HHA) was developed.

Dr. Leppink's chapter, then, discusses the development and construction, use, and interpretation of the instrument in a clear, straightforward manner with case illustrations on interpreting the computer printout. Dr. Leppink points out that a one-to-one interpretation of the printout between physician, health advisor, or health professional and consumer-participant or patient is essential.

Looking into the future, the author points out that the missing ingredient is a national commitment to the primary prevention of noncommunicable diseases. Although there does appear to be a dawning of such a commitment in the Surgeon General's Report "Healthy People," Leppink believes that not until primary prevention is dignified by third-party reimbursement will it really be applied in the mainstream of medical care.

These three chapters provide the reader with a broadly based comprehensive overview of the field of health promotion, of the key concepts and theoretical underpinnings of the emerging field of health promotion. Together, they serve as a stimulating introduction to the area of risk reductions methods found in Part Two.

1 / Risk Reduction Goals Throughout Life

Jonathan E. Fielding, M.D, M.P.H.

With the evolution of civilization has come major alterations in our expectations of health and longevity. As one medical historian wrote, "Primitive man's life expectancy was probably little more than thirty years, daily menaced by falling boulders and trees, ravines and bogs, by the slashing horns and fangs of cornered beasts."[1]

By 1977 average longevity at birth had increased to 73.2 years in the United States.[2] Today even the major causes of death at the turn of the century—influenza, pneumonia, diptheria, tuberculosis, and gastrointestinal disease—are far down the list of killers. Combined mortality rates for these diseases declined from 580 per 100,000 per year in 1900 to 30 per 100,000 per year in 1977.[3] Diseases that take many years to develop and are characterized by chronicity have supplanted infectious diseases as the primary causes of death. Cardiovascular disease and stroke together account for about one half of all deaths, with cancer being responsible for an additional 20 per cent. Among the young and through early middle age accidents are the primary cause of serious injury, disability, and death.[3]

In terms of mortality, we have made progress in reducing mortality for most of the feared killers. Only cancer mortality continues to climb, with the 1977 adjusted rate 6 per cent higher than in 1950.[4] Table 1 portrays changes in age-adjusted death rates from 1950 through 1977.

Too much, however, cannot be generalized about the health of Americans from mortality data. In 1977 about 25.5 million Americans had some degree of activity limitation defined as inability to carry out a major activity appropriate to one's age group such as working, attending school, keeping house, participating in desired recreational, regional, or civic activities. In the same year illness or injury caused an estimated 3.8 billion restricted activity days, an average of 17.8 days per person.[2] Almost 12 per cent of the population assessed their health as fair or poor, based on data from the National Health Interview Survey.[2]

Dental health, important to quality of life, is likewise poor. Three-fifths of Americans 65 to 74 have fewer than half their permanent teeth, and a random sample of the population surveyed by dental examination revealed about 40 per cent needing work on decayed teeth.

Although we all desire to improve health, finding agreement on its definition has been difficult. Rather than attempt to achieve consensus on what health is, it may be preferable to define the objectives of programs to improve it. At a minimum these might include (1) avoiding preventable death; (2) reducing avoidable morbidity; and (3) minimizing disability that interferes with usual functioning.[5]

When physicians are asked to chronicle the advances that have led to objective improvements in gross indicators of health status, we frequently invoke improvements in mechanistic medicine—improved diagnostic techniques, the advent of antibiotics, a broader range of therapeutic weapons against disease. A more careful look at history is humbling. Available evidence strongly suggests that the greatest improvements in health

TABLE 1. Age-Adjusted Death Rates[a] and Average Annual Percentage Change, According to Leading Causes of Death in 1950: United States, Selected Years 1950–1977.[b]

		Cause of Death				
Year	All Causes	Diseases of the Heart	Malignant Neoplasm	Cerebrovascular Disease	Accidents[c]	Tuberculosis
		Deaths per 100,000 resident population				
1950	841.5	307.6	125.4	88.8	57.5	21.7
1955	764.6	287.5	125.8	83.0	54.4	8.4
1960	760.9	286.2	125.8	79.7	49.9	5.4
1965	739.0	273.9	127.0	72.7	53.3	3.6
1970	714.3	253.6	129.9	66.3	53.7	2.2
1975	638.3	220.5	130.9	54.5	44.8	1.2
1976	627.5	216.7	132.3	51.4	43.2	1.1
1977	612.3	210.4	133.0	48.2	43.8	1.0
		Average annual percentage change				
1950–77	–1.2	–1.4	0.2	–2.2	–1.0	–10.8
1950–55	–1.9	–1.3	–.1	–1.3	–1.1	–17.3
1955–60	–0.1	–0.1	0.0	–0.8	–1.7	–8.5
1960–65	–0.6	–0.9	0.2	–1.8	1.3	–7.8
1965–70	–0.7	–1.5	0.5	–1.8	0.1	–9.4
1970–77	–2.2	–2.6	0.3	–4.5	–2.9	–10.7
1975–77	–2.1	–2.3	–.8	–6.0	–0.5	–0.9

[a]*Note:* Age-adjusted rates computed by the direct method to the age distribution of the total U.S. population as enumerated in 1940, using 11 age intervals.
[b]*Source:* Division of Vital Statistics, National Center for Health Statistics: Selected data. Data are based on the national vital registration system.
[c]Includes motor vehicle and all other.

have derived from better housing, improved sanitation, water purification and sewage disposal, enhanced techniques of food preservatives, and changes in reproductive behavior.[6] Reviewing English data McKeown makes a convincing case that for most infectious diseases (polio is an important exception) these general public health measures made a much larger contribution to the reduction in incidence and prevalence than did specific vaccines or pharmacological agents. Even for tuberculosis, which benefited from the availability of streptomycin from 1947 and B.C.G. vaccination starting in the 1950s, only 3.2 per cent of the deaths prevented during its decline from 1948 to 1971 were attributable to these specific therapies.

Approaching risk reduction in the 1980s requires a broad view of the determinants of health and illness. The Surgeon General recently summarized the causes of the major killers in these words:

We are killing ourselves by our careless habits.
We are killing ourselves by carelessly polluting the environment.
We are killing ourselves by permitting harmful social conditions to persist—conditions like poverty, hunger and ignorance—which destroy health, especially for infants and children.[3]

Risk reduction requires looking at not only what medicine can do but what public health and public policy can contribute. An important contribution to setting organized rational strategies for health improvement is dividing the life cycle into coherent stages and addressing the risks and their potential reduction separately for each stage. This approach was termed "lifetime health monitoring" in a 1977 article by Professors Lester Breslow and Anne Somers. Their Lifetime Health Monitoring Program divided the life span into ten periods based on changing life-styles, health needs, and problems: pregnancy and perinatal period; infancy (first year of life); preschool child (1-5 years); school-age child (6-11); adolescence (12-17); young adulthood (18-24); young middle age (25-39); older middle age (40-59); elderly (60-74); and old age (75 and over). For each of these ten periods, the authors formulated brief general goals and professional services requirements related to these goals.[7]

For each period to which specific health goals can be assigned there are a number of types of interventions which may reduce health risk. One possible set of interventions deals with economic issues. It has been proposed that the most effective way to decrease drug abuse among urban black youths is to provide relevant education and meaningful jobs. Aging dilapidated housing stock increases the risk of lead poisoning among children living in houses where many layers of lead paint are ubiquitous and accessible because of peeling paint and falling plaster, Inadequate financial resources for the elderly as a result of inflation eroding the purchasing power of fixed pensions may lead to inadequate nutrition, which increases the risk of disease.

Another set of interventions relate to environmental controls. Many obvious opportunities are being missed. Continued emission of chlorofluorocarbons and aircraft exhaust appear to be contributing to an increase in the short ultraviolet light reaching the earth that causes skin cancer.[8] Thousands of new chemicals are manufactured each year without careful pretesting of adverse health effects. Air pollution has adverse health effects on virtually all inhabitants of the Los Angeles area, yet a requirement for annual auto emission checks to reduce pollution perennially goes down to defeat in the California legislature. Fluoridation can reduce dental caries by 50 to 60 percent and has a cost/benefit ratio in the range of 1/35 to 1/65.[9] Still many communities do not fluoridate their water supply.

Intervention to reduce health risk can also concentrate on the work, school, and home environments. The National Institute of Occupational Safety and Health estimates that there are 100,000 yearly deaths in America due to occupational illnesses and almost 400,000 new yearly cases of occupational disease. They also report that nine out of every ten American industrial workers are inadequately protected from exposure to at least one of the 163 most common hazardous industrial chemicals.[3] Many school children are exposed to asbestos in their schools.

Among the many health risks of the home environment is the risk to a toddler of a swimming pool without a surrounding fence. Another risk is the placement of medicines and household cleaners where a young child can reach them. Smoke detectors can reduce the risk of injury and death from fire in all age groups. Smoking parents may not only increase the risk of respiratory infections in their young children but increase the risks that their children will become smokers. A bathtub with a slippery bottom and no handrail increases the risk of hip fractures in the older age groups.

The more subtle and difficult risks involve family relationships. Parental neglect creates a high risk for emotional dysfunction in children. Overt potential physical abuse may threaten life but more frequently is manifest by burns, other "accidents," and deep emotional scars. A deprived sociocultural environment is thought to increase the chance of mild mental retardation (IQ 50 to 70).

Another set of interventions focuses on human behavioral patterns. Particular health habits such as smoking, alcohol and drug consumption, and poor nutrition confer great increases in risk to the growing fetus. Parental examples are very important determinants of their children's habits in such vital areas as nutrition, exercise, risk-taking behavior, and drug use (including cigarettes and alcohol). Use of seatbelts reduces risk of serious injury or death for all children over 40 pounds and all adults; infant carriers and child restraints help protect smaller children. Motorcycle travel is more than seven times as dangerous, mile for mile, as automobile travel. Whereas education regarding the relationship of health habits and health is important, behavioral techniques are essential when trying to make lasting changes in ingrained behavior. The major clear-cut risk factors for cardiovascular disease are smoking, high cholesterol levels, and blood pressure, all to some extent under individual control. Periodontal disease, the major cause of tooth loss in adults, could be reduced by simple regular brushing and flossing.

Increasing the availability of effective but underutilized risk reducing services involves yet another set of approaches. For example amniocentesis, useful in identifying fetuses affected by serious genetic disease prenatally, is being used by only a minority of women who could benefit from its availability coupled with sensitive genetic counseling. Immunization levels are still inadequate in many areas and early screening for sensory defects that could be ameliorated if detected early is not uniformly available. Financial barriers prevent many older citizens from obtaining two pieces of equipment which can make the difference between simply existing and enjoying life—dentures and hearing aids.

In some cases risk could be reduced through more judicious use of medical interventions. There are many drug reactions from overprescribed prescription drugs. Most technological diagnostic therapeutic procedures confer some risk. Excessive x-rays increase risk of cancer and genetic mutation; hospitalization confers a risk of infection; idiosyncratic reactions to chemicals used for diagnosis, anesthesia, or specific therapeutic techniques and agents can cause death or severe impairment. In clinical medicine risk and benefit must always be weighed.

While risks appear ubiquitous, many successful efforts to reduce specific causes of morbidity, mortality, and "unhealthy" feeling have been successful and can be considered models of preventive strategies. Some successful strategies in dealing with each of the three major causes of death—accidents, heart disease, and cancer—have been chosen as illustrations.

Auto Safety: Auto accidents are the leading cause of death in this country from infancy to early middle age. The public has been perennially barraged by auto safety educational campaigns designed to instruct people to slow down because "speed kills." For some years, variations on this message virtually monopolized "public service" advertising. Hence, auto safety should have been uppermost in the public mind; but the mind seemed far from the heavy foot, which continued to propel the car in excess of every posted speed. Other factors, however, combined to accomplish what education and exhortation had not—a decline of over 42 per cent in the national fatality rate from motor vehicle crashes between 1966 and 1976 (from 5.7 per 100,000,000 passenger miles to 3.4).[9] An important contribution to this improvement was the reduction of the speed limit to 55 mph coupled with the federal government's pressure on states to enforce this limit. Although motivated by the energy crisis, this change would have been equally defensible as a safety measure. Unfortunately, consumer acceptance of high gas prices and less vigorous speed limit enforcement have since eroded much of the improvement noted.

A second factor in the improved mortality statistics has been the requirement, effective January 1968, that every car be equipped with lap belts and shoulder harnesses for all passenger positions. Other factors responsible for reducing the fatality rate in the United States include the enforcement of federal motor vehicle safety standards, enactment of motorcycle helmet use laws (now unfortunately being repealed in many states in the name of individual liberty), improvement of highway design, and provision of emergency medical services. Although seatbelt usage rates of 10 to 15 per cent nationally can be construed as indicating public apathy, attention can as easily be focused on the millions of Americans who routinely wear seatbelts and thus reduce their chance of death or serious injury by 35 to 50 per cent.[10,11] In other countries, particularly Australia and in some Canadian provinces, belt usage has been required by statute. Where such laws have been mandated, studies show reductions in occupant fatalities of 17 to 39 per cent and in occupant injuries of 15 to 32 per cent.[12]

Cervical Cancer Mortality: Cancer is the most dreaded category of diseases. The Papanicolaou (Pap) smear has become an accepted part of medical practice, and an early diagnosis of precancerous lesions can assure both patient and physician that its progression can be halted by a minor operation. The incidence of cervical cancer in the United States declined from 44 per 100,000 women in 1947 to 8.8 per 100,000 in 1970,[13] and the mortality rate from cervical cancer fell from 9.3 per 100,000 women in the period 1950-54 to 6.2 per 100,000 women from 1963 to 1969. In the absence of clear evidence of any change in the natural history of this disease, it is reasonable to infer that this marked reduction results mainly from earlier treatment made possible by earlier detection through Pap tests. Conservative estimates of the number of Pap smears performed annually today are over 15 million; 75 per cent of women over age 17 have had at least one Pap test.

Although articles questioning the effectiveness of screening on the reduction of cervical cancer mortality abound, a recent extensive and careful review article concluded: "Therapy based on confirmed positive smears can reduce the incidence and mortality rates of invasive cervical cancer, as shown by declining rates before screening began, lower rates for geographic areas and occupational groups having less screening and lower rates among screened women than unscreened women."[13] One study of the effect of Pap smears estimates that the increase of annual screening from 0 to 30 per cent of the women at risk over a 35-year period has added 3 years to the life expectancy of women diagnosed as having cervical cancer.[14]

The controversy over the effectiveness of cervical screening in reducing cervical cancer mortality illustrates some of the problems of risk reduction progress. At first, the Pap smear was hailed as a paradigm of clinical preventive medicine, and a major selling job by the American Cancer Society and the medical profession convinced adult women of its indispensability. Then researchers reviewing its impact had difficulty confirming its contribution to the declining cervical cancer mortality rate. Despite some lingering uncertainty about effectiveness and efficiency in screening programs, most public health professionals feel that cervical cancer screening (followed by treatment when needed) is correctly counted as a prevention success. Few physicians would dare suggest to a woman that she cease having the test performed at regular intervals. After a careful review of the natural course of cervical cancer and the costs and effectiveness of screening the American Cancer Society has modified its recommendation from annual Pap smears for all women to Pap smears every 3 years after two negative tests, one year apart and limited to women over 20 and those under 20 who are sexually active.[15]

Smoking Cessation: In the 15 years following the original Surgeon General's Report on Smoking and Health in 1964 the proportion of adult American men who smoke decreased from 52 to 38 per cent and of women, from 39 to 30 per cent. Twenty-nine million Americans stopped between 1964 and 1975. Of physicians, dentists, and pharmacists who ever smoked, 64, 61, and 55 per cent, respectively, have quit, and the proportion who smoked in the mid 1970's was reported to be to 21, 30, and 28 per cent several years ago and has probably further declined since.[16]

Analysis of smoking trends suggests that the antismoking advertising on the electronic media in the late 1960's contributed to significant annual declines in cigarette consumption. Per capita tobacco consumption from 1960 to 1970 declined 10.5 per cent in the United States compared to increases of 4.2 per cent for Canada, 11.9 per cent for Belgium, 17.1 per cent for Finland, and 19.6 per cent for West Germany. Since smoking cessation begins to reduce individual risk for coronary heart disease with almost no time lag, the fact that mortality from coronary heart disease, the leading cause of death in the United States, began its pattern of decline at mainly the same time as the first Surgeon General's Report appears to be more than coincidence.[18]

Concern by smokers over the health effects of their habit has led to an increase in the use of filter cigarettes; by 1974 they were smoked by 61 per cent of male and 54 per cent of female smokers. Health concerns have also fostered the development and successful marketing of low-tar and low-nicotine brands (15 mg or less tar, 1.5 mg or less nicotine) whole sales increased from 11 per cent of the total sales in 1975 to an estimated 25 per cent in 1977,[19] and it is likely that the majority of smokers are currently smoking these brands with an additional 10 % smoking ultra low tar (0.6 mg) brands.

Smoking cessation clinics have achieved a 12- to 18-month success rate of 13 to 37 per cent and an approximately 20 per cent success rate in 4- to 5-year follow-up studies.[20] Newer techniques promise to push 1-year success rates to 40 to 60 per cent.[21,22]

Why smoking has experienced such a marked decline is unknown. Persistent warning plus teaching by example on the part of health professionals and an overwhelming fear of cancer on the part of smokers and their loved ones are frequently proposed reasons, but the answer probably has at least as much to do with a changing social climate where nonsmoking is the norm and with an increased interest in feeling healthy. Opinion leaders have increasingly abandoned smoking, and their quitting has been presented to the public as a success story. Family pressures, including those from children, to quit or not start have intensified. The millions starting to exercise strenuously and regularly find it difficult if not impossible to do so if they smoke. Smoking is no longer chic or socially required. In fact, it is increasingly regarded, at least by most adults, as a socially unacceptable habit, in much the same way as spitting started to be viewed several generations ago. (Part of the early campaign to control tuberculosis involved reducing the spread of the tubercle bacillus by portraying spitting as ill mannered. A public not well versed in disease etiology came to view spitting as antisocial and abandoned it primarily for that reason.) Nonsmokers have also become more militant; smoking is legally restricted in more and more public places, and nonsmokers are demanding enforcement. Courts are starting to declare that workers are entitled to a smoke-free environment. The silent non-smoking majority has become vocal. In addition, there is growing concern about the adverse health effects of second-hand smoke. One widely publicized study showed that nonsmoking patients with angina pectoris experienced reduced exercise tolerance after several hours' exposure to secondhand cigarette smoke.[23] Release of results from this type of study and one showing reduced performance in pulmonary function tests in those with long term exposure to secondhand smoke may intensify pressures for government and industry action to discourage and restrict smoking.[24]

An important advance has been the development of effective smoking prevention curricula that can be integrated into existing health education classes. Several studies have found that incorporating effective behavioral techniques into such curricula leads to a reduction in the age-specific adoption of smoking behavior by up to one half.[25,26]

One of the most difficult questions is the degree to which risk identification and reduction can and should be integrated into the clinical practice of medicine. It is difficult to get agreement on what preventive services meet criteria that suggest the benefits outweigh the risk. Also hotly debated is what should be the role of the doctor and other health professionals, especially in helping individuals change health habits.

A composite of criteria developed by a number of medical groups for routine application of specific preventive services to the well population is as follows:[27,28,29,30,31]

1. The condition screened for is an important cause of morbidity, disability, or mortality.
2. The disease or condition has an asymptomatic period during which detection and treatment can substantially reduce morbidity, mortality, or both.
3. The natural history of the disease is sufficiently well known, treatments are sufficiently effective, risks resulting from the screening are low enough, and efficacy in reducing morbidity, disability, or mortality is high enough to conclude that screening-initiated diagnosis of the disease will lead to a net benefit to the target population.
4. The tests used in screening are acceptable to the target population and have acceptable characteristics with respect to false negatives and false positives.
5. Appropriate follow-up of positive findings is assured. The first results of a screen are usually to designate "suspects" for having a disease and links to sources of care for follow-up are essential.
6. Compliance among asymptomatic patients for whom an early diagnosis has been reached is at a level effective in altering the natural history of the disease.
7. The procedure is relatively easy to administer, preferably by paramedical personnel with guidance and interpretation by physicians, and is generally available at reasonable cost.

An *ad hoc* advisory group of the Institute of Medicine was convened to develop a list of preventive services which met these general criteria, further distilled as follows:[32]

• The importance of the disease or disability to be prevented, in terms of the number of persons afflicted or severity of the disease.
• Scientific proof or efficacy of the intervention in preventing or altering the natural history of a disease (as with immunizations for childhood diseases and blood pressure determinations) or, in the absence of scientific proof, prudent interpretation of available evidence concerning potential benefits, costs, and risks (as with determination of serum cholesterol in adolescence or breast examination for women under 50).
• Feasibility of application of the preventive measure—technical, economical, and sociocultural.

The resultant packages of services were organized by the ten periods of the life span mentioned by Breslow and Somers.[7] The *ad hoc* advisory group did not cover preventive mental health or preventive dental services, nor did it consider prevention services which might be appropriate to various high-risk groups because of genetic predisposition, occupational exposure, or membership in a specific racial, social, cultural, geographic, or economic group. With the exception of the counseling component the list is very sparse compared with the content of many routine physicals. The lists in Tables 2, 3, and 4 are consensus lists and do not represent the conclusion of any group member. However, they do serve as a point of departure for further discussion and refinement.

TABLE 2.   Preventive Services for the Well Population—Pregnant Women and Fetus

Services	Initial Visit[1]	Subsequent Visits[2]
History		
General medical	*	
Family and genetic	*	
Previous pregnancies	*	
Current pregnancy	*	*
Physical examination		
General	*	
Blood pressure	*	*
Height and weight	*	
Fetal development		*
Laboratory examinations		
VRDL	*	
Papanicolaou smear	*	
Hemoglobin/hematocrit	*	
Urinalysis for sugar and protein	*	*
Rh determination	*	
Blood group determination	*	
Rubella HAI titer	*	
Amniocentesis (for women over 35)[3]	*	
Counseling with referrals as necessary and desired		
Plans for pregnancy continuation	*	*
Nutrition during pregnancy	*	*
Nutrition of infant, including breast feeding	*	*
Cigarette smoking	*	*
Use of alcohol, other drugs during pregnancy	*	*
Sexual intercourse during pregnancy	*	*
Signs of abnormal pregnancy	*	*
Labor and delivery (including where mother plans to deliver)	*	*
Physical activity and exercise	*	*
Provisions for care of infant	*	*
In response to parental concerns	*	*

Labor and delivery[4]

Postpartum visit (including family planning counseling and referral, if desired)

[1] Initial visit should occur early in the first trimester.

[2] Subsequent visits should occur once a month through the 28th week of pregnancy; twice a month from the 29th through the 36th week; once a week thereafter.

[3] If desired, amniocentesis should be performed at about the 13th or 14th week for women who are over 35 or who have specific genetic indications.

[4] Although not a "preventive" service, labor and delivery should be included in a package of pregnancy-related services.

Source: Institute of Medicine, Ad Hoc Advisory Group on Preventive Services, Washington, D.C., April 13, 1978.

TABLE 3. Preventive Services for the Well Population—Normal Infant

Services	Birth Visit	Second Visit[1]	Subsequent Visits[2]
History and physical examination			
Length and weight	*		*
Head circumference	*		
Urine stream	*		
Check for congenital abnormalities			*
Development assessment			*
Procedures			
PKU screening test		*	
Thyroxin T4		*	
Vitamin K		*	
Silver nitrate prophylaxis	*		
Immunizations			
Diphtheria			*
Pertussis			*
Tetanus			*
Measles			*
Mumps			*
Rubella			*
Poliomyelitis			*
Parental counseling, with referrals as necessary and desired			
Infant nutrition and feeding practices (especially breast feeding)		*	*
Parenting		*	*
Infant hygiene		*	*
Accident prevention (including use of automobile restraints)		*	*
Family planning and referral for services		*	*
Child care arrangements		*	*
Medical care arrangements		*	*
Parental smoking, use of alcohol, and drugs		*	*
Parental nutrition, physical activity, and exercise		*	*
In response to parental concerns		*	*

[1] Second visit should occur within 10 days or before leaving the hospital.
[2] Four visits during the rest of the first year, or enough to provide immunizations on schedule.
Source: Institute of Medicine, Ad Hoc Advisory Group on Preventive Services, Washington, D.C., April 13, 1978.

The Canadian government has recently supported the development of recommendations for periodic health assessment for persons of different ages using similar criteria for inclusion.

Lists such as these must be considered in light of a host of accompanying caveats regarding level of evidence regarding efficacy, problems of quality control, education and appropriate skills of those providing services, difficulty in finding appropriate financing vehicles, and problems in deciding on appropriate settings for provisions of the listed services. Particularly perplexing is how to make counseling components effective. While some of the counseling elements are frequently addressed in clinical practice, others are not. How often do physicians discuss sexual adjustments with their patients, especially older ones, or sleep problems or the importance of seatbelt usage? Few studies have tackled either the content or effectiveness of physician counseling in changing patient's behavior. Even in those cases where there are clear end points that can be considered educational objectives (weight reduction, cessation of smoking, seatbelt use), the behavior change occurring may be due to entirely different factors (a loved one who says, "you'd look better thinner," a friend dying of lung cancer, a serious auto accident injury to an unbelted family member). In many cases, practitioner counseling may catalyze a patient's will to change but may be effective only in combination with other forces (peer pressure, messages through the mass media, self-perception of symptoms arising from unhealthful habit or in combination with support groups in the community such as Weight Watchers or organized smoking cessation groups).

For other items covered under counseling such as sexual adjustment, nutrition, and problems surrounding retirement, educational objectives and behavioral objectives defy sharp definitions. Yet these are all important health issues and deserve increased attention if health promotion is to be strengthened as an objective of practice.

There are some data that suggest the importance of physicians in influencing one specific behavior, smoking, especially through delivering strong admonishments at times of illness related to smoking.[33] Physician advice may have an enhanced chance of being needed if provided at times of life when individuals are willing to modify behavior to avoid harming a loved one, such as during pregnancy, or when trying to promote good health habits in their children. In one study, 35 per cent of women smokers, ages 18 to 35, quit during pregnancy and 32 per cent cut back.[34] A preliminary report suggests the willingness of pregnant smokers to enter and benefit from a smoking cessation behavior modification program.[36]

If packages of preventive services are to be available as benefits, it will be important to make explicit how much is expected of the physician and for how much time he or she will be paid for this component of the package. In many cases, a midlevel health professional can assume significant responsibility for parts of the counseling responsibilities. But, regardless of provider, limitations of the practice setting need to be recognized. The provisions of carefully conceived pamphlets or audiovisual materials that provide necessary factual information on a number of counseling topics and/written instructions can be useful adjuncts to oral communication but not substitutes. Finally, one of the most important services provided to a patient can be an up-to-date list of community resources that specialize in assisting people to improve specific health practices.

Effectiveness of preventive service packages requires considerable cooperation by the public. Some of the limitations for any proposed services to improve health are (1) patients may not present for preventive services at suggested intervals, (2) patients with possible or definite problems amenable to intervention may not present for further diagnostic testing or initiation of therapies, and (3) patients may not adhere to the therapeutic recommendations (including the taking of medications) of health care practitioners. When insurance policies cover "routine " physicals, usually a minority of those covered take advantage of that service and most of those individuals present less frequently than the minimum covered interval. Although a greater proportion of those covered might take advantage of preventive services if the rationale was clearer, if their practitioners strongly recommended conformance to a particular frequency of examinations, and if the patient was sure that all these preventive services were covered, there is little likelihood that utilization would even be close to the maximum covered.

TABLE 4. Preventive Services for the Well Population

Services	Preschool[1]	School Child[2]	Adolescent[3]	Adult Entry[4]	Years[5]	Years[6]	Older Adults[7]	Old Age[8]
History and physical examination and referrals when necessary								
Height and weight	*	*	*	*	*	9*	*	*
Developmental assessment	*	*	*					
Blood pressure		*	*	*	*	9*	*	*
Vision	*	*	*	*		9*	*	*
Hearing	*	*	*			9*	*	*
Speech	*	*	*					
Screening for scoliosis (girls, 9–10 years, or at first visit)			*					
Skin		*	*					
Breast examination in women				*	*	9*	*	*
Rectal examination						*	*	*
Mammography (women over age 50)						*	*	*
Electrocardiogram (one baseline value at 40 or 45)						*		
Laboratory examinations								
Serum cholesterol (once during age periods specified			*			*		
VDRL, if not otherwise required or obtained recently				*				
Papanicolaou smear (women)				*	*	*	*	
Gonococcal culture (women)				*				
Rubella titer (women)				*	*	9*		
Blood glucose						*	*	*
Hematocrit						9*	*	*
Urine analysis for sugar and protein						9*	*	*
Stool guaiac						9*	*	*

Immunizations

Completion of immunization schedule	*						
Tetanus				*			
Diphtheria				*			
Against influenza, when and as required (especially over age 65)						*	*

Counseling with referrals as necessary and desired

Nutrition	*		*	*	*	*	*
Hygiene	*		*	*	*	*	*
Accident prevention	*		*	*	*	*	*
Physical activity and exercise	*		*	*	*	*	*
Alcohol, other drug use	10*		10*	*	*	*	*
Family relations, social problem, sexual development and adjustment	*		*	*	*	*	*
Family planning (contraception if appropriate)			*	*	*	*	
Sleep				*	*	*	*
Obesity	*		*	*	*	*	*
Antecedents of adult disease	*		*	*	*		
Teaching breast and skin self-examination				*	*	*	*
Retirement						*	*
Living arrangements						*	*
In response to parental or individual concerns	*		*	*	*	*	*

[1] Two health visits, one at 2 to 3 years and one at school entry.
[2] Two health visits, one at 6 to 7 and one at 9 to 10 years of age.
[3] Two health visits, the first preferably about age 13.
[4] One health visit.
[5] Three health visits, about age 25, 30 and 35.
[6] Four health visits, about age 40, 45, 50, and 55.
[7] Health visit at age 60, and every 2 years thereafter.
[8] Annual health visits.
[9] To be performed once during the interim between examinations.
[10] Counseling about effects of parental use on children.

Source: Institute of Medicine, Ad Hoc Advisory Group on Preventive Services, Washington, D.C., Apr. 13, 1978.

A considerable body of literature explores the lack of continuity between screening and follow-up. Even if we assume good organizational and logistic linkages (e.g., same locus, same practitioner or practitioners), asymptomatic patients may react to news of potential problems by ignoring them. Symptomatic of the problems is the observation that, for all types of appointments, ambulatory care facilities report broken appointment rates of 16 to 44 per cent.[37] In fact, appointment-keeping behavior is a problem in all practice settings. Symptomless patients may fail to keep follow-up appointments up to 50 per cent of the time.[38] Four large-scale studies of hypertension awareness and control between 1971 and 1975 revealed that between 10.8 and 22.7 per cent of those with hypertension were aware of their condition but were not on therapy.[39]

Adherence to therapeutic regimens by an asymptomatic individual is likely to be difficult when

- The need for the therapy is not reinforced by clinical symptoms.
- Therapy is required over a long period of time.
- Therapy requires significant changes in strongly ingrained habits.
- Therapy produces undesirable side effects.
- Therapy is very time consuming.
- The patient lacks future orientation.
- The patient does not understand the need for the therapy and the consequences of nonadherence or has strong self-destructive feelings.

Adherence rates of asymptomatic individuals with problems such as rheumatic fever, tuberculosis, and hypertension may be as low as 40 per cent,[40] although practitioner attention to improving adherence can significantly improve the results. Good communication between practitioner and patient, including repetition in explaining why it is important to take the medicine, is essential. Improved communication should prevent duplicating the disappointing results of one recent interview study of adherence which found that of those hypertensives who had stopped taking their medication, 33 per cent reported stopping "on the advice of their physician" and 28 per cent reported stopping because they believed they no longer had high blood pressure.[41]

Some promising approaches to improving adherence include (1) enlisting the assistance of allied health personnel, such as pharmacists (2) providing the personal physician with patient-education strategies and (3) financial incentives for nurse counseling.[40,41,42,43] Changes in the cultural environment that would provide external reinforcement for healthful behavior are also important.[44]

Opportunities abound for risk reduction throughout the life cycle. In addition to incorporating preventive services into medical practices there are opportunities for government regulation (e.g., childproof containers, requiring clothing to be inflammable, passive automobile restraints), for financial incentives (e.g., life insurance premium reductions for nonsmokers, joggers, thin people), and for technically-oriented education and skill building to teach and reinforce healthful habits as well as to help individuals maintain good interpersonal relationships.

REFERENCES

1. Marti-Ibanez, F., *The Epic of Medicine*, New York: Clarkson N. Potter, 1962.
2. *Health United States 1979*, Washington, D.C.: Department of Health, Education and Welfare, 1980.

3. *Healthy People, The Surgeon General's Report on Health Promotion and Disease Prevention*, Washington, D.C.: Department of Health, Education, and Welfare, 1979.
4. Fingerhut, L., Wilson, R., and Feldman, J., "Health and Disease in the United States," *Annual Review of Public Health*, 1 (1980).
5. Fielding, J., "Successes of Prevention," *Health and Society*, 56: 3 (Summer 1978).
6. Mckeown, T., *The Role of Medicine*, London: Nuffield Provincial Hospitals Trust, 1976.
7. Breslow, L. and Somers, A., "The Lifetime Health Monitoring Program," *New England Journal of Medicine*, 296 (1977).
8. Urbach, F., "Ultraviolet Radiation and Skin Cancer in Man," *Preventive Medicine*, 9:2 (March 1980).
9. Haddon, W., Jr., President, Insurance Institute for Highway Safety, Washington, D.C. Personal communication, 1978.
10. *Safety Belt Usage: Survey of Care in the Traffic Population–November 1977– June 1978. Performed by Opinion Research Corporation, National Highway Traffic Safety Administration, Department of Transportation, Washington, D.C., 1979.*
11. Robertson, L. S., "Factors Associated with Safety-Belt Use in 1974 Starter-Interlock Equipped Cars." *Journal of Health and Social Behavior* 16: 2 (1975).
12. Department of Transportation, "Effects of Safety Usage Laws Around the World." *Traffic Safety Newsletter*, February 1, 1977, p. 9.
13. Guzick, D. S., "Efficacy of Screening for Cervical Cancer: A Review," *American Journal of Public Health* 68: 2 (1978).
14. Dickinson, L., Mussey, M. E., and Kurland, L. T., "Evaluation of the Effectiveness of Cytologic Screening for Cervical Cancer. II: Survival Parameters Before and After Inception of Screening." *Mayo Clinic Proceedings* 47 (1972).
15. *American Cancer Society Report on the Cancer-Related Health Checkup*, New York: American Cancer Society, 1980.
16. U.S. Public Health Service, National Clearinghouse for Smoking and Health. *A Survey of Physicians, Dentists, Nurses and Pharmacists: Their Behavior and Attitudes Concerning Tobacco.* Washington, D.C.: U.S. Government Printing Office, 1977.
17. Warner, K. E., "The Effects of the Anti-Smoking Campaign on Cigarette Consumption." *American Journal of Public Health* 67: 7 (1977).
18. Walker, W. J., "Changing United States Lifestyle and Declining Vascular Mortality: Cause or Coincidence?" *The New England Journal of Medicine* 297: 3 (1977).
19. "Cigaret Companies Vie for Low-Tar Smokers, a Fast-Growing Breed," *The Wall Street Journal*, March 21, 1978.
20. West, D. W., et al., "Five Year Follow-Up of a Smoking Withdrawal Clinic Population." *American Journal of Public Health* 67: 6 (1977).
21. Danaher, B., "Innovative Directions for Smoking Research." Paper presented at the Annual Meeting of the Association for Advancement of Behavior Therapy, Atlanta, Ga., December 1977.
22. Landow, H., "Successful Treatment of Smokers with a Broad Spectrum Behavioral Approach." *Journal of Consulting and Clinical Psychology* 45: 3 (1977).
23. Aranow, W.S., "Effects of Passive Smoking on Angina Pectoris." *The New England Journal of Medicine* 299: 1 (1978).
24. White, J. R., and Froeb, H. F., Small-Airways Dysfunction in Nonsmokers Chronically Exposed to Tobacco Smoke,
25. McAlister, A., Perry, C., and Maccoby, N. "Adolescent Smoking: Onset and Prevention," *Pediatrics* 63 (1979).
26. Botvin, G., Eng, A., and Williams, C. L., "Preventing the Onset of Cigarette Smoking Through Life Skills Training," *Preventive Medicine* 9 (1980).
27. *Preventive Medicine U.S.A.*, New York: Prodist, 1976.

28. World Health Organization, *Mass Health Examinations*, Public Health Paper 43. Geneva; World Health Organization, 1971.
29. Frame, P. S. and Carlson, S. J., "A Critical Review of Periodic Health Screening Using Specific Screening Criteria," *Journal of Family Practice* 2 (1975), pp. 29–36, 123–129, 189–194, 283–289.
30. U.S. Department of Health, Education, and Welfare, Public Health Service, National Institutes of Health, National Cancer Institute. "Report of the Working Group to Review the National Cancer Institute/American Cancer Society Breast Cancer Detection Demonstration Projects," Washington, D.C., 1977.
31. U.S. Department of Health, Education, and Welfare, Prevention Task Force, Services Work Group. "Preliminary Report and Working Paper of the Services Work Group, Prevention Task Force, Department of Health, Education and Welfare," Prepared for the National Academy of Sciences. Institute of Medicine Conference of Health Promotion and Disease Prevention, Washington, D.C., February 16,1978.
32. National Academy of Sciences, Institute of Medicine, Ad Hoc Advisory Group on Preventive Services. *Preventive Services for the Well Population.* Washington, D.C., 1978.
33. Lichtenstein, E. and Danaher, B. G., "Role of the Physician in Smoking Cessation." In *Chronic Obstructive Lung Disease*. R. E. Brashear and M. L. Rhodes, eds. St. Louis: Mosby, 1978.
34. U.S. Department of Health, Education, and Welfare. *Cigarette Smoking Among Teenagers and Young Women.* DHEW Publication Number (NIH) 77-1203, Washington, D.C.: U.S. Government Printing Office, 1977.
36. Danaher, B. G., Shisslak, C. M., Thompson, C. B., and Ford, J. D., "A Smoking Cessation Program for Pregnant Women: An Exploratory Study," *American Journal of Public Health*, 68 (1978), pp. 896–898.
37. Hertz, P. and Stamps, P. L., "Appointment Keeping Behavior Reevaluated." *American Journal of Public Health* 67 (November 1977), pp. 1033–1036.
38. Greenlick, Merwyn et al. "Comparing the Use of Medical Care Services by a Medically Indigent and a General Membership Population in Comprehensive Prepaid Group Practice Program." *Medical Care* 10 (May–June 1972), pp. 138–200.
39. Haynes, R. B. et al., "Manipulation of the Therapeutic Regimen to Improve Compliance: Conceptions and Misconceptions." *Clinical Pharmacology and Therapeutics* 22: 2 (1977), pp. 125–130.
40. Ward, G. W., "Changing Trends in Control of Hypertension." *Public Health Reports* 93 (January–February 1978), pp. 31–34.
41. Podell, R. N., "Physician's Guide to Compliance in Hypertension." In *Preventive Medicine U.S.A.*, New York: Prodist, 1977.
42. McKinney, J. M. et al., "The Effect of Clinical Pharmacy Services on Patients with Essential Hypertension." *Circulation* 48 (November 1973), pp. 1104–1111.
43. Inui, T. S., Yourtree, E. L. and Williamson, J. W., "Improved Outcomes in Hypertension After Physician Tutorials: A Controlled Trial." *Annals of Internal Medicine* 84 (1973), pp. 646–651.
44. Task Force on Consumer Health Education, National Institutes of Health, Amercan College of Preventive Medicine. *Promoting Health: Consumer Education and National Policy*, A. R. Somers, ed. Germantown, Md.: Aspen Systems, 1976.

2 / Social Perspective on Risk Reduction

Henrik L. Blum, M.D., M.P.H.

"Health promotion and maintenance through risk reduction" is a broad-ranging style of intervention that is widely believed to hold major well-being benefits for most of us as individuals, and as a consequence, for our society. In turn we generally assume that what is "good" for our society will further promote the long-term well-being of individuals.

Risk reduction will be presented as emanating from two sources. One, which I will call *micro*, embraces the efforts made by individuals to so comport themselves as to minimize their exposure to health hazards. The other, which I will call *macro*, embraces the efforts made collectively by a society to preclude or minimize the possibility of its members being exposed to health hazards. I believe that the interdependence of these two approaches is poorly understood at this time and will make the case that significant risk reduction can only be built upon intermeshing the micro and macro approaches, for each is dependent on the stimulation and actions of the other.

To understand the concept of risk reduction one must first explore the nature of health and what affects it. Then we can understand when, where, and how to apply risk-obviating interventions. Having examined what risk minimization involves, we will then be able to identify our assignment, the social concerns that arise as a result of applying various risk-reduction strategies.

FORCES THAT DETERMINE HEALTH

A Brief History and the "Canadian Breakthrough"

The multitude of forces at work in shaping the state of health were well appreciated in many ancient cultures and have been restated from time to time. Hippocrates made clear the relationship of various forces to the occurrence of various forms of ill health.[1] McKeown[2] and others[3] presented a well-supported thesis of how the environment affected health in both general and specific ways.

In 1968 and again in 1969 and 1974 the author vigorously promoted an enlargement and clarification of the concept of forces that affect health so that health planners could see more clearly how to intervene rationally and effectively to reduce the risks that presaged ill health.[4-6] (See Figure 1.) For a number of reasons, this idea did not catch on.

Fortunately, however, beginning with a sociopolitical reconnaissance of the "facts of life" as part of its quiet but overwhelming social revolution, the Canadian province of Quebec created the Castonguay-Nepvue Commission (1966–1972), which documented many of the same concerns.[7] This was followed in 1972 by the Hastings report on "The Community Health Centre in Canada"[8] and the 1973 formulation by

Family and Community Health, 3:1 (May 1980).

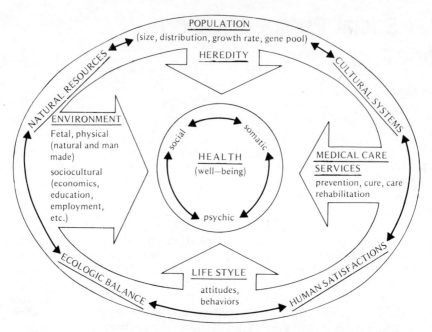

FIGURE 2-1.   The force-field and well-being paradigms of health. (Source: Blum, H. L. *Planning for Health* 2nd ed. New York: Human Sciences Press, 1980.)

Laframboise of the basic importance to well-being of the environmental and behavioral risks.[9]

The classic text of Lalonde put the force-field of risk factors of Laframboise into political orbit by converting it into Canadian national health policy.[10] The subsequent worldwide popularization of what is portrayed in Figure 1 was immensely aided by growing worldwide public and political disenchantment with larger doses of increasingly more expensive traditional medical care which was also perceived as becoming decreasingly effective in improving health.

Force-Field Paradigm

Figure 1 conveys the nature of the field of forces that affect health. The width of the arrows, portraying the four major types of forces, is symbolic of the relative importance the author attaches to the influence of each set of forces on the well-being of human beings.

Environment: By far the most potent and omnipresent set of forces is the one labeled "environmental." In it are included such elements as education, affluence, culture, form of political governance, peace, adequacy and safety of food and water, and the state of the *homo sapiens*-affected natural environment and the *homo sapiens*-created physical environments. The evidence that the environment is far and away the major determinant of health has been martialed time and time again.[11]

Behavior: The second most powerful force to affect health is undoubtedly beharioral. The documentation prepared in Canada for the Lalonde report was certainly not the first, but it was one of the most telling compilations of the contributions made by ill-advised behaviors and life-styles to the morbidity and mortality of the people of a modern and affluent nation.

Medical Care: Medical care is shown as the third major force affecting health. The decisive technologies that are represented by such basic breakthroughs as immunizations are remarkably effective.[12] Once understood and made available, these may require little or no traditional medical activities. In innumerable traumatic and infectious conditions, and to a lesser degree in metabolic, carcinogenic and degenerative ones, medical interventions play key restorative or ameliorating roles. But they are predominantly applied only after disease occurs and therefore are often too late and at a great price.

Beyond some basic minima, medical care seems to add only modestly to wellness or to survival. It also adds its own disturbances of wellness, particularly as more potent and more heroic measures introduce more risks stemming directly from the elements of care themselves (iatrogenesis).

Heredity: The fourth force is that of genetic endowment. Although they are critical shapers of each of our destinies, many genetic configurations achieve their guiding potential only in the presence of certain environmental forces. Others may be neutralized or activated by various medical interventions.

Interaction Among the Four Forces: The peripheral ring shown in Figure 1 points up the effects of each of the forces on one another. The contributions made by environment and medical care to genetically potentiated disease have been noted. Individual behavior is most markedly affected, if not generated, by various aspects of the environment.

Human behavior is further affected by contact with medical care which may teach individuals how to live more sanely or utilize preventive procedures. Inadvertently, the same care may promote such behaviors as waiting for symptoms of illness, and dependence on and use of professional care to overcome disease once it has occurred rather than living in such a way as to avoid it.

Well-Being Paradigm

There is a second paradigm built into Figure 1—one of an indivisible state of well-being. Psychic, somatic, and social health are intertwined and inescapably transmutable facets of health. Ill health, in any of the three artificially separated aspects of health, metamorphoses from one to the other regularly and rapidly. The literature to support this view is extensive and overwhelmingly consistent.[13] Accidents are only rarely accidental. Even illnesses are predictably related to life changes and stresses,[14-16] even if the form they will take remains unpredictable.

It is important to understand this paradigm so it is not thought that only somatic forces create somatic problems, psychic forces the psychic ones, or social forces the social ones. Some of the newest evidence of force-field relationships emphasizes the overall role of social networks in maintaining all aspects of well-being,[17] and presumably its utility for risk reduction.

Those wishing a better understanding of these two paradigms should study Brody's fascinating picture of the *homo sapiens* hierarchy of systems which provides the ability to explain the empirical evidence[18] summed up by the two paradigms presented in Figure 1.

THE NATURE OF RISK REDUCTION STRATEGIES

The general tenor of risk reduction strategies at the moment seems to be that of getting people to *behave* so as to avoid the inevitable hazards around them and not to provoke additional hazards by such behaviors as smoking or drug abuse. This set of risk reduction strategies encompasses only a small fraction of the routes to risk reduction and does not stand alone without significant support from major societal mechanisms. Because it is necessary to view the whole subject in some reasonable perspective, this article will utilize the idea of *micro* or individually based and *macro* or collectively based risk reduction approaches to examine the nature of risk reduction possibilities. (See Figure 2.)

Micro Approaches

Micro approaches are by far the most popular ones currently proposed. (*Micro* because they require behavioral changes on the part of individuals, each of whom provides the driving force and undertakes the activities that will result in risk reduction.) The micro approach takes several forms. One may be called *creative* behavior. This avoids or minimizes omnipresent hazards by such means as careful driving, provision of fire and smoke detectors in one's home, taking suitable exercises, and so on (box 7 in Figure 2). The

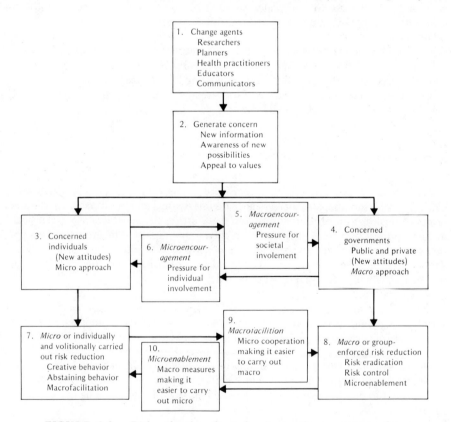

FIGURE 2-2.   Risk reduction through micro and macro approaches.

second micro form consists of *abstaining* behavior such as not smoking, not abusing drugs, not overeating, not selecting fatty foods and so on, in order not to *add* new hazards (box 7 in Figure 2).

These two forms are commonly used together for self-protection, as in obtaining immunizations for enteric diseases and avoiding nonpotable water. The critical ingredient in common is that the individuals use their own personal interest, know-how, ingenuity, and resources to achieve the risk reduction. This means that they use the personal "wiggle room" made available to them by chance, inheritance, education, resources, physical strength, security or whatever is involved in the behaviors called for. The individuals have to be informed about the risk potential for them as individuals; they have to generate concern over their risk potential, be knowledgeable about the correct means for avoidance, be motivated to make the necessary efforts, and have the resources relevant to the behavioral efforts called for.

A third micro form is shown as emerging from box 7, going via box 9 to box 8. It is one of facilitating the operation of macro type measures by personal cooperation with them. It can be called *macrofacilitation*.

A fourth micro form is similar to the one just described. It is shown as emerging from box 3, going via box 5 to box 4. It is one of creating pressures for one or another kind of relevant macro action. It can be called *macroencouragement*.

People are constantly being told that the micro approaches should suffice, that no one will be involved twice in a DC 10 failure (which is likely to be true), that no one should patronize a food dealer who distributes botulism or buy from a car company that makes dangerous cars. The latter two examples, which are more typical situations, should make it clear that food dealers cannot be expected to avoid distributing botulism if there are no well-established food controls, or that car producers will not be able to keep cars free of dangerous defects if there is not a strong official surveillance-and-recall mechanism. Examination of matters such as lead poisoning of young children in the ghetto, or asbestosis at work (and even at home and at school) also suggests small likelihood that micro or personal approaches alone can be effective.

Macro Approaches

The *macro* forms of risk reduction by means of group action are also shown in Figure 2. They can be seen to consist of two major entities that share the common framework of organized group or governmental action (box 8). The first is the simplest: A hazard to health is *eradicated* or eliminated. Single-level railroad-highway crossings are not built, or, if present, are replaced by crossings with underpasses or overpasses. Exposed and explosion-prone gas tanks are not permitted in cars, or, if present, would presumably be required to undergo safety proofing.

The second major macro form is one where society creates a form of surveillance or *control* for conceivable defects that have yet to appear, as in new automobile models; or those mechanisms which check for evidence of weakening in the face of known hazards, as routine airplane examinations; and for known exacerbated hazards, such as DC 10 motor mounts. Water, meat, poultry, milk, other food inspections and so on are traditional examples of risk-reducing surveillance. Highway patrolling for speed and safety is another highly organized control mechanism, as is policing in general.

A third macro form is shown as emerging from box 8, going through box 10 to box 7. This is one of enabling various micro activities to take place (e.g., forced creation of better quality breadstuffs from which individuals can then choose). It can be called *microenablement*.

A fourth macro form is similar to this. It is shown as emerging from box 4 and going through box 6 to box 3. This is one of creating more pressures or encouragement for motivation of individuals to carry out various micro acts. It can be called *microencouragement*. This macro form of effort includes the mass campaigns directed toward changing personal safety practices, diet, rest, exercise, and other health-affecting behaviors.

Mixture of Micro and Macro Approaches in Risk Reduction

WHERE MICRO RESORTS TO MACRO ACTION

Figure 2 shows that researchers, health planners, health workers, and various communicators and educators (box 1) set in motion waves that set off public concern (box 2). These waves reach different ears, some belonging to individuals (box 3) who develop an active interest in risk reduction. Some of these persons press right on to do whatever their understanding and resources allow in the way of micro or personal behavioral changes (box 7). Some individuals may see in a given issue no sensible way of taking micro action alone or no way in which purely micro action is relevant. In these cases—such as meeting the need for safer transport, avoiding air pollution, guaranteeing safe water, and so on—highly motivated individuals exercise their micro initiative to join with others to force macro concern to initiate what is called for (boxes 3 → 5 → 4 → 8). In other situations, where there are relevant macro institutions at work which need individual support, such as 55 mph speed limits, individuals exert their micro initiative by wholehearted personal cooperation and put pressure on others (boxes 3 → 7 → 9 → 8), such as law enforcers, to to their job.

WHERE MACRO RESORTS TO MICRO ACTIONS

Just as micro approaches often need a macro base, so macro approaches typically need a strong micro base. Food poisoning, for example, cannot be avoided *just* by what is done by the inspected and complying food producers, processors, and distributors. Individuals make the final food preparations and can undo the entire safety pattern simply by inadequate use of heat and cold. Similarly, if otherwise reasonably well people put continued pressures on physicians for antibiotics to treat the common cold, such ministrations will ultimately result in dangerous reactions as well as increased bills (but little good). Thus it can be seen that macro-based institutions must also call for widespread individual or micro action if a good job is to be done (boxes 4 → 6 → 3 → 7).

A second set of related strategies may also be involved. If, for example, there are no desirable baby foods, cereals or breadstuffs, or if there are widely publicized and misleading advertisements, how do even strongly motivated individuals identify the suitable products, or perhaps even find such a product on the shelves? To be able to exercise their micro-risk reduction impulses, they must get society to ensure that there are suitably advertised and available low-risk products. This pathway of concerns, stimulated by individuals to get group action which then allows the individual to exercise suitable micro behavior, is shown by boxes 3 → 5 → 4 → 8 → 10 → 7.

Long-Range Mutually Reinforcing Micro-Macro Strategies

Democracy does not often allow for clear-cut public or macro action until there is a strong and widespread individual understanding of a situation that calls for macro action and any subsequent micro actions. Public action to require use of seat belts or non-smoking in set-aside, smoke-free, public places will not succeed until a majority of people feel that they as individuals would be better off under those circumstances. And then they will have to initiate such macro action (boxes 3 → 5 → 4 → 8) by pressuring their elected decision makers or will themselves have to vote on such proposals as whether to have required seat belts, enforced no-smoking areas, and so on. It is foreseeable to planners, enforcers, and favorably disposed individuals that macro enforcement of speed limits or no-smoking areas also aids those already favorably inclined to "do better," and even forces those who are unfavorably inclined to do likewise.

Canada has had a very strong governmental push (albeit with many apologies[19]) to change individual attitudes about such matters as safety, smoking, and drinking. The avowed purpose is to change habits. But planners with long-range goals in mind are hoping to achieve a change in outlooks sufficient to create demand which in turn will secure votes for new macro measures, which will then require that seat belts be worn, forbid smoking in public places, and so on. Thus micro shifts in attitudes allow macro measures which in turn assist and "force" micro or individual behavioral shifts. The long-range strategy may be seen as boxes 4 → 6 → 3 → 5 → 4 → 8 → 10 → 7.

Is this too Machiavellian to be called public planning? Perhaps some people do not believe that public purposes should allow vigorous dispensation of honest information (boxes 4 → 6 → 3 → 5 → 4) because of the way in which people's attitudes might be swayed for or against various macro or public undertakings. But if so, what are our corresponding feelings about private dispensation of factual information (or even of distorted or false information) over the media? Who gets to present which kinds of information to the public?

Choice Among Alternative Risk-Minimizing Options: Criteria

There are some risk factors (including many of the major casualty producers) that can probably be effectively controlled only by macro eradicative approaches.[20] Some can be controlled in any one of many ways. For example, cigarette smoking responds modestly to education geared to micro action. It also responds to macro taxing schemes and would probably respond comparably to other causes of price increases, such as withdrawal of government tobacco subsidies. It also responds to the macro technique of extending nonsmoking areas. It is unfortunately true that one can expect the different kinds of interventions to work to different degrees in different social groups, and probably to differ in their effectiveness or outcomes from substance to substance (e.g., alcohol, hard drugs, or tobacco).

In some conditions the laying-on of hands by professionals—as in prospective medicine for adults[21] or for children[22] or for lifetime monitoring[23]—has been a modestly effective micro-bolstering macro-type intervention. But it is one of significant cost and of limited availability. The most powerful interventions are macro interventions which focus on the socioeconomic environment, such as taxing, general prohibitions, or general provisions. But their ultimate outcomes are hard to predict. There is little doubt that how a society views major problems (e.g., use of illicit drugs, prescribed medications, or modes of transport) will be critical to how society acts on the problems. The acceptance of hard drugs in America at the turn of the century, when alcohol was being denounced (and was well on its way to being outlawed), is part of a fascinating historical saga. However, as potent as the antialcohol crusade was, the intervention known as prohibition not only did not curtail alcohol abuse but carried with it gross, if unintended, incentives for violence and organized lawbreaking. In due time, alcohol became very socially acceptable while hard drugs became associated with organized crime and law breaking.

Others have described suitable problem analysis schemes that attempt to clarify major precursors of and consequences to problems and point up (1) the many places at which we might intervene and (2) the kinds of interventions that might work at each of these places.[24-26] What must be pointed up here are the means by which the probably value of alternative kinds of interventions (programs, activities) are judged. It takes significant analysis to determine the probability of achieving the desired outcomes, of inducing other desirable secondary results, and of inducing those that are undesired. And all of this also has to be viewed in relation to the proposed levels of investment.

The issue of choice is not wisely one of debate about whether to concentrate on micro, macro, or mixed micro-macro methods of mounting interventions; the issue is the likelihood of specific success, the overall prices to be paid, and the overall consequences to be faced, if one or another proposed intervention is used. It is not just the years-of-life type of gains but the effects on all major values—such as liberty or security— that must also be considered. Many persons would, for example, forgo an effective and efficient mode of immunization if it required presenting a certifying card or tattoo whenever they crossed a state border.

As has been seen, successful intervention will involve serious prior consideration of many types and mixtures of interventions. What is needed next is some guidance as to how to choose from the welter of possibilities. Prospective or anticipatory evaluation of alternative interventions to indicate what they are likely to do if they are carried out is at the very heart of planning or policy analysis. Because prospective evaluation is infrequently carried out adequately, it is critically in need of reviewing. Here the following major sets of criteria are always relevant:[27]

TECHNOLOGIC FEASIBILITY
This set of concerns is a bounding one for it tells if a proposal is technically possible or if a new tool (e.g., immunization against venereal disease) must be invented before it can be used.

HEALTH GAINS
This set of concerns of criteria requires a prediction of what savings in lives, disability, illness or other health gain will be achieved. It forces a realization that some savings (e.g., years of life) may be at the price of many more years of varying levels of disability or distress.

POLITICAL FEASIBILITY AND PLANNER SURVIVAL
This set of criteria requires facing the political feasibility of any proposal and the political gains and losses (survival issues) for those involved in examining or promoting any given intervention.

SOCIETAL PRIORITIES GENERALLY
This battery of criteria is as diverse as what alternative interventions are likely to do (1) for equity, (2) for promoting democracy, or (3) in terms of cost per unit of specifically desired health gains. Three areas stand out as being of special concern:

Class Disadvantaging: Using the current fad for micro risk reduction approaches as an example provides an illustration of how class disadvantaging takes place. Usually it is the better off and better educated who have the required personal "wiggle room" to learn what is better, who have the time and know-how to search out the wiser buys or patterns, who have the money and the time to obtain a safer car, a better diet, a prospective checkup or health appraisal, or who can take more enjoyable exercises. The sickest and generally neediest elements of a society will not only be too poor to make the initially often more costly choices, but are too laden with chores and cares to give extra thought, time, or money to do what is involved.

Meaningful macro behavior is required as an enabler or inducer for most good micro behaviors. On the job and community sponsorship and leadership—for periods for exercise and nutritious low-cost meals at work, good public transport, safe sidewalks and streets, and opportunities for nominal-cost adult education and recreation—are examples of macro-based, micro-enabling efforts whose utility far transcends that of macro-based exhortation.

The post-Proposition 13 era may mean a diminishing involvement by government in such macro-sponsored micro ventures. However, the potential for increased health and the avoidance of unnecessary health care costs would seem to justify renewed efforts on the parts of management, labor, and government to go past the class-distinguishing micro blandishments and into tangible macro measures which allow all socioeconomic levels to join into a widespread micro rejuvenation. (In all fairness, it should be pointed out that it will probably take such basic macro measures as "full" employment and "decent" living conditions for all if there is to be useful micro involvement of the bottom socioeconomic quarter of our society which has the most adverse health behaviors as well as environment, and consequently the most health failures.)

Cost-Utility: Cost-utility type criteria or measurements are then applied to those alternative interventions that appear to offer predominantly highly desired consequences. Potentially useful and desirable interventions need to be compared with one another for costs per unit or degree of gain. Gain may be measured in terms of health to provide *cost-effectiveness* ratings, or in terms of monetary savings overall, as for avoided costs of care and avoided production losses (*cost-benefit* ratings).

- Outputs—This prospective check will be for the probable outputs of alternative interventions (e.g., how many messages will be put out, how many persons will be reached, how many cars will be halted or ticketed, how many seat belts will be installed, and so on). Of course, output measures say nothing about how many risks are averted or how many casualties will be avoided. It is a measure of actual jobs done, irrespective of quality or meaningfulness. In a few cases, such as certain immunizations, just getting the right persons inoculated does guarantee certain desired results—that is, they will not get those diseases. (It does not, per se, consider the degree of risk from those diseases to begin with.) When the outputs are related back to probable costs, they become efficiency measures which by themselves still do not tell much about cost-utility.

- Outcomes—The second and infinitely more important set of criteria contains estimates of what will happen to those who will be affected by each of the competing interventions: How many fewer cigarettes will be smoked, how many persons will stop smoking, how many who would have started will not, and so on. If one cannot be sure that a lessening of smoking is paralleled by a corresponding level of decline in various diseases, then the intervention must be regarded as an experiment in which the actual relationship of less smoking to factors such as less lung cancer, emphysema, and heart disease will have to be ascertained.

  Cost-utility criteria also take into account predictable losses or damages of any kind that the interventions are likely to create. Since so many impacts and outcomes are likely to occur with a major measure (micro or macro directed), and since gains and losses often go to different parties, just getting overall benefit-cost ratios or net gains of benefits does not usually provide enough guidance. The economic, and thus the political, implications of who gains what and who loses what need to be examined. It is particularly important to see who are to lose and whether they can be treated fairly out of the gains for others. Measures that modestly increase the well-being of large groups but economically wipe out a smaller one and plunge it into the ill health to be born of poverty, abandonment, migration, or ghettoization (e.g., fighting inflation with unemployment) spell trouble.

Impacts: Each alternative intervention has to be examined for its longer term impacts on society as a whole and on any groups especially liable to feel its consequences.[28]

A very effective "hard" macro program (such as prohibition) may, as observed, lead to extensive law-breaking attitudes and the growth of organized crime irrespective of its outcomes initially on curtailing a certain action. By contrast, a determined but "soft" macro-sponsored micro effort might get few tangible initial outcomes but create strong ultimate support and demand for "hard" macro programs—for which there will then be cooperation and ultimately good outcomes with no significantly adverse impacts.

Macro campaigns for micro action, when meaningful micro action is all but unattainable, may breed more broadly directed hatred and distrust than healthier lifestyles. Examples of such campaigns would include promotion of good diets in ghettoes and reduction in smoking and drug abuse in minority areas with high teenage and young adult unemployment.

Some impacts, such as those spawned by brilliantly designed and brilliantly publicized medical technology (and accompanied by prepayment for care) have resulted in people depending overwhelmingly on professionals for sickness care rather than depending on themselves for wellness-oriented behavior, and even in avoiding self-care for the simplest things. The subsequent increase in costs of care is equally impressive and can be expected to continue for a long time. There is presently, however, both a healthy rebound reaction to the impact of such follies and a growing concern for healthy behavior and more self-care.

THREATS TO EFFECTIVE RISK REDUCTION AND HEALTH PROBLEM SOLVING

Conceptual anemia, wishful thinking, and social irresponsibility are very much a part of this nation's current way of life and its unrelenting search for pain-free and quick "fixes." There must be a sensitization to the capacity of these three traits for misdirecting and subsequently discrediting risk reduction.

It should be said that risk reduction is not new. Developing effective risk reduction (whether in the micro form of "let people change themselves," in the macro form of "have society make the key moves," or some mixture of the two) is nothing more than competent problem analysis directed toward attacking precursors to problems, such as risks. This problem-solving approach must include a suitable search for problem precursors among each of the four force-field factors—environment, behavior, medical care and genetics (Figure 1).[29]

Feeble conceptualization, wishful thinking, and lack of concern for the general welfare make up a formidable set of barriers to designating and implementing effective risk reduction, the proper name for which is health problem solving. It takes no great perspicacity to surmise that social irresponsibility (special interest vestedness) will narrow conceptual involvement and that wishful thinking can do likewise. Conceptual weakness and wishful thinking will in turn lend themselves to proposals that unguardedly support hopes for a quick answer that will easily blend in with social irresponsibility.

This triumvirate of "evil forces" not only directs attention to wrong issues and spurious solutions but has a high likelihood of sponsoring failures (and unhappy side effects) which justifiably discredit the involved scientists, therapists, planners, and policy makers, as well as the bureaucrats of private and public enterprises. No country can afford these negative forces, for in the times ahead all of the public trust that can be earned must be.

What are the failures that loom on the horizon if "risk reduction" is to be offered as a simplistic do-it-yourself substitute for the real thing (i.e., suitable problem analysis)?

Failure to Analyze Problems Adequately

The popular slogans of risk avoidance and risk reduction intentionally slight the major societal and environmental inputs to health in favor of the behavioral inputs which for the most part are themselves nothing but a response to the same societal and environmental forces. As it is now being popularized, risk reduction has somehow been reduced to its micro aspect. This ersatz risk reduction has been perceived as a new approach to solving problems and thus as an excuse for not looking at the real origins of problems or at their consequences. (It must be remembered that for some problems the only currently available answers are to attack the consequences, and that in others, attacking the consequences—e.g., treating a case of tuberculosis—is also the eradication of a precursor to future cases.)

Conceptual anemia further allows one to overlook the examination of each type of problem that has its very own set of precursors which also may vary from group to group and place to place. All of the major health problems, and even the minor ones, are "wicked problems"[30] for which there can be no rote reliance on doing the "obvious" or conventionally accepted "wise" thing[31]—which nowadays is often presented in the form of micro risk reduction.

It is heartening to see that Califano, as departing Secretary of Health, Education, and Welfare, (HEW) in mid-1979, brought major macro concerns back to the risk reduction fold.[32] And in a powerful new book Nancy Milio presents the innumerable macro policy forces in and out of the health sector that affect health and the possibilities for risk reduction.[33] Perhaps efforts such as these will restore to risk reduction a meaningful macro as well as micro outlook.

Most of the larger problems (such as strokes, heart disease, lung cancer, alcoholism, or auto accidents) do not imply simple, clear-cut, cause-and-effect systems. Unfortunately a little more scrutiny of the "simple" polio situation of new cases among the unimmunized tells more than that victims are not immunized. A little further "upstream" in the cause-and-effect chain,[34] it soon becomes evident that many factors conspire to prevent polio immunization: poverty and the absence of free immunizations; isolation and lack of inexpensive transportation; ignorance, fear or unconcern (even for a service that is readily available and free); anomie, frustration, and concomitant distraction from basic health concerns—all of these, and more, enter into the problem in varying degrees among different groups. But enter they do. A single intervention such as education through the media or in the schools may do little. Free weekly clinics in the neighborhood may do little more.

The problem has to be understood well enough to identify the key underlying obstacles to favorable action in a given situation. This may not be hard to do. But then again, people may not wish to deal with the responsible societal ways and gerrymandered or benighted policies that perpetuate gross class discrimination in employment, income, education, housing, and other opportunities that appear to underlie even such simple matters as failure to be immunized (as well as most other grossly adverse health situations).

Failure to Examine and Compare Relevant Possible Interventions

An earlier section indicated how competing alternative interventions must be checked out and compared in advance of implementation. All around are skeletons of earlier programs failures as well as ongoing monsters because these interventions were never checked out before being implemented.

Failure to Become Conversant with the Implementation Pathways

Many of the change agents who so vigorously search out the causes of problems, and even those who design the solutions to them, are typically not politically or programmatically oriented. Their personal rewards come from their exploratory efforts. Even the majority of planners who try to integrate the findings of the researchers into action seem to be satisfied with describing impressive goals but remain rather unconcerned about how to obtain them, or what else will happen if they are obtained.

One of the most obvious implementation failures is due to an inability to educate the public and the policy makers. Part of that failure is the sincere and well-financed opposition of the special interests that are threatened. And part surely lies in the change agents' lack of concern and skill in getting their views into the policy arena or to support risk reduction-oriented agencies that try to do so. (Porter warns that many of the macro-oriented risk reduction measures that have taken so long to be put into place—such as the Federal Trade Commission—seem headed down the tube, as are consumer affairs programs generally.[35]

The change agents often also do not know how or care to work with opposed vested interests (including workers) who cannot be expected to tolerate eradication of their source of existence. Change agents, equally, do not know how or care to work with organizations and administrators who are to carry out the new interventions once adopted. Thus good ideas get lost, hopelessly gerrymandered or operationalized into oblivion.

Is it possible to influence the public policy makers and bureaucrats if the media, policy makers, and bureaucrats have to respond to the highest bidders? This may be the failure that is ineradicable in a society that is committed to policy making by a pluralism of vested interests.[36] However, major significant public agency macro risk reduction efforts have been created under adverse circumstances and are still effective.[37] Risk reduction efforts will, of course, continue to be initiated and energized by the never-ending procession of bigger and better disasters which force private business and governments to keep moving in the direction of macro eradication, macro control, and macro-based micro-enabling efforts, as well as micro stimulation (Figure 2).

Blaming the Victim

Blaming the victim[38] is a neat trick that distracts attention from the origins of a problem by heaping disapprobation on those who fail to see or are incapable of sidestepping the problem and thereby become its victims. Holding the victims responsible for not undertaking suitably evasive behavior assumes that each person is a free actor and minimally enmeshed in environmental forces. It says that people behave as they do, not as a result of the impingements of our suprasystems (family, friends, communities, culture, societal institutions with their schooling, advertising, rewards and punishments, and survival needs), but out of pure self-determination.

This belies everything that is known about behavior.[39,40] Programming based on such folly can have but limited positive effects. It is more likely to insult and alienate those with the highest potential for becoming victims, for they often know or sense all too well the macro forces that guide or force them into antihealthful behavior—the very forces which victim-blamers carefully ignore—and thereby proclaim their own intellectual or moral bankruptcy.

The fact that the three-city micro-oriented (boxes $4 \rightarrow 6 \rightarrow 3 \rightarrow 7$ in Figure 2) experiment works to a significant degree[41] is the very kind of evidence that is used by the victim-blamers who demand that the nonresponders should be doing what the health-gaining responders have done. What the victim-blamers overlook, however, is why and how the environments of the responders differ from those of the nonresponders. The limits to responding to this kind of macro manipulation are not grounds for stopping such programs, but suggest that there is a lot more to learn about macro efforts at changing environments and that there is small cause to blame the nonresponders.

SOCIAL RESPONSIBILITY FOR PLANNING AND IMPLEMENTING EFFECTIVE RISK REDUCTION

Because health planners in the health-planning agencies are intentionally trained and placed in positions where knowledge and values are to be turned into political, social, and economic guides for health programs, they should be at the center of concern over social responsibility for planning and implementing effective risk reduction. Other parties may equally fail to look for precursors to problems, perversely or blindly convert data into false logic, or submerge public well-being under pressure or blandishments from special interests. But these others have not accepted the formal responsibility for making intelligent and equitable conversions of information into relevant public proposals for action. The social irresponsibility of planners who fail at their task is total. The same failures in the hands of scientists, practitioners, or politicians is a deplorable, although a natural enough, propensity for those unfamiliar with guiding public action by widely held values (the scientists and practitioners) or those unfamiliar with guiding public action by scientific understanding (the politicians).

The responsibilities inherent in various groups in the area of risk reduction follow.

Professionals

It has already been indicated that planners who succumb to the "easy fix," which is neither easy nor much of a fix, fail to analyze issues and thereby produce or tolerate such sad cost-containment proposals as are contained in the 1978 National Guidelines for PL 93-641[42] and the National Health Planning and Development Law (which do not even include a mention of risk reduction).[43]

The other health professionals involved, primarily the researchers and the practitioners, rarely analyze the public application aspects of problem resolution. They tend to focus their energies on the problems of either "science" or clients who bring them satisfaction, status, and resources. The practitioners take the most frontal, probusinessas-usual stance for they see their judgment as the key tool by which to take care of the only problems of which they are aware—the immediate ones brought to them by their clients.

There presently are few tangible returns or rewards for all but a few categories of health professionals to carry out risk-reduction efforts. As a result, the medical community may even look with grave misgivings when someone else offers to undertake only the simplest and least socially threatening micro-promoting and enabling programs.[44] This situation is not likely to change until professionals are appropriately and even preferentially paid and applauded for performing risk-minimizing tasks. Whether their training and inclination to work directly with the more physical tools will change to participation with social tasks involving collective action is open to question. However, there are more practitioners turning to family care careers, and that carries a heavy commitment to family well-being that is overwhelmingly dependent on collective action for macro changes such as steady income, safe dwellings, and so on, which have to go well beyond micro stimulation and enablement.

The dominant educators of health professionals are themselves mostly health professionals and seem to be even more isolated from the health facts of life than are their practicing brethren.

The professional educators of the public, although existing in many shapes and forms, seem unlikely to be a great deal different from those they educate and are the recipients, if not the victims, of the same conventional teachings and messages. It seems that at any level they are not too adept at teaching how to examine information and problems. Rather, they seem much more attuned to providing established answers for dealing with problems—answers that seem to strike out more and more frequently as the world changes faster.

If one were to list some general responsibilities to be borne by professionals they would be an echo of the professionals' own credo of the search for fact, for interpretation, for verification, for educating those dependent on them, for clarifying misinterpretations and, above all, for mediating among the divergent interpretations. But these are not the day-to-day realities for professionals.

Policy Shapers and Makers

The mass media are probably the major shapers of policy for most issues, usually at the behest of their major advertisers who are their major source of support. Other shapers are those who are formal members of planning bodies, for they are specifically designated to shape policy. Those who are on policy-making bodies are shapers as well as the designated makers of policies for the groups they represent.

In general, it can be said that policy makers are very much a part of their society. Mavericks or independent thinkers have a limited constituency and thus usually have a short span of office. Will has painted the anomaly well: our representative leadership cannot *take* its sense of direction from the masses and at the same time *invent* new and more relevant paths and persuade their constituents to follow them. Unfortunately, exploring and popularizing meaningful macro and micro risk minimization will involve our policy makers in "difficult and perilous tasks."[45]

The situation is not entirely bleak. The world situation will probably not allow business-as-usual, but this is no guarantee that new styles of operation will be better. Progress is being made in some democratic countries where the endlessly overlapping problems of energy, pollution, agriculture, food, and health are being examined—each in the light of the ramifications of the other.

If one were to list some general responsibilities of policy shapers and makers, the list would include integrity in preparation of agendas, giving priority to the most pressing well-being problems, giving hearing to the victims, pressing for relevant explanations, and searching for solutions that do not prejudice the survival of small or large groups. That these are a long way from being realized is all too evident.

Individuals as Independent Entities and as Members of a Collectivity

No matter how the issues raised in this chapter are viewed, it must be concluded that it will take individuals to conceive of and popularize new ways of examining and proceeding. Yet if they are not meshed with a receptive society that creates collective action, their efforts are likely to be resisted, forgotten, or lost.

It is heartening to observe that many millions of individuals as independent entities who have the educational, intellectual, social, and economic resources to do so have (under collective endorsement) moved into various aspects of micro health involvement as soon as they were made aware of the possibilities. In spite of accompanying excesses and irrelevancies in many directions, the heart of the movement seems sound and may well already have made a significant contribution to America's recently decreased mortality rates (a rate of decrease that is not paralleled by all countries that enjoy comparable affluence and socioeconomic-political environment).[46] The commercial interests that are profiting from various phases of the micro movement offer the usual tangible, and far from negligible, economic, social, and political support to such movements.

It is important to note that it is not just in the United States—that while involvement with micro risk reduction spreads, there is a growing and not necessarily unrelated erosion of collective concern for the macro forces which (1) stimulate various micro activities, (2) facilitate pursuit of micro enablement, and (3) undertake out-and-out macro eradication of some, and control of other, risk-creating situations.

Halting traditional growth patterns, declining productivity, increasing reluctance to be taxed, inflation, and continued high levels of unemployment—all powered by such overshadowing issues as fuel shortages and rising costs—seem to have undermined the spirit to pursue sensible macro-based solutions.

Yet these problems are no longer the kind that are amenable to bargaining by special interests. They require major collective responses[47] which must undoubtedly be preceded by vigorous and gifted leadership. Because leadership appears to have shrunk at least as much as problems have enlarged, there may be emerging a go-it-alone mentality that is manifested, on one hand, by the health-enhancing new behaviors and on the other, by the hedonistic health-destroying ones. And both are accompanied by a loss of concern for and belief in the macro or collectively-based endeavors (which in many cases undeniably offer only problematic outcomes).

The professionals and academics are still in the best position to provide the leadership for impartial examination of this nation's major problems, with a view to what is likely to be best for the general welfare as well as for the individuals. High on their list of things to do should be careful examination of the micro, macro, and joint strategies for risk minimization (i.e., suitable individual and collective interventions for our worst well-being problems). Unfortunately, there is no reason to expect more from them than the occasional outbursts from splinter groups and mavericks. Their risks from pursuing traditional patterns or inaction are still little more than a long-term erosion of status.

The policy makers continue to be vulnerable to the maladroit advice of the professionals and academics, as well as to be afflicted by continued subscription to special interest bargaining on one hand and dependency on adversary strategies on the other. They will have to learn more about the tradeoffs or considerations required by the interests of those whose activities will have to be curtailed (the cigarette interests, the energy interests, and so on). The directionless wearing down of collective resources by potentially lethal, intersectoral blood-lettings is no longer affordable. Nor can new groups of displaced, unemployed, discouraged and less-than-well workers be contemplated because a battle was won by the "good" or the "bad" team and no collectively meaningful action was directed to the well-being of the group that "lost" out.

It is also important to learn about new ways of gaining conformance through sensibly employed incentives rather than continuing in our traditional way of using perverse ones and then depending on expensive exhortation, surveillance, and harassment to get much less conformance (at much greater cost) than is desired or achievable.[48,49]

As has been stated, risk reduction is an attractive way of looking at problem solving if one is not party to its misinterpretation or does not abort it into calls for purely individual action. But to keep it in a legitimate and useful individual and collective focus is not going to be easy.

REFERENCES

1. Dubos, R., *Man, Medicine and Environment*. New York: Praeger, 1968.
2. McKeown, T. and Lowe, C. R., *An Introduction to Social Medicine*. Philadelphia: F. A. Davis Co., 1966.
3. McKinlay, J. B. and McKinlay, S. M., "The Questionable Contribution of Medical Measures to the Decline of Mortality in the United States in the Twentieth Century." *Milbank Memorial Fund Quarterly* (Summer 1977), pp. 405–428.
4. Blum, H. L. et al., *Notes on Comprehensive Planning for Health*. San Francisco: Western Regional Office APHA, October 1968.
5. Blum, H. L. et al., *Health Planning 1969*. San Francisco: Western Regional Office APHA, December, 1969.
6. Blum, H. L., "Health and the Systems Approach," in *Planning for Health*. New York: Human Sciences Press, 1974.
7. *Report of the Commission of Inquiry on Health and Social Welfare*, Vols. 1–7. Quebec: Government of Quebec, 1967–1972.
8. *Report of the Community Health Centre Project to the Conference of Health Ministers*. Ottawa: Information Canada, 1972.
9. Laframboise, H. L., "Health Policy: Breaking the Problem Down into More Manageable Segments." *Canadian Medical Association Journal* 108 (1973), pp. 388–393.
10. Lalonde, M, *A New Perspective on the Health of Canadians*. Ottawa: Government of Canada, April 1974.
11. Blum, H. L., "Evidence Supporting a General Systems View of Health," in *Expanding Health Care Horizons*. Oakland, Calif.: Third Party Associates, 1976.
12. Thomas, L., *The Lives of a Cell*. New York: Bantam Books, 1974, pp. 35–42.
13. Blum, "Health: The Quality of Functioning of Person Level System," in *Expanding Health Care Horizons*. Oakland, Calif.: Third Party Associates, 1976.
14. Holmes, T. H. and Masuda, M., *Life Changes and Illness Susceptibility in Stressful Life Events: Their Nature and Effects*. New York: Wiley-Interscience, 1970.
15. Slote, A., *Termination: The Closure of Baker Plant*. Indianapolis: Bobbs-Merrill, 1969.
16. Levi, L., ed., *Society, Stress and Disease*, Vol. 1. London: Oxford University Press, 1971.

17. Berkman, L. F. and Syme, S. L., "Social Networks, Host Resistance and Mortality: A Nine Year Followup Study of Alameda County Residents." *American Journal of Epidemiology* 109:2 (February 1979), pp. 186–204.
18. Brody, H., "The Systems View of Man: Implications for Medicine, Science and Ethics." *Perspectives in Biology and Medicine* 17:1 (Autumn 1973), pp. 71–92.
19. Lalonde., *A new Perspective.*
20. Etzioni, A. "Individual Will and Social Conditions: Toward an Effective Health Maintenance Policy." *Annals of the American Academy of Political and Social Science* 437 (1978), pp. 62–73.
21. Robbins, L. C. and Hall, J. H., "How to Practice Prospective Medicine." Indianapolis: Methodist Hospital of Indiana, 1970.
22. Williams, C. L. et al., "Chronic Disease Risk Factors Among Children: The Know Your Body Study." *Journal of Chronic Disease* 23 (1979), pp. 505–513.
23. Breslow, L. and Somers, A. R. "The Lifetime Health-Monitoring Program." *The New England Journal of Medicine* 296:11 (1978), pp. 601–608.
24. Stokey, E. and Zeckhauser, R. *A Primer for Policy Analysis.* New York: W. W. Norton, 1978.
25. Quade, E. S. *Analysis for Public Decisions.* New York: American Elsevier, 1955.
26. Blum, H. L., ed., "Design, Analysis and Comparison of Alternative Interventions," in *Planning for Health*, 2nd ed. New York: Human Sciences Press, 1981.
27. Ibid.
28. Churgin, A., "Evaluation," in Blum, ed. *Planning for Health.*
29. Blum, "Problem and Goal Analysis," in *Planning for Health.*
30. Weber, M. W. and Rittel, H., "Wicked Problems, Dilemmas in a General Theory of Planning." *Policy Sciences* 4:2 (June 1973), pp. 155–169.
31. Forrester, J. W., *World Dynamics*, Cambridge, Mass.: Wright Allen Press, 1971.
32. Califano, J. A., *Healthy People.* Superintendent of Documents Pub. No. 017-001-004162. Washington, D.C.: U.S. Government printing Office, July 1979.
33. Milio, N., *Making Health: Toward a Health Policy Strategy for Prevention.* Philadelphia: F. A. Davis Co., 1981.
34. Ardell, D. B., *High Level Wellness*, Emmaus, Pa.: Rodale Press, 1977, pp. 179–180.
35. Porter, S., "Drive on to Paralyze the FTS." *San Francisco Chronicle* (August 21, 1979), p. 50.
36. Lowi, T. J., *The End of Liberalism.* New York: W. W. Norton, 1969.
37. Sabatier, P., "Social Movements and Regulatory Agencies: Toward a More Adequate—and Less Pessimistic—Theory of Clientele Capture." *Policy Sciences* 6 (1975), pp. 301–342.
38. Ryan, W., *Blaming the Victim.* New York: Pantheon, 1971.
39. LaBelle, T. J., *Non-Formal Education and Social Change in Latin America.* Los Angeles: UCLA Latin American Center Publications, 1976.
40. Inkeles, A. and Smith, D. H., *Becoming Modern.* Cambridge: Harvard University Press, 1974.
41. Stern, M. P. et al. "Results of a Two Year Health Education Campaign on Dietary Behavior: The Stanford Three Community Study." *Circulation* 54:5 (November 1976), pp. 826–833.
42. HEW, Health Resources Administration, *National Guidelines for Health Planning.* DHEW Pub. No. 78-643. Washington, D.C.; U.S. Government Printing Office, March 28, 1978.
43. Diamond, K. J., "Trying to Take the National Guidelines for Health Seriously: Issues for Thought." *American Journal of Health Planning* 3:2 (April 1978), pp. 28–35.
44. Mabley, J., "From Brownies to Carrot Sticks: A Community Health Education Story." *Trustee* 32:8 (August 1979), pp. 21–28.
45. Will, G., "Showboat Politics." *Newsweek* (September 3, 1979), p. 76.

46. Epstein, F. H. and Piza, Z., "International Comparisons in Ischemic Heart Disease Mortality." Mimeograph for the "Conference on the Decline in Coronary Heart Disease," Washington, D.C., 1978.

47. Dahl, R. A. and Lindblom, C. D., *Politics, Economics, and Welfare*, 2nd ed. New York: Harper Torchbooks, 1976, Preface.

48. Lindblom, C. D. *Politics and Markets.* New York: Basic Books, 1977.

49. Schultz, C. L., *The Public Use of Private Interest.* Washington, D.C.: Brookings Institution, 1977.

3 / Health Risk Estimation

Harold Leppink, M.D.

In the 1970s preventive medicine embraced a new direction—a new era. There were significant rumblings of the impending change in the 1950s and 1960s spurred by the Surgeon General's Report on Smoking and Health and the Framingham Prospective Study on Risk Factors and Heart Disease. It slowly dawned that the challenge was shifting from communicable disease prevention and control to the chronic or noncommunicable diseases. And, too, it dawned that this was a very different problem. These were multi-causal diseases, insidiously spawned in our life-style.

All the data in the fifties were telling us that a dramatic shift in morbidity and mortality had taken place. The leading health problems were of a different kind, one might say diseases of choice—personal or societal choice. The top four were now diseases of the heart, mainly atherosclerotic coronary disease; cancer, with cancer of the lung leading all others; brain infarction, strongly related to hypertension; accidents, particularly automotive; and coming into fourth place in some large metropolitan areas, cirrhosis of the liver, positively related to the consumption of ethyl alcohol. Significantly, just below these leaders were suicide and homicide.

These leading diseases—cardiovascular disease, cancer, hypertension, accidents, and cirrhosis—easily accounted for 60 per cent of deaths in the United States. It should be noted that these are not deaths in advanced age. Ominously, 5.5 per cent of white males age 40 would die within the next 10 years. Fifty to 60 per cent of these deaths would be due to the half-dozen diseases or catastrophies previously mentioned. The mortality pattern for the average white female in her 40s was similar in that no communicable diseases appeared in the list. Her principal chance of death was from cancer of the breast, followed by heart disease and stroke.[1,2,3]

Interestingly enough, more current data project that cancer of the lung is rapidly increasing, and it is likely in the 1980s to surpass cancer of the breast as the principal killer of females in the prime of life.

The noncommunicable diseases do lend themselves to primary prevention, but almost all preventive efforts grind down to effecting individual or, ultimately and ideally, societal behavioral changes. For years public health and prevention had relied heavily on laws and regulations and the provision of services to prevent or control communicable disease. Now with the modern diseases it has become a matter of individual and societal choice. In a free affluent society people have to make informed choices. Therefore the question is, assuming they want to, How do we go about helping them to do it?

This chapter will suggest that health education may be the best method we have for implementing the primary prevention of noncommunicable diseases. After accepting this, the first step is to inform people of the problems, that is, create awareness. The second is to identify those people with high risk; and the third is to offer those so identified the benefits of what we know about motivating and supporting behavioral change. In this chapter we will discuss the rationale for the shift of emphasis to education, an

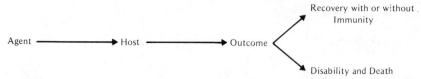

FIGURE 3-1. Communicable disease model. Usually within a relatively short time span. Onset to outcome is usually a transient episode in life.

instrument for finding persons at risk, and some of the barriers to finding them and offering them educational experiences which may affect their choices.

Sickness and wellness are recognized as parts of a continuum of life. It has become clear that for most people the quantity and quality of wellness may be enhanced or prolonged. However, with the noncommunicable diseases, primary prevention or intervention must occur before the irreversible and anatomical changes of sickness have happened. Prevention prior to the key transition point or phase is vital. After the sickness phase has begun, usually total anatomical restoration is impossible.

Over the years we developed a medical care system and an approach to primary prevention that was geared to the control of communicable diseases. We operated on the communicable disease model which was simple in its concept and served our purposes reasonably well. Involved was a single causative agent acting upon a host to produce a disease from which full, or nearly full, anatomical restoration was usually possible. Equally important, from the onset of disease to outcome, with a few exceptions, the time span was short, a matter of days or weeks. Medical practice based on specific point crisis intervention evolved to deal with these communicable disease problems. The ill person's role was largely a passive one and there was little need to understand the disease process, only to accept the ministrations of the healer (Figure 1).

Traditionally, in public health or preventive medicine we have directed our efforts toward either separating the potential host from the causative agent or doing something to the host to increase its resistance to the agent. This communicable disease model, with its simplistic prevention and intervention concept, does not apply well to the chronic noncommunicable diseases. We need a new model characterized by multiple factors, precursors, or agents impinging upon the host to produce a disease and an outcome which is rarely complete recovery but usually involves some permanent residual disability and possibly death (Figures 2 and 3).

The noncommunicable disease model must also convey a different time relationship, that is, a very long incubation period and variable durations of agent impingement

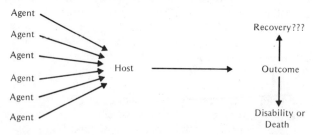

FIGURE 3-2. Non-communicable disease model. Varying amounts of time. Usually a very long time. Often a life time.

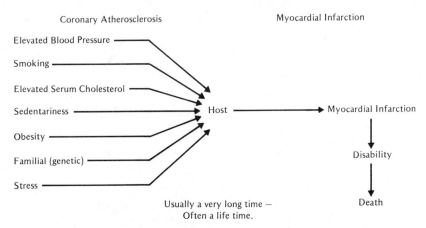

**FIGURE 3-3.   Non-communicable disease model. Usually a very long time.
Often a life time.**

upon the host. Beyond this, it should be noted that various combinations of the factors or agents are likely to have more than a simple additive effect in the production of disease outcome. This was demonstrated in the Framingham Prospective Study of Cardiovascular Risk Factors[4] (Figure 4).

In order to better understand the concept of noncommunicable disease, we also can think in terms of the stages in the natural history of most chronic diseases. We can divide the history or the progression of most noncommunicable diseases into six stages [1] (Figure 5).

1. The first stage is a period of time in an individual's life when he or she is at "no risk" of developing the disease. This period may vary from a few to many years.

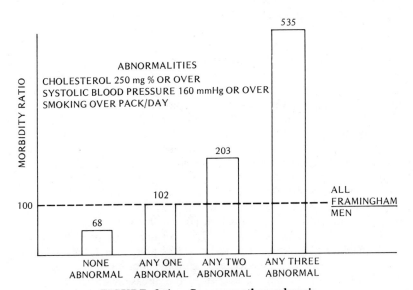

FIGURE 3-4.   Coronary atherosclerosis.

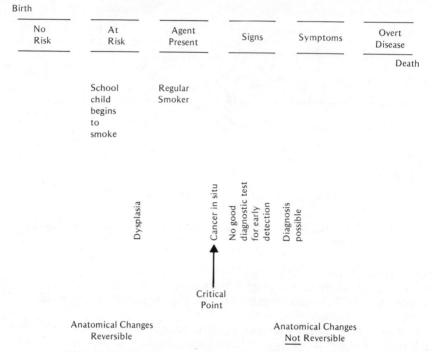

FIGURE 3-5. The natural history of cancer of the lung.

2. Following this there is a period of life when risk is encountered. One or more of the causative agents or factors becomes a part of the host's living experience or environment.

3. During this stage the causative agent or agents can be shown to be definitely active in the individual's life even though no symptoms or sign of overt disease can be detected by any known diagnostic means.

4. Here the critical point is passed and we move into the area of the natural history of disease called *signs*. This is the crucial transition stage from wellness to sickness. Prior to this point elimination of the offending agent from the environment would likely reverse or significantly decelerate the disease process. After this point, with special diagnostic equipment the earliest biological or anatomical changes of overt disease may be detected. The patient, however, is as yet completely unaware that any disease process is underway. Even here behavioral change relative to the offending agent or agents, or some specific intervention may have some effect in arresting the progress of the disease or reducing the seriousness of its complications. It may still be possible to significantly enhance longevity.

5. This next stage is called *symptoms*. Here the patient becomes aware for the first time that something is wrong and it is usually at this point that he or she becomes engaged with the sickness care system. Even so the diagnosis of the overt disease may still be elusive. However, it is likely by this point that behavioral change will have no effect, or at most a palliative effect, on the course of the disease.

6. In the final stage of the natural history of the disease, we encounter evidence of overt disease, and a definitive diagnosis is usually readily established. At this point

the person invariably has some degree of disability and, with rare exceptions, little can be done to effect reversal or regression of the anatomical changes.

Most of conventional medicine is practiced in the final two stages of symptoms and overt disease. Minimal efforts are now made to engage the patient at the level of signs but almost no effort is being made to engage the disease process in the first three stages of the natural history of disease.

We may cite many disease examples in which this natural progression of events can be identified. Cancer of the cervix and cancer of the lung are excellent models, and coronary atherosclerosis likewise fits the model well.

In the case of cancer of the lung it is obvious the individual is at negligible risk until the time cigarette smoking is undertaken. At some point in response to the carcinogens in cigarette smoke there develops dysplasia of the epithelial cells of the bronchi giving evidence that the agent is active. Intervention at this point by cessation of smoking will prevent the disease and allow for reversal of the anatomical changes.

The next stage is a localized cancer in situ some place in the bronchial tree, which, if it could be discovered, might be eliminated. However, usually the disease progresses to the point of symptoms and, from this point on, the rate of cure and survival is indeed dismal.

One can see a similar pattern in the development of cerebral vascular accidents or brain infarction. The progress is from an individual with normal blood pressure and at no risk to asymptomatic changes in the blood pressure. When the elusive critical point is passed, the progression from symptoms to disability may be quite rapid and is usually irreversible due to target organ anatomical changes.

Putting these diseases into the model makes it clear that prevention or reduction of morbidity is usually possible by changing some behavior or activity during the first three stages of the disease. Therefore, our health care delivery system must find new ways of encountering people while they are still well and well within these early stages. The old communicable disease model suggested that crisis intervention would produce a reasonable possibility of a favorable outcome, but the natural courses of the noncommunicable diseases affords no such outlook. Yet in our health care system there are no good tools or instruments with which we can readily, easily, or comfortably encounter the well individual with the risk factors or precursors of disease prior to the time that he or she passes the critical or transitional point. It seems clear that we need to look at well people, not for overt disease, nor for signs or symptoms, but for the risk of developing disease. We need to look for the agents, the factors, and the precursors of disease.

Thus, if we hope to increase useful life expectancy by reducing morbidity and mortality from the noncommunicable diseases, we must (1) screen the population to identify those persons who are at risk of developing these diseases, (2) offer them comprehensive individualized risk reduction–oriented health education, and (3) ideally, follow the individual at risk to ensure some continuity of support for the changes undertaken.

Traditionally, as we have said, the relationship of the patient to the sickness care system has been one of passivity. The patient was seldom required to be an active participant or knowledgeable actor in his or her own behalf. In past public health efforts directed at prevention, the participant has passively carried out certain dictums of the health department or submitted to certain procedures and services which had the effect of preventing disease. In the old system public health, like the doctor, was a parent figure and the patient was a child. In the new model if we are to effectively engage the noncommunicable diseases, the doctor or significant health advisor/counselor must be an adult relating to an active, knowledgeable adult patient/participant. Our education efforts must be designed to fit this new philosophy. This is the dawning of the age of individual responsibility for health.

Another old idea of preventive medicine was the concentration on early detection of disease. Such detection was based on the discovery of signs and symptoms, theoretically at a point where some secondary prevention or delay of disease and disability was still possible. This approach was costly and discouragingly ineffective. We might describe the old kind of medical care or preventive medicine as "retrospective" medicine. In retrospective medicine we ask what has happened to the patient and how can we prevent further progression of the condition by some type of treatment or manipulation. The new concept that we need could be called "prospective" medicine, in which we ask the question, What may happen to the patient and how can I prevent it from happening?[1]

Prospective medicine is quite different from the traditional preventive techniques for early disease detection. Prospective medicine involves detecting precursors and operative risk factors in the patient's life and attempts to reduce these risks by some type of intervention which has behavioral change as the expected outcome.

In summary, the steps in prospective preventive medicine are these: screening for risk factors, agents of disease, or precursors rather than for symptoms and signs of overt disease; quantification and appraisal of the degree of risk, systematic risk reduction planning; risk-specific health education aimed at permanent behavioral change; and, finally, societal support to sustain change.

In order to implement prospective preventive medicine and its concomitant health education, we need for well people at least an efficient, dignified, credible screening instrument capable of identifying, quantifying, and appraising risks to continued wellness or health. The instrument to quantify risk must measure reasonably well the individual's risk of death or morbidity. It must, if it is to be cost effective in the public health preventive medicine arena, be designed for efficient application to large numbers of people at reasonable cost and produce a significant impact upon the participants' health value system and, of course, enhance favorable sustained behavioral change.

In the late 1940s and early 1950s Dr. Lewis Robbins conceived the idea of risk appraisal which we can also call risk quantification or estimation. In the 1960s Robbins joined Dr. Jack Hall at Indiana Methodist Hospital, and they developed a risk estimation instrument which they called Health Hazard Appraisal (HHA) and began to use it in the family practice residency program at Indiana Methodist. Two key contributions to Health Hazard Appraisal were made by Harvey Geller, statistician, and Norman Gesner, consulting actuary. The former developed the Geller Mortality Tables for cohorts of ten years for males and females of black and white races. These tables list the dozen leading causes of death in order of decreasing significance for each ten year cohort [1,3,5] (Figure 6).

Evidence from many sources provided the agents or precursors, but Gesner devised a formula for quantifying the morbidity impact of precursors, singly and in combinations. His work became the risk factors which gave weight in terms of reduced longevity to the agents or precursors in the participant's life-style. We may define risk factor as the mortality ratio of a population with a specific precursor compared to the population average or the mortality ratio of a group with the agent precursor compared with otherwise similar group without the agent precursor.[1] With the Geller Mortality Tables, the Gesner computed risk factors, and the Robbins-Hall data base question-

White male Age 20		White female Age 20	
MVA	581	MVA	119
Suicide	126	Suicide	40
Homicide	63 56%	RHD	27 38%
Drowning	40	CVA	23
Aircraft acc.	39	Ly.Sar.	20
Ly. sar.	39	Neph & Neph	20
Other	693	Other	411
Total deaths per 100,000	1581	Total deaths per 100,000	660

White male Age 30		White female Age 30	
ASHD	329	Ca breast	91
MVA	302	MVA	88
Suicide	178	Suicide	71 36%
Cirr	68 47%	Ca uterus	68
CRHD	64	CHRD	61
CVA	55	CVA	56
Other	1123	Other	785
Total deaths per 100,000	2119	Total deaths per 100,000	1220

White male Age 40		White female Age 40	
ASHD	1877	Ca breast	351
MVA	285	ASHD	297
Suicide	264 56%	CVA	200 43%
CVA	222	Ca uterus	181
Cirr	222	CRHD	133
Ca Lung	202	Cirr	133
Other	2453	Other	1725
Total deaths per 100,000	5525	Total deaths per 100,000	3020

White male Age 50		White female Age 50	
ASHD	5764	ASHD	1313
Ca lung	860	Ca breast	631
CVA	717	CVA	548 49%
Cirr	488	Ca Int & Rec	343
Suicide	345	Ca uterus	302
MVA	345	Hy heart dis	246
Other	5764	Other	3468
Total deaths per 100,000	14283	Total deaths per 100,000	6850

FIGURE 3-6.   Geller Tables—Probability of death within 10 years from the six most common causes for a cohort group.

naire, any individual could have his or her chances of surviving for the ensuing 10 years appraised or estimated.

The question of validity of the risk factors is often raised. Do we precisely know the negative impact on longevity of a sedentary life-style, or a serum cholesterol exceeding 250 mg, or smoking 20 cigarettes per day? The answer is we do not precisely know this in any case. However, we do know from good epidemiological evidence that the precursors appear to be very important determinants of disease. We also know that some are more potent determinants of disease than others and that in combinations they have more than a simple additive effect.[4] Robbins and Hall, supported by input from many others, made a diligent effort to have their instrument reflect a conservative reasonable and credible result. It can be readily argued that medicine is not an exact science, and if our intervention efforts were always to be staid until we had precise knowledge we would be severely handicapped. Medicine has very often had to go with "the best we can do," the "state of the art." We have had to risk empirical interventions and therapies when sound reason gave support to them and evaluation of results was unceasing. Estimating risk is a noninvasive, modestly intrusive, nonlife-threatening event in a participant's life. Certainly some anxiety may be raised, but the doctor-patient relationship is almost always fraught with anxiety. The art of medicine is heavily involved with constructively and effectively dealing with anxiety—the doctor's and the patient's. So, in health-risk quantification we are dealing rationally with imprecise measures, but our best judgment supports the contention that we are not giving the participant a dishonest picture of the risks he or she is running or their significance to continued good health.

At this juncture we should also deal with another often raised question about risk quantification. Is it legitimate to apply group data to the individual? Hippocrates put great emphasis on prognosis in disease. Prognosis was central to practice in his day and is in ours too, if we think about it. Risk-factor quantification in terms of longevity is giving a kind of prognostic consultation to the still well person. Prognosis is always based upon some knowledge of group experience, often only the physician's experience in years of practice with similar cases. Nonetheless, properly we should in our counseling remind the participant that he or she is a part of a group which will experience certain consequences, not that the individual himself or herself will surely suffer those unfortunate consequences. What we are in effect urging upon a participant with a high risk estimation is to get out of the group and into a safer population.

With the basic development done by Robbins, Hall, Geller, and Gesner, the instrument was ready for wider application. However, there are a great many well people with and without risks. To encounter them in a cost-effective fashion has always been the problem of preventive medicine whether private or public. It was apparent that for mass application the data base had to be acquired from a largely self-administered instrument and the computations made by computer with the production of a readily interpretable printout. In the private sector one of the earliest practical efforts to accomplish this was made by Dr. Charles Ross in California, and in the public sector by Dr. Harold Colburn of the Ministry of Health and Welfare of Canada using Canadian mortality data. The author, working with an advisory committee of physicians and health educators, and with consultation and advice from Drs. Robbins and Colburn, did the same thing in a county health department in the United States.

It is not possible to describe every instrument that has been developed. Therefore, as author I will be presumptuous and choose our own. Let it be said at the outset that it is basically similar to those of Colburn, Ross, and others. Every risk-quantification instrument gathers from the participant epidemiologically relevant data to answer the key questions of prospective medicine, what may happen, and how can such disaster be prevented or delayed for this participant? The data base involves a health history: physical measurements limited to height, weight, body build, and blood pressure, and measurement of serum cholesterol.

The data is computer-processed to a printout which graphically displays the data, giving weight to the leading causes of death for the participant's age, sex, and race. Probably the most significant information on the printout from the participant's point of view, is the chronological/appraised/achievable age construct. In effect, we are saying of the participant that he or she has three ages: the first, a chronological age, is obvious; second, an appraised age, which is more important for it is the age group, or population group, into which the participant is placed as the result of the risks operating in his or her lifestyle. The risk or appraisal age may be greater or less than the chronological age. If less it indicates that the individual's chances of death in the next 10 years are less than average, or standard. If it is more it suggests that the individual is a part of a group experiencing a higher mortality rate. The achievable age represents the challenge and the motivation to behavioral change and suggests the group the individual could join with appropriate elimination or reduction of the risks under his or her control.

To illustrate the Health Risk Appraisal printout we may look at John Doe's appraisal as a sample (Figures 7 and 8). John Doe is a 43-year-old white male who gets little exercise, smokes a pack plus a day, has high blood pressure, is 15 per cent overweight, and so on. These characteristics are called risk factors or precursors.

The first page of the printout is the computerized bar graph (Figure 7). The second page is a detailed summary of the data which is displayed in the bar graph (Figure 8).

Following are explanations for each numbered area on bar graph (1–19):

1. *Patient Name–Doe,* John–Name of participant.
2. *Patient Number, 008587–Birthdate, 12/15/35*–Participant number assigned to individual. Birthdate–individual's date of birth.
3. *Prov/Phys–Well Person Center/Duluth*–The provider, or physician where the individual had the appraisal done. If done through a company or organization, this would be indicated here.

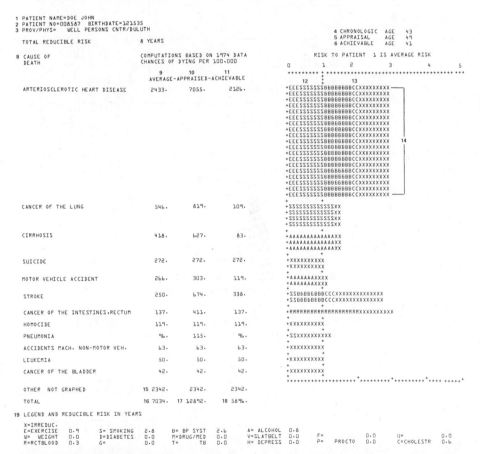

FIGURE 3-7.   Health appraisal–a program of the Health Departments of St. Louis and Lake Counties, Minnesota.

```
20 FOR HEIGHT 68 INCHES AND MEDIUM FRAME, 172 LBS. IS APPROXIMATELY 15 PERCENT OVERWEIGHT  DESIRABLE WEIGHT IS 149
                          --- ACHIEVABLE ---
21 YOUR HEALTH RISKS WILL BE REDUCED BY MAKING ANY OR ALL OF THE FOLLOWING CHANGES IN YOUR BEHAVIOR---
              EXERCISE   FROM:    LOW MODERATE      TO:    EXERCISE PROGRAM
              SMOKING    FROM:    STILL SMOKES 20+  TO:    STOPPED-SMOKING
              BP SYST    FROM:    180 MM.           TO:    146 MM.
              BP CIAS    FROM:    94 MM.            TO:    90 MM.
              ALCOHOL    FROM:    7-15/WEEK         TO:    1-2/WEEK
              WEIGHT     FROM:    172 LBS.          TO:    149 LBS.
              CHOLESTR   FROM:    220 MGS. PERCENT  TO:    196 MGS. PERCENT
              RCTBLOOD   FROM:    BLOOD IN STOOL    TO:    BLOOD IN STOOLODIASV
```

****
                * * * DETAIL * * *   FILE NO: 41

22 CAUSE OF DEATH	23 PRECURSORS	24 APPRAISAL YOUR CURRENT CHARACTERISTIC	25 RISK FACTOR	26 COMP R-FAC	27 ACHIEVABLE YOUR POTENTIAL CHARACTERISTIC	28 RISK FACTOR	29 COMP R-FAC
ARTERIOSCLEROTIC HEART DISEASE	BL.PRESS	PH(0/ 0) 180/ 94	2.2/1.3		146/ 90	1.5/1.1	
	CHOLESTR	220	1.00		196	0.70	
	DIABETES	NOT DIABETIC	1.00		NOT DIABETIC	1.00	
	WEIGHT	172	1.00		149	1.00	
	EXERCISE	LOW MODERATE	1.00		EXERCISE PROGRAM	0.50	
	SMOKING	STILL SMOKES 20+	1.50		STOPPED SMOKING	0.70	
	FAM/HIST	NO	0.90	2.90	NO	0.90	0.87
CANCER OF THE LUNG	SMOKING	STILL SMOKES 20+	1.50	1.50	STOPPED SMOKING	0.20	0.20
CIRRHOSIS	ALCOHOL	7-15/WEEK	1.50	1.50	1-2/WEEK	0.20	0.20
SUICIDE	DEPRESS	SELDOM OR NEVER	1.00		SELDOM OR NEVER	1.00	
	FAM/HIST	NO	1.00	1.00	NO	1.00	1.00
MOTOR VEHICLE ACCIDENT	ALCOHOL	7-15/WEEK	1.50		1-2/WEEK	0.70	
	MIL/YEAR	8000	0.80		8000	0.80	
	SEATBELT	75-100 PERCENT	0.80		75-100 PERCENT	0.80	
	DRUG/MED	NONE BEFORE DRIVING	1.00	1.14	NONE BEFORE DRIVING	1.00	0.45
STROKE	BL.PRESS	PH(0/ 0) 180/ 94	2.2/1.3		146/ 90	1.5/1.1	
	CHOLESTR	220	1.00		196	0.70	
	DIABETES	NOT DIABETIC	1.00		NOT DIABETIC	1.00	
	SMOKING	STILL SMOKES 20+	1.20	2.70	STOPPED SMOKING	1.00	1.35
CANCER OF THE INTESTINES, RECTUM	POLYP	HAS NOT HAD	1.00		HAS NOT HAD	1.00	
	PROCTO	NOT HAD IN PAST YEAR	1.00		NOT HAD IN PAST YEAR	1.00	
	RCTBLOOD	BLOOD IN STOOL	3.00		BLOOD IN STOOL (DIAG)	1.00	
	ULCEROOL	HAS NO SYMPTOMS	1.00	3.00	HAS NO SYMPTOMS	1.00	1.00
HOMOCIDE	ARRESTS	NO ARRESTS	1.00		NO ARRESTS	1.00	
	WEAPONS	DOES NOT CARRY	1.00	1.00	DOES NOT CARRY	1.00	1.00
PNEUMONIA	ALCOHOL	7-15/WEEK	1.00		1-2/WEEK	1.00	
	BACTPNEU	HAS NOT HAD	1.00		HAS NOT HAD	1.00	
	SMOKING	STILL SMOKES 20+	1.20		STOPPED SMOKING	1.00	
	EMPHYSEM	DOES NOT HAVE	1.00	1.20	DOES NOT HAVE	1.00	1.00

```
*  RISK FACTORS ADAPTED FROM HOW TO PRACTICE PROSPECTIVE MEDICINE, DRS. ROBBINS AND HALL, METHODIST HOPPITAL OF INDIANA.
*  ACKNOWLEDGEMENT TO H.N. COLBURN, MD-MPH HEALTH AND WELFARE CANADA AND J.W. TRAVIS, MD-MPH U.S. P.H. SERVICE BALTIMORE,MD
*  THE COMPUTER PROGRAM THAT PRODUCES THIS PRINTOUT WAS DEVELOPED BY, IS THE PROPERTY OF, AND IS USED WITH PERMISSION OF,
*                       ST. LOUIS COUNTY HEALTH DEPT., DULUTH, MINNESOTA.
```

FIGURE 3-8.

4. *Chronological Age—43*—John Doe's present age.

5. *Appraisal Age—49*—Because of John Doe's health risks, he has the same statistical chances of dying in the next 10 years as persons who are in a 49-year-old cohort. It does not say he will die 6 years earlier, but that his chances of dying are the same as a person 6 years older than he actually is. Risk is converted to years only to make it easier for participants to understand.

6. *Achievable Age—41*—The risk age John Doe could have if he made all the recommended behavioral changes, that is, reduced risks to the lowest level possible. He would then have the same statistical chances of dying in the next 10 years as persons who are in a 41-year-old cohort.

7. *Total Reducible Risk—8 Years*—This is the difference between the appraisal and the achievable age, and is the sum in terms of years gained that the health behavior changes would afford.

8. *Cause Of Death*—This column lists in rank order from the Geller Tables the 12 leading likely causes of death for John Doe in the next 10 years.

9. *Average Deaths/100,000*—These are the number of expected deaths associated with each disease. The data are taken from the National Center for Health Statistics and reflect the 1974 United States mortality experience. This shows that 2,433

deaths from arteriosclerotic heart disease can be expected per 100,000 white male 43 years old in the next 10 years. Similarily, 546 deaths from lung cancer, and so on.

10. *Appraised Deaths/100,000*—This column shows the adjusted mortality figures for John Doe. This shows that because of his increased risks to heart disease, John Doe is in the same group that might expect 7,055 heart disease–related deaths per 100,000.

11. *Achievable Deaths/100,000*—This column reflects the expected deaths per 100,000 for John Doe, assuming modification of *all* risk-reducing behavioral changes are made.

12. *EEESSSSSSSSBBBBBBBBBCC*—This represents the reducible risk explanation of letters found at the bottom of the first page of the printout.

13. *XXXXXXXXX*—This is the irreducible component of John Doe's health risks, for example, family history. The combined irreducible and reducible risk make up the total risk multiplier for arteriosclerotic heart disease and is read as 2.9 from the horizontal scale.

14. The height of the bar graph reflects the relative significance of each cause of death in terms of its contribution to the total number of expected deaths for an average 43-year-old white male.

15. *Other*—All other causes of death are lumped together. Individually, none accounts for more than 1 per cent of the total deaths.

16. *Total 7034*—The sum of this column shows that the average risk for 43-year-old white males for all causes of death is 7,034 deaths per 100,000 over the next 10 years.

17. *Total 12892*—The sum of this column shows that John Doe's health risks place him in a group which would have 12,892 deaths per 100,000 individuals, giving him an appraisal age of 49 years.

18. *Total 5896*—The sum of this column shows that by complying with recommendations made, John Doe can reduce his risk equal to the group which has 5,896 deaths per 100,000 individuals, giving him an achievable risk age of 41 years.

19. *Legend And Reducible Risks In Years*—This is the legend for the letters used in the bar graph. Each is followed by an expression (in years) of its contribution to the total reducible risk.

   *Stopping smoking reduces risk of dying from heart disease, lung cancer, emphysema, pneumonia, and strokes by 2.8 years.

   *Following a prescribed exercise program reduces risk of dying from heart disease by 0.9 years.

   *Stopping alcohol consumption, or limiting consumption of it, with no drinking before driving, reduces risk of dying from motor vehicle accidents, cirrhosis of the liver, and pneumonia by 0.8 years.

   *Reducing serum cholesterol reduces risk of dying from heart disease and stroke by 0.6 years.

   *Having a rectal examination to diagnose blood in stool reduces risk of dying from cancer of rectum by 0.3 years.

   *Reducing blood pressure to 146/90 reduces the risk of dying of heart disease and stroke by 2.6 years.

By complying with all of these recommendations an achievable risk age of 41 years may be attained.

The following are explanations for Figure 8 (20-29):

20. This describes John Doe's frame, weight, and height. This shows he is 15 per cent overweight (based on Metropolitan Life Insurance Company desirable weight tables for adult males) and that his desirable weight is 149 pounds.
21. The changes recommended are those John Doe shoud make in order to achieve the same risk of dying within 10 years as a person 41 years old.
22. *Cause Of Death*—This column lists causes of death for which there are precursors or factors.
23. *Precursors*—For each cause of death, the contributing factors or precursors are listed, such as for *arteriosclerotic heart disease*: blood pressure, cholesterol, diabetes, weight, exercise, smoking, family history.
24. *Appraisal—Participant's Current Characteristics*—This section provides the participant data. For example, for arteriosclerotic heart disease, the participant's blood pressure is 180/94, and his cholesterol is 220 Mgs. He is not diabetic, his exercise level is low moderate. He has no family history of heart disease. He smokes 20 plus cigarettes a day and weighs 172 pounds.
25. *Appraisal—Risk Factor*—This column lists the risk factors for each precursor. The risk factor answers the question, To what degree does the individual with this precursor deviate from average? For example, this patient's blood pressure is 180/94 which corresponds with the risk factor 2.2/1.3. His cholesterol, being 220, is average or 1.0, while his smoking behavior gives him a risk factor of 1.50 or one and a half times average risk. Risk factors are from Robbins and Hall.
26. *Appraisal—Composite Risk Factor*—Each composite represents a combination of all the single risk factors in a particular disease category. If a disease category has only one precursor, this risk factor is used as the composite.
27. *Achievable—Your Potential Characteristic*—This column lists the participant's precursors as they would be if recommended changes were made.
28. *Achievable—Risk Factor*—This column lists the risk factors for each precursor assuming the recommended behavioral changes have been made. By decreasing blood pressure from 180/94 to 146/90, John Doe reduces his risk from 2.2/1.3 to 1.5/1.1.
29. *Achievable—Composite Risk Factor*—Indicates the combination of all the single *new risk* factors after recommended behaviors have been modified. This column indicates the individual's achievable risk in that disease category.

The foregoing described the graphic computer printout. Its purpose is to quantify and dramatize "risk." With a modicum of explanation, the participant gets a picture of his or her health risks and what they may mean for his or her personal longevity. It is designed as a bar graph to get attention and, hopefully, to have a better impact on the participant's value system.

The second printout sheet (Figure 8) is informational, a composite of the data base upon which the risk estimation was made, and systematically suggests the value of behavioral changes which might be made by the participant. This sheet is useful primarily to the significant health counselor who interprets the graphic printout to the participant.

The objective of all these instrument design efforts was to place in the hands of the participant's significant health advisor a credible dignified prop, like an ECG, a brain scan, or a chemistry profile, to be used to interpret important health-related information to the participant/patient. Trying to avoid any suggestion of gadgetry, game playing, or mail order appraising, we have insisted that counseling the well human being is a serious undertaking. We have insisted on one-to-one interpretations for all who evidence a significant risk, allowing small group interpretations for those participants whose risks are negligible and whose greatest need is support and reinforcement of an already health-enhancing life-style.

This health-risk quantification procedure alone appears to provide significant and probably sustained positive health behavioral changes in many participants. Our evaluations have been based on participants' surveys which suggest significant impact.[7,8] Considering that health educators have long accepted that behavioral change is usually a stepwise process, it is reasonable to assume that participants in health-risk quantification could well motivate a person to mount a step or two and await a further motivating input to move on to full commitment to change, the final step. These intermediary steps are very hard to measure in an evaluation of the impact of the instrument. It is reasonable to assume that a person with a risk to health seldom moves directly from awareness to definitive behavioral change as a result of one motivational nudge.

For this reason, risk-specific health education based on computer retrieval of risk-specific groups of participants has to be a part of a health risk intervention program. We must be able to select, out of the population groups, individuals with specific risks and combinations of risks; for example, all males 40 to 45 years old with family histories of heart disease who smoke a pack of cigarettes a day and have a serum cholesterol over 250 mg. Or maybe we just want to isolate a group of smokers, male or female, any age, to offer them participation in a Lung association "Stop Smoking" support group. In every community there are health-related risk-reducing efforts going on. The key is to offer them to the people who need them the most. It may be this risk-specific health education effort that moves the participant at risk from simple awareness to definitive change.

Beyond this, the computer allows us easily to do two more manipulations. In the Geller Tables for the younger under 30 group, the dismal pattern of deaths from health risks is not yet evident and the printout of a participant under 30 could well mask the eventual impact of the precursors already operative in the individual's life-style. The computer can be programmed to provide participants under age 30 with a second printout projecting his or her risk status to age 45. In the chronic diseases we need to allow for a long incubation period. At age 45 the disease impact of smoking, obesity, lack of exercise, and other factors becomes much more dramatic. The participant in effect gets a look into the future to the risk group he or she may one day be a part of.

Beyond this the computer program can provide another useful service, group profiling. Suppose an employer offers health risk appraisal to employees. At the outset it is always understood that the data and printouts of all participants are confidential. However, the employer and the employees have a vested interest in the composite outcome of the program. The employer may want to offer employees some opportunities for risk reduction. We can have the computer give the employer a risk profile of all employees. Usually, such a profile reveals the areas in which company-sponsored or encouraged risk-specific health education would afford the greatest rewards in behavioral change. Beyond this one can envision the day when an employer, profile in hand, bargains with the unions and the health insurance providers for contract conditions and premiums tailored to the health needs and risks of the employee group.

Having just alluded to the use of health-risk quantification with employee groups, we should consider briefly our experience thus far in finding a place for health-risk quantification in the health care delivery system. At the outset we conceived of health-risk appraisal as a primary care modality and a part of the routine health maintenance effort that primary care physicians would want to offer their patients. Therefore, our opening effort was to offer our health-risk appraisal instrument to primary care physicians. Its reception was enthusiastic. The deep reasons for this can only be surmised, but at least these, we feel, are part of the reason complex leading to rejection or non-interest:

1. The procedure was perceived as too time consuming by the physicians and as a needless "burden" by their ancillary staffs. They see their job as caring for the sick and from that effort come their strokes.
2. They did not know how to price it, or they were uncomfortable charging a fee for a nondisease-related procedure, that is, pure prevention and health counseling.
3. The educational role it required caught them unprepared and thus unsure and uncomfortable. Many physicians appeared to be uncomfortable in providing health counseling to the well person.
4. There was no third-party reimbursement; therefore, whatever fee was established the patient had to pay it.

Probably physician attidudes could be summed up generally as nihilistic or skeptical in the area of the worth of primary prevention in chronic diseases. They could identify well with a "cure" oriented practice but could not fathom having a primary prevention oriented modality integrated into it.

Next we tried opening a "wellness center" or "well peoples' clinic" in the outpatient section of a medical center. It was staffed with public health nurses and public health educators trained to administer and interpret the health risk appraisal instrument. We encouraged physician referrals and received a modest number. We advertised for participants and solicited employee groups. There was an initial flurry of interest and then it waned. Likely its failure was due to an old public health dictum: if you want to encounter the population of well people you cannot expect them to seek out your service at your convenience and in your place. Rather you must reach out to places and times convenient to the population at risk. Probably the one positive lesson we learned from the wellness center was that participants were very accepting of health counseling from a nurse or a health educator. They relished this opportunity to ask questions and to learn about their well-being.

Our next effort was to approach community groups, employee groups, and industry.[9] This area seems most promising for it solves the logistical problems of moving people to a distant screening site. It often solves the problem of reimbursement and very often affords continuing opportunities for risk-specific group health education and intervention. Larger industries with onsite medical service staff offer the best sites for applying a health-risk quantification instrument and integrating it into their existing ongoing health maintenance program. Industries without medical staff or programs must depend on an outside contractor to come in periodically to administer, interpret, and , hopefully, follow up on the program.

Gaining the interest of employers has not been difficult. Many have had long-time commitments to fostering the health of their employees through various efforts to screen or to examine for disease and, hopefully, to detect them early and thus effect cures. However, some have become disillusioned with this approach, realizing that the cost of such a program is great and the results in actually cured diseases is disappointing. Whether risk-factor quantification and intervention efforts will do better at less cost is still to be answered by critical evaluation.

By way of evaluation we can say that the risk appraisal procedure appears to motivate behavioral change. We studied at 1-year intervals 366 of our early participants and found that 71 per cent of the respondents stated they had made at least one health risk-related behavioral change.[7,8]

Blankenbaker studied the cost effectiveness of health-risk quantifications showing that in one study 2,141 diagnostic tests were performed on 474 persons using a battery of nine different screening examinations. The effort produced 1267 clinical problems at an average cost of $22.23 per problem. He showed that a single risk quantification test conducted on each of the participants at the same time disclosed 2,616, clinical problems—67 per cent of all the problems detected—at any average cost of $1.36 per problem.[10]

What of the future? It seems the missing ingredient is a national commitment to the primary prevention of non-communicable diseases. In the latest Surgeon General's Report on "Healthy People" there appears to be a dawning of such a commitment, but not until primary prevention is dignified by third-party reimbursement will it really be applied in the mainstream of medical care.[11]

And what can we say of outcome evaluation? These diseases have long incubation periods and multiple causal factors and a great array of variables all along the way. All we can say is that the data suggest a decline is underway in heart disease in white males, a tipping or a flattening of the lung cancer curve in males, and an ominous continuing climb in females, probably to surpass cancer of the breast in the next few years. Maybe the clues to the worth of primary prevention in these life-style diseases are beginning to turn up. Historically our efforts at prevention, often modest, have paid off more handsomely than our prodigious and expensive efforts to cure, even when we have had to go with less than immutable epidemiological evidence that we were solidly on the right prevention track, or that we had the ideal instrument with which to effect our program. Health-risk estimation is far from perfect, but our evidence suggests that it does have a favorable impact upon a large number of the people who participate in the program and favorably influences some of their decisions about their own health. Needless to say, health-risk estimation is not the only weapon we should use in combatting non-communicable disease. We need in our armamentarium a myriad of weapons to bring to bear on our target diseases.

REFERENCES

1. Robbins, Lewis C. and Hall, Jack H., *How to Practice Prospective Medicine*. Indianapolis: Slaymaker Enterprises, 1970.
2. U.S. Department of Health, Education, and Welfare, Public Health Service, Center for Disease Control, *Leading Causes of Death and Probabilities of Dying, United States, 1975 and 1976*. Washington, D.C.: March 1976.
3. Geller, Harvey and Steele, Greg, *Probability Tables of Death the Next Ten Years from Specific Causes*. Indianapolis: Health Hazard Appraisal, Methodist Hospital of Indiana, 1972.
4. Kannel, William B., *Cardiovascular Risk Factors: The Framingham Study*. St. Petersburg: Proceedings of Fifteenth Annual Meeting Society for Prospective Medicine, October 1979, pp. 8–10.
5. Robbins, Lewis C. and Petrakis, Nicholas L., *Converting Ratios to Risks, A Foundation for Prospective Medicine*. San Diego: Proceedings of Twelfth Annual Meeting Society for Prospective Medicine, October 1976, pp. 48–50.
6. DeGrassi, Antonion, et al., *Reference Manual for Health Risk Appraisal and Health Risk Reduction*, Rev. ed. Duluth: St. Louis County Health Department, 1973.
7. Leppink, Harold B. and DeGrassi, Antonio, *Changes in Risk Behavior: A Two Year*

Follow Up Study. San Diego: Proceedings of Thirteenth Annual Meeting Society for Prospective Medicine, September 1977, pp. 104–107.

8. Lauzon, Richard R. J., *Randomized Controlled Trial of Ability of HHA to Stimulate Appropriate Risk Reduction Behavior.* San Diego: Proceedings of Thirteenth Annual Meeting Society for Prospective Medicine, September 1977, pp. 102–103.

9. Durfee, Jean A. and DeGrassi, Antonio, *Health Hazard Appraisal in the Workplace.* St. Petersburg: Proceedings of Fifteenth Annual Meeting Society for Prospective Medicine, October 1979, pp. 71–73.

10. Blankenbaker, Ronald, *Total Care the Cost-Effective Way.* San Diego: Proceedings of Twelfth Annual Meeting Society for Prospective Medicine, October 1976, pp. 103–107.

11. U.S. Department of Health, Education, and Welfare, Public Health Service, *Healthy People, the Surgeon General's Report on Health Promotion and Disease Prevention.* Washington, D.C.: U.S. Government Printing Office, 1979.

PART II
Risk Reduction Methods

The concepts, strategies, and techniques associated with primary prevention and health promotion are most easily applied to the early years of life and up through middle adulthood, though behavioral life-style changes can reap significant health benefits even during late middle age. For these reasons, we have chosen to focus the text's coverage of risk reduction methods from a developmental point of view.

The first four chapters of Part Two are devoted to a discussion of Risk Reduction for Childbearing, Risk Reduction from Birth to Kindergarten Age, Risk Reduction in the Middle Childhood Years, and Risk Reduction in the Adolescent Years. The author of these four chapters is Naomi M. Morris, M.D., M.P.H., who is professor and director of the Community Health Sciences Program, School of Public Health, University of Illinois at the Medical Center. The four chapters authored by Dr. Morris provide comprehensive and detailed coverage of risk reduction strategies, methods, and techniques that can be effectively implemented in preventive strategies and in promoting wellness for childbearing women and children into the teenage years.

Mental Health Risk Reduction for Children, Chapter 8, has been contributed by Jules R. Bemporad, M.D., William Beardslee, M.D., and Felton Earls, M.D. Precursors of future mental illness or childhood mental health risk factors are extremely difficult to clearly delineate during childhood. Dr. Bemporad and coauthors observe that many factors operate concurrently so that it becomes arduous, if not impossible, to isolate the discrete action of any one precursor life event. Thus, the authors have selected the option of dividing factors into the categories of (1) inborn, (2) intrafamilial, and (3) extrafamilial. In addition, the authors have described the complications that arise from conducting or interpreting research in this area.

Finally, the authors have reported the pertinent literature describing coping strategies of children in high-risk situations. Dr. Bemporad and coauthors believe that the study of coping strategies is indeed most pertinent as it may eventually lead to methods of intervention and remediation.

Chapter 9 focuses on Promoting Mental Health and Reducing Risk for Mental Illness and is contributed by psychiatrist Paul C. Mohl, M.D. In agreement with Dr. Bemporad et al., Dr. Mohl points out that mental health promotion and the clear-cut identification of mental health risk factors is exceedingly difficult because mental illnesses are highly variable in their forms and complex in their etiologies. The exact risk factors are difficult to define and change. Adding to these complexities, the effectiveness of various intervention strategies is not well researched. Dr. Mohl reviews in this chapter the four major forms of intervention: (1) mental health consultation, (2) crisis intervention, (3) group support, and (4) stress management. The focus is on how these forms of intervention may assist high-risk individuals in coping with stresses. Examples of the application of these interventions are offered along with references for more detailed descriptions. Dr. Mohl points out that no comprehensive mental illness risk-reduction program employing all of these interventions has been reported in the literature.

In Chapter 10, R. G. Troxler, M.D., discusses Stress Reduction Programs for Business and Industry Employees. In the past year particularly many health promotion programs, including programs specifically devoted to stress reduction, have been initiated throughout a growing number of businesses. It is hoped that careful evaluation of these programs will be undertaken in all settings in order to provide health professionals with some substantial scientific documentation of the results of such programs.

Turkan K. Gardenier, Ph.D., Health Statistician, U.S. Environmental Protection Agency, has contributed a concise and highly informative chapter (Chapter 11 detailing methods of data collection, assessment of significant factors, data analysis, methodology, interpreting, and relating findings to identification of environment-related health effects. The author also covers in detail data banking, retrieval and correlation, computer mapping and graphics, and dissemination of risk date—all of these methods have aided in the awareness of etiology identification and control of environmental risk factors.

Chapter 12 focuses in detail on the relationship between nutrition and risk reduction. The author is Christopher Hitt, M.S., who succinctly discusses the relationship of life-style, nutrition, and degenerative disease. The chapter outlines life-long principles and practices by which Americans can improve their chance of remaining healthy.

4 / Risk Reduction
for Childbearing

Naomi M. Morris, M.D., M.P.H.

Being well-born provides a good start for a healthy life. If an individual could pick his or her parents, surely among the criteria used would be the absence of strongly inheritable detrimental traits and any condition which might compromise the physical and emotional strength needed by the parents for childbearing and child-rearing. Optimal health of the mother at the time of conception, during pregnancy, and at childbirth is particularly important since she provides the environment in which the vulnerable growing new life develops. Parental health and well-being have been related to the outcome of pregnancy in many ways, the most important of which will be discussed in this chapter.

CHILDBEARING RISKS

Risks conventionally associated with childbearing include mortality and morbidities of the mother and child. Adverse social and economic consequences of childbearing may also be conceptualized as morbidities, since they are handicaps to optimal family life and child development.

Risks to the Mother

MORTALITY

The national maternal mortality rate reached an all-time low in 1978, approximately one per 10,000 live births.[1] A study of 149 maternal deaths from 1970 to 1976 in New York State concluded that 80.5 per cent were preventable.[2] Preventable maternal deaths were defined as due to inadequate care of facilities, adverse conditions in the community, or the patient's failure to seek or accept advice or treatment. Nationwide, in the 1970s, hypertensive states of pregnancy, hemorrhage, and sepsis were the main causes of maternal deaths. Modern prenatal and delivery care are almost always successful against these problems. Nonpreventable maternal deaths are due to irreversible causes such as advanced kidney or heart diseases; these may preexist in the mother and are aggravated by the physiologic effects of pregnancy.

MORBIDITIES

Serious permanent complications of childbearing are rare; but varicose veins, relaxation of the pelvic floor, and genitourinary tract symptoms are common. Physicians do not usually worry about these problems, but maternal energies may be drained by them. They may have consequences for subsequent pregnancies, such as embolism, GU tract infections, and fetal loss or premature delivery. The relationships of sustained hypertension and the development of diabetes mellitus to pregnancy are not clear, but high parity(many pregnancies) may augment the tendency of predisposed women to develop these conditions.[3] Any morbidity reduces the mother's capacity for investment of energy in child care, so prevention of maternal morbidity is in her children's interest.

Risks to the Infant

MORTALITY

Fetal: Fetal losses may occur at any time during pregnancy. The earliest ones are usually undetected, occurring during what appears to be a normal menstrual period.[4] The proportion of conceptions lost is unknown, but based on animal studies and some human research, it may be between 30 and 50 per cent.[5] The main causes for the earliest losses are chromosomal anomalies and abnormal development of the embryo. Other causes of early loss (miscarriages) include maternal infection, irradiation, and physical or chemical trauma. Maternal insults which do not result in fetal deaths may damage the fetus, causing congenital anomalies. The anomalies reflect the nature, timing, and severity of the insult. Late fetal losses or stillbirths may result from fetal abnormalities or from maternal complications such as diabetes, toxemia of pregnancy, or placenta previa. Good prenatal care has led to reduction of the late fetal loss rate through improved therapy for maternal complications.

Infant Mortality: Infant mortality is defined as the death of a live-born baby before one year of age. The national infant mortality rate went steadily down in the 1970s, and as of 1978 was 13.6 deaths per 1,000 live births.[6]

The main causes of infant mortality include problems related to immaturity, congenital defects, birth-associated problems, influenza and pneumonia, and sudden infant death syndrome (SIDS).[6,7] *Immaturity* as a cause of death reflects the inability of the very small baby born too soon to adapt to life outside the womb. Respiration is the most critical function. The newborn's lungs may not be prepared to remain open and allow adequate gaseous exchange.

Birth-associated accidents which result in infant mortality include such problems as the cord wrapped around the infant's neck, sudden hemorrhage of the mother, leading to anoxia of the baby or trauma resulting from the difficult delivery of a baby lying in an unusual position within the uterus.

About 3 per cent of newborns have *congenital defects.*[7] Some congenital defects, such as abnormally constructed hearts of grossly malformed nervous systems, may be incompatible with survival after birth. Other congenital defects may be marginally functional but may predispose the baby to death from overwhelming infection or failure of the affected system later in the first year of life (or beyond).

Sudden Infant Death Syndrome (SIDS) occurs most often in infants two to four months of age. Its etiology is not understood, but a defect in control of the regularity of breathing, particularly when the baby is asleep, is currently suspected.[8]

Neonatal Mortality: Neonatal mortality is the death of a live-born infant before 28 days of age. Two thirds of all infant deaths occur during the neonatal period. In fact, half of all infant mortality occurs during the first 24 hours. The causes are condisered essentially prenatal. Most neonatal deaths occur to low-birth-weight babies. The U.S. neonatal death rate in 1978 was 9.4 per 1,000 live births.[6]

Postneonatal Mortality: Postneonatal mortality is defined as deaths from 28 days of age up to one year. These deaths are more and more attributable to the effects of the environment the further one gets from the time of birth. For example, a child may survive the neonatal period with an underlying congenital defect, but an infectious agent from the environment may later become the direct cause of death. Even an apparently normal baby, subjected to an upper respiratory infection passing through the family, may succumb to an overwhelming pneumonia. Deaths from environmental causes are considered more preventable than deaths from intrauterine or perinatal causes, yet in recent years postneonatal mortality has declined less rapidly than neonatal mortality. The U.S. postneonatal death rate in 1978 was 4.2 per 1,000 live births.[6]

MORBIDITY

Prematurity: The rate of prematurity in the United States in 1976 was 7.3 per cent.[7] This rate has not varied much over the last 15 years. For the purpose of statistics, all live-born babies weighing under 2,500 gm are classified as premature. Technically, babies weighing less than 2,500 gm at birth are currently referred to as "low birth weight," and the more precise concept of prematurity includes birth at a gestational age of less than 37 weeks. The use of 2,500 gm as a rough dividing line between babies at increased risk of problems and babies at average risk has been valuable. Babies weighing less than 2,500 gm have 20 times the risk that larger babies have of dying in the first of life.[7] Factors associated with infant neonatal and postneonatal mortality are usually correlated with low birth weight. Since the birth of low-birth-weight babies is more common than mortality, low birth weight makes a useful measure of poor pregnancy outcome.

Survivors of Perinatal Anoxia: Anoxia around the time of birth may affect the central nervous system. Some survivors of perinatal anoxia have lasting neurological damage. The damage may be widespread and lead to paralysis, seizures, or other apparent deficit. Some damage may be far more subtle and result in spotty evidence or "soft" neurological findings such as dyslexia or other circumscribed learning disorders which are not apparent until the child is a toddler or of school age.

Survivors with Birth Injuries: Some birth injuries are apparent from early infancy onwards. One example is a bleeding event within the brain, possibly the result of trauma to the head during delivery. This may cause a stroke, with subsequent weakness of one side of the body. Although the individual may recover enough strength for ambulation, there may be asymmetry of the legs and some persistent neurological abnormality of the reflexes and strength of the affected leg muscles. The affected arm may also be functional, but will never have the dexterity nor be maintained in the posture characteristic of a normal arm. The individual is handicapped for life. Other birth injuries may heal and leave no trace. One example is Erb's palsy, due to excessive traction on certain arm nerves during delivery.

Children born with congenital heart disease and congenital deformities of other critical organs have elevated risks of mortality throughout their lives. Although affected children may not succumb during infancy, congenital problems are the second leading cause of mortality from the age of one to four years, and the third leading cause during the ages five to 14.[7] Survival has been lengthened by improved medical and surgical treatment, but serious congenital defects are apt to remain a lifetime handicap. Congenital defects are often used as a measure of pregnancy outcome, but differences in definitions and detection rates make them more suspect in statistical comparisons than mortality and birth weight.

PARENTAL FACTORS WHICH AFFECT
PREGNANCY OUTCOME

Genetics

SYNDROMES

Down's Syndrome: Down's syndrome, a well-known cause of severe mental retardation, occurs in approximately 1 per 1,000 births.[7] The risk of having a Down's syndrome child increases with parental age. The syndrome is associated with the presence of an extra chromosome; the father contributes the extra chromosome in about one-fourth of all cases.[7] Sampling intrauterine fluid (amniocentesis) can detect Down's syndrome.

Neural Tube Defects: Neural tube defects occur in about 2 per 1,000 births, approximately half dying in the newborn period.[7] Neural tube defects include spina bifida (incompletely formed vertebral column) and anencephaly (incompletely formed brain). Neural tube defects can be detected furing pregnancy. Families with a previous history of the defect are at high risk.

Metabolic Disorders: Phenylketonuria (PKU) occurs in 1 of every 15,000 births and can lead to severe mental retardation.[7] Treatment with a special diet compensates for a genetic liver enzyme deficiency. Most newborns in the United States are currently tested for this disorder.

Congenital hypothyroidism (cretinism) occurs in 1 of every 5,000 births.[7] This condition can cause mental retardation. Some cases are genetically determined, but others may result from maternal iodine deficiency during pregnancy. Many states currently screen newborns for congenital hypothyroidism. Early treatment can prevent the retardation.

Defects Characteristic of Certain Population Groups: Tay-Sachs disease occurs most commonly among Jewish families of eastern European descent. Children die by age five with severe mental retardation and progressive neurologic deterioration.[7] The responsible gene is recessive. Both parents must be carriers for their children to be at risk. A screening test can identify carriers before pregnancy.

Sickle cell anemia is the most frequent serious genetically determined disease seen in blacks. The condition may lead to years of pain and death from possible complications. Potential parents wich sickle cell trait can be identified before pregnancy.

Cystic fibrosis occurs in about 1 of every 2,000 white births.[7] Abnormal mucus production causes chronic lung obstruction and disability during early life. Afflicted individuals survive longer than they used to due to contemporary treatment and many reach adulthood.

Sex-Linked Defects: Certain congenital disorders affect the sons of mothers who carry an abnormal sex chromosome. Hemophilia and muscular dystrophy are two serious examples.[7] Color blindness is also transmitted this way.

ERYTHROBLASTOSIS FETALIS (RH OR ABO BLOOD INCOMPATIBILITY)

Blood type (Rh or ABO) incompatibility between the mother and baby can lead to jaundice in the newborn of a severity which damages the brain. Exchange transfusion has been a helpful procedure to reduce dangerous levels of jaundice. Recently, prevention of the Rh-related condition has become possible through predicting which mothers are at risk of sensitization and giving them RHOGAM, an antibody against the baby's Rh type, immediately following any pregnancy termination. This prevents the mother's immune system from constructing its own antibodies against the baby's blood cells, which would endanger later babies with the same blood type. It is necessary to know the blood types of the mother and father with regard to the Rh factor in order to predict first pregnancies at risk.

IN GENERAL

Although some 2,000 genetic problems are known, fewer than 20 cause most genetic disease in the United States, and 5 types are responsible for most of the illness and death.[7] Amniocentesis, as noted, can be used to detect Down's syndrome plus many less common conditions. Amniocentesis is not without risk. It is a procedure best carried out in a medical center. Careful selection of candidates for the procedure is necessary because of the risk, expense, and technical aspects involved. Further refinement can be expected in biological tests for genetic disorders. Genetic histories of the parents are useful in calculating risks, but cannot give the positive answer concerning a current pregnancy which can come only from a more direct test.

Parental Age

As noted previously, increasing parental age is associated with the occurrence of Down's syndrome. There is more than one genetic mechanism responsible for the appearance of trisomy 21, the condition in which an extra chromosome is associated with the Down's syndrome. Young mothers may also give birth to a trisomy-21 child; in this case the extra chromosome can sometimes be detected in the cells of the mother or father. The genetic mechanism responsible for the extra chromosome in older parents is more often an abnormality in the process of cell division, rather than a result of the parents' genetic makeup. Older paternal age is a major factor in other anomalies due to fresh gene mutations.[9]

The mother's age also correlates with prematurity, fetal loss, and neonatal and post-neonatal death rates.[10] Very young mothers and older mothers have higher rates of these poor pregnancy outcomes. Part of the correlation is due to interaction with social variables such as education and marital status, also highly correlated with the outcomes. Mothers who reproduce at the extremes of age tend to be less well-educated and of lower socioeconomic status. The youngest mothers are generally unmarried. Research suggests that with adequate social support, age alone is not as great a handicap as it appears in simple correlations between young age and pregnancy outcome.[11] The absence of health care, inadequate diet, and social stress characterize many early teenage pregnancies.

Age, parity, and spacing interact to associate with an elevated risk of low-birth-weight babies. When pregnancies are very close together, with less than 3 months between the end of one and the beginning of the next, the subsequent child is apt to be of low birth weight.[12] Rapid childbearing at an early age may influence birth weight through depletion of mothers' nutritional stores.

Maternal Habits

Many maternal behaviors and habits have been found to have direct biological effects on the developing fetus.

NUTRITION

Diet and nutritional status of the mother correlate with the birth weight of the baby.[10] Historically, maternal height, as well as weight, has also predicted birth weight. The implication of average or greater maternal height is in part that her childhood nutrition was adequate. Of course, height is also related to the absolute size of the pelvic girdle and the body. Larger mothers tend to have larger babies. Genetic factors may play a role, as well as nutrition. Current diet, as well as dietary or nutritional status at conception, is related to adequate nutrition for the fetus. The NINDB collaborative study of 50,000 pregnancies plus data from other studies have led to the recommendation that maternal weight gain during pregnancy should average 24 pounds, and that dieting to lose weight should never occur at this time.[13] If the mother was underweight before pregnancy began, gaining more weight during pregnancy is appropriate.[14]

SMOKING

Many studies have shown that smoking mothers have smaller babies.[15] It is believed that smoking causes exposure of the fetus to carbon monoxide and relative lack of oxygen. The placenta of such a baby is smaller than usual, and exhibits gross and microscopic vascular abnormalities. The amount of food and oxygen which can reach the baby is limited by underperfusion from the uterus.[16] It is not clear whether the smaller babies of smoking mothers are less healthy, but the small size is a definite handicap in the perinatal period, especially when combined with other factors leading to premature births.

ALCOHOL

Alcohol-induced birth defects occur at the rate of approximately 1 for every 100 women consuming more than 1 ounce of alcohol daily.[7] A fetal alcohol syndrome has been defined which includes low birth weight and mental retardation. In addition, there may be behavioral, facial, limb, genital, cardiac, and neurological abnormalities. The risk and degree of abnormality are directly related to the amount of alcohol consumption. The only amount of alcohol consumption unquestionably safe during pregnancy is zero.[17] Since early pregnancy is a critical time, this implies that women exposed to the risk of pregnancy, whether or not they intend to become pregnant, should not consume alcohol.

DRUGS

Mood Altering: Drugs taken as intoxicants comprise as-yet ill-defined hazards to the fetus.[18,19] It is believed that there is a potential for harm from any drug, especially during the first trimester of pregnancy. To foster optimal fetal health and well-being, it seems prudent to try to prevent the use of any of these drugs by women who are exposed to the risk of pregnancy, pregnant, or lactating.

Medications: It is unclear the extent to which common medications may harm the fetus. Certain drug hazards are known. Thalidomide is the classic example. Available over the counter in Europe in the 1960s, it was taken during early pregnancy as a mild sedative and to decrease nausea. It led to developmental defect, particularly of the arms and legs, in about 35 per cent of infants born to the mothers using it.[7] Another well-known example is diethylstilbestrol (DES), taken by high-risk mothers during pregnancy presumably to help them carry the child. DES has been linked to abnormal vaginal tissue growth in daughters during adolescence, with some malignancies.[20] Abnormalities have also been seen in some of the sons' genitourinary tracts.[21]

In general, any medication should be avoided during pregnancy, especially during the first trimester, unless there are overriding health considerations. Many studies documenting the large number of drugs consumed by pregnant women have resulted in surprise and dismay.[22]

Maternal Health

CHRONIC ILLNESSES AND THEIR CONTROL

Diabetes: Diabetes has long been known to have an effect on fertility and pregnancy outcome. Juvenile diabetics prior to the discovery of insulin did not survive to reproduce, or if they were afflicted furing adolescence, often were not fertile because of their illness. With the availability of insulin, overt diabetics were able to conceive, but had a high rate of late fetal loss and a high rate of congenital defects in the live-born offspring. Because of oversize babies and unexplained stillbirths, diabetic mothers have been subjected to caesarean section more often than other mothers.[23] Increasing control of the disease has led to better and better pregnancy outcome for diabetics. It is currently possible for diabetics to experience the same risk as other women in reproduction, providing they maintain very close control of their blood glucose level through frequent daily blood testing and multiple shots of insulin.[24]

Heart Disease: Maternal heart disease affects the baby through reduction of oxygen delivered to the placenta. The mother may be inadequately oxygenated herself. Or there may be reduction of circulation to the placenta, secondary to stress on the mother's heart during the period of pregnancy when the blood volume is at its greatest. Mothers with this severe degree of heart disease are currently put to bed to assist the heart in coping with the increased load. Mothers with severe heart disease, nevertheless, currently have higher rates of infant mortality and congenital defects.[3, 25]

Kidney Disease: Mothers who have kidney transplants have been known to conceive and deliver normal children. Nevertheless, mothers with severe kidney disease are facing a high risk when they undertake pregnancy, since they add to the load which their kidneys must handle. To the degree that their kidneys are unable to remove the body wastes, the abnormal metabolic state may create defects in the baby or fetal loss and early infant death.[26]

Hypertension: Mothers with preexisting hypertension before pregnancy are at greater risk for hypertensive states of pregnancy, which include marked edema, loss of protein in the urine, and associated signs of toxemia, leading to convulsions and coma. If the mother's health declines into the eclamptic state, it may be necessary to deliver the baby before term. The baby thus may be prematurely born, and suffer the risks related to premature birth. If the baby remains in the mother's uterus while she goes into a convulsive state, the baby may then suffer the complications of anoxia. Maternal hypertension is associated with higher rates of fetal loss, premature birth, and congenital defect.[25, 26]

Seizure Disorders: The natural history of mothers with seizure disorders and pregnancy is not too well-known, since controlled studies of mothers not receiving medication have not been possible. However, syndromes associated with the use of epilepsy medications have recently been discussed. Diphenylhydantoin, trimethadione, and other anticonvulsants may be teratogens for fetuses in the early months of pregnancy.[27,28] For some mothers there is no choice but to use these medications. The development of new medications may eventually make possible substitutions which create less risk to the fetus.

Mental Health: There is no evidence of a connection between maternal mental health and fetal health.[25] There is a realtionship between anxiety late in pregnancy and complications during labor and delivery. The mechanism for this association is not clear. It is possible that women whose anxiety is manifest to the caretakers will receive more anesthesia and analgesia, resulting in greater depression of the newborn and related complications.[29]

ACUTE INFECTIONS
Rubella: German measles (rubella) infection in the first trimester of pregnancy may result in damage to the fetal heart and other organs. Fetal loss may occur, or a damaged baby may be born.[10,30]

Herpes: Herpes simplex infection of the female genital tract at the time of delivery is a danger to the newborn, who may become infected and seriously damaged by overwhelming viral infections.[30]   To avoid infection from active herpetic lesions, babies by be delivered by cesarean section.

Cytomegalovirus: Antibodies against cytomegalovirus in our adult population are fairly common. However, the timing of the infection in women of childbearing age may be critical. A child infected in utero may experience central nervous system (CNS) damage and subsequent mental retardation.[30]

Other Live Viruses: Other live virus infections occurring during the first trimester of pregnancy may result in fetal loss or fetal damage.[30] Later infections may not cause morphological changes but are capable of retarding growth and development.

Sexually Transmitted Diseases: Syphilis has long been known to cause congenital defects in fetuses.[3] For this reason, efforts are made to detect syphilis early in pregnancy and again later. Adequate treatment before the spirochete is able to cross the placenta protects the baby. Other sexually transmitted diseases may also influence fetal well-being. Gonorrhea, Chlamydia, and Herpes simplex may be transmitted sexually. Gonorrhea, like herpes, is a danger to the child as it passes through the birth canal. Gohorrhea infection of the eyes can be adequately prevented by using silver nitrate drops at birth, as is common practice. Chlamydia may cause pneumonia in newborns.

Infections of the genital tract must be carefully treated during pregnancy and between pregnancies. Certain sexually transmitted diseases, especially gonorrhea, are also threats to future fertility.

Tuberculosis: Tuberculosis is an illness which threatens the newborn (and infant) with overwhelming infection.[3] During pregnancy, however, if the maternal nutritional state is adequate, the baby may develop normally. Certain antituberculosis medications may damage a fetus. For this reason, physicians need to know about the pregnancy when selecting drugs for the treatment of tuberculosis.

Malaria: Drugs (containing chloroquine) used for the suppression of malaria infection may be harmful to the fetus. The desease also poses a hazard. For this reason, the timing of pregnancy and travel to a malaria-infected area should be considered.

Other: Since any infection and any treatment may potentially affect the fetus either in early pregnancy or at the time of delivery, it is clear that all efforts possible should be made to protect a woman planning to become pregnant, or already pregnant, from sources of infection.

Other Environmental Exposures

RADIATION

Irradiation of the embryo during the first trimester may cause fetal loss or fetal structural damage. Children presenting with leukemia or other cancers more frequently have a history of prenatal irradiation or x-ray in infancy than children presenting with other illnesses. It is therefore believed that exposure to x-ray at any time during pregnancy or early life should be kept to an absolute minimum and, if possible, avoided.[3]

OCCUPATIONAL AIR POLLUTANTS

In occupational settings, mothers may be exposed to air pollutants which may cause fetal loss or damage. Women working in operating rooms, breathing small amounts of anesthetic gases, have a higher rate of spontaneous abortion than other women. Exposure to factory atmospheres containing lead is known to cause infertility; whether lead in the air can reach the fetus and cause central nervous system damage, as it is believed to do in infants and older children, has not been demonstrated, but it is a logical hypothesis.

Previous Pregnancy Outcomes

It has been observed that mothers tend to repeat the types of pregnancy outcomes they have experienced previously.[10,26,31] Some women will have many early fetal losses. Some will have many late fetal losses. Women who have one low-birth-weight baby are at greatly elevated risk of having another. In some cases the etiology of these repeat performances is clear, such as the incompetent cervix which leads to late fetal loss. A temporary surgically placed drawstring can overcome this problem. In other cases, the reasons are unknown. Nutrition, birth-spacing, or general health may need attention.

Social and Psychological Factors

MATERNAL IQ AND EDUCATION
Women with more education and with a higher IQ, which in general is correlated with more education, are seen to have infants of higher birth weight, that is, a lower rate of low-birth-weight births, and lower infant mortality.[10] It is possible that education influences physiological well-being by assisting the woman to take better care of herself and to obtain more adequate health care.

MARITAL STATUS
In general, the unmarried mother is socially disadvantaged in that she has less income and fewer social supports as she tries to provide food, clothing, and shelter for herself and her offspring.[10] Unmarried social status and higher rates of infant mortality are most highly correlated for young mothers, although the differential exists at all ages.

INCOME
Lower income is associated with higher rates of infant mortaility and low birth weight.[10]

RACE
Compared with whites, nonwhites have higher rates of infant mortality and low birth weight, but if one breaks this down by subgroup and socioeconomic status, within-race differences appear. Income, marital status, and education create expected patterns. In general, American Indians and Orientals have average birth weights. Women with Spanish surnames give birth to babies weighing between those of blacks and whites. Blacks have the lowest mean birth weights.[32]

GEOGRAPHIC MOBILITY
Rural-born babies are heavier than urban-born babies. Poor women living in urban areas who were born on the farm have larger babies than women who have always lived in the urban areas.[10] This may relate to childhood nutrition of the mothers or to selection of the group moving to urban areas.

SOCIAL MOBILITY
Women born into lower socioeconomic status homes who achieve middle-class status by marrying a middle-class husband or entering a middle-class occupation have larger babies than similar women who remain within lower socioeconomic class status or women who start in middle socioeconomic class status and move into lower-class

status through marriage or occupation.[33] This finding has not been totally explained, but seems to suggest something about basic health and personal endowment of the individual involved.

USE OF HEALTH SERVICES, INCLUDING PRENATAL CARE
It has been long observed that groups of women who use health services and prenatal care less tend to have smaller babies and higher infant mortality. They also have less education, are more apt to be unmarried, and live in poverty. Because of the confluence of factors, it is difficult to attribute an appropriate amount of importance to the health services for an individual woman, especially when there are no health problems prior to the time of delivery. Within high-risk population groups, continuous comprehensive prenatal care offers the advantage of early detection and control of complications for those women who develop the problems.[10]

SOURCE OF PRENATAL AND MATERNITY CARE
An important study in New York has illustrated that the sources of prenatal and maternity care play important roles in pregnancy outcome. Women from approximately similar backgrounds who selected private care as opposed to public or municipal hospitals had better pregnancy outcomes than women who went to the municipal hospitals.[34]

ANXIETY
As mentioned earlier, there are correlations between measures of anxiety in late pregnancy and complications of delivery. Education for childbirth has been demonstrated to reduce certain kinds of anxieties but to create others.[35] To the extent that the education appears to reduce the need for analgesia and anesthesia, this has been helpful.

PARENTING SKILLS
Since infant mortality is a measure of the rate of deaths during the first year of life, how well the mother cares for the baby during that time may be relevant to the pregnancy outcome. Young mothers with many babies born close together at times are seen to neglect their infants. Postneonatal mortality rates are higher in such families.[12]

ACTIONS TO PROMOTE HEALTHY CHILDBEARING

Actions to promote healthy childbearing are based on reducing the risks revealed in the previously mentioned associations.

Lifelong Health Education

The knowledge necessary to bring parents to a stage of optimal health at the time they begin childbearing must be part of the basic knowledge accumulated from early childhood. Habits of nutrition and hygiene are influenced by patterns at home and at school. Peers and teachers play a very important role in reinforcing individuals' health habits. The lifelong exposure must not only be to explanations and exhortations concerning what one should do, but to the modeling behaviors of others important in the child's life.

Sex Education

Sex education similarly is an education to be derived over a lifetime. It occurs continuously in the home and in the school through contacts with parents, peers, and teachers. The school system must definitely plan ways to incorporate the topic. It does not have to stand by itself in a course labeled "sex education" or "family life education," nor is it apt to be meaningful or effective when offered in this form at the last moment in high school. In literature, art, music, biology, botany, zoology, history, or any subject dealing with life of people, there are interactions of males and females which can be related to reproduction and human ecology.

Ideally, sex education becomes more and more concrete and more and more explicit as the child approaches puberty. Discussions of conceiving children only when desired and the use of birth control methods cannot be timed according to grade level or chronological age. They must be introduced when the child is ready, which in general will be at the time of development of secondary sexual characteristcs. The physician and the parent need to discuss the subject beforehand so that the parent can acquire the proper vocabulary and reinforcement for useful attitudes. Sex education can be done best by the parents in terms of timing and sensitivity. They need to be informed about the situation in present-day society in the United States. Their own behavior will provide the modeling for their own values. By making it possible for the multiple brief discussions related to this subject to occur in the home, the parents provide a context within which the child can utilize information acquired from other sources. By becoming expert themselves, the parents can assist the child in interpreting what he or she hears elsewhere. When the parent cannot function in this manner, the physician and teacher must try to play the role of counselor insofar as possible.

Education Concerning Family Formation and Parenting

Parenting skills are modeled within one's family of origin. However, many variations on the theme of "family" exist, and the school setting is an appropriate place to make possible discussions of these various forms. The sociology of family formation and the tasks and roles of parents are necessary topics within the general area of family life education starting in grade school. Children are educating themselves along these lines when they play "house" as 5-year-olds. As the details of the complex roles of parents are elaborated, it is to be hoped that parenting is not a role a child would choose too early in life.

In high school, associated day care facilities make possible concrete learning experiences concerning the care of young children. This is of value for children who have not had the experience of caring for younger brothers and sisters. It also provides a convenient service for young parents who wish to continue attending high school.

Planned Pregnancies: Advantages

Deferring the parental role until one has completed education and selected and prepared for an occupation is one obvious reason from a professional viewpoint for planning the first pregnancy as opposed to just letting it happen. Advantages for deferring the first birth or the first pregnancy are best presented to the adolescent in terms of the advantages to herself or himself. In 1976 only 25 percent of all births to teenagers,

(15 to 19) were unplanned or unwanted.[36] The figure is over 75 percent for never-married females, however, and is higher for the younger girls.[37]

Reasons for the wanted births include the assumption of adult status, leaving the parental home or acquiring a new status within that home, and leaving an unsatisfactory school situation. For some girls, the assumption of the maternal role in this social sense decidedly betters their living situation. The positive advantages for those who choose to delay the first birth must be real and of equal validity. Education and occupational training must lead to attainable futures if they are to be meaningful goals.

Let us consider other advantages of delaying parenthood. The youngest mothers have poor pregnancy outcomes, as discussed already. In addition, ultimate family size is larger when childbearing begins earlier. The early pregnancies tend to be closely spaced. There are more advantages for child development within smaller sibships. Both infant health and parental opportunities for personal development seem better when pregnancies are planned and well-spaced.[12] Economic advantages of delayed childbearing and small family size have been widely stressed.

Accessibility of Family-Planning Services

Of course, services to make birth control possible must be available in order for young people to avoid too-early childbearing. Education concerning what to do is not enough. The means must exist for the individuals to act. When society makes this difficult, education will not succeed in influencing behavior.

Education Concerning Use of Health Services

Not only the use of birth control services but also the use of health services in general must be subjects for teaching. Appropriate use of services is a matter of education and knowledge. To the extent possible, individuals must learn self-care. They must know when it is appropriate to consult a professional for advice and assistance. They must also know what kinds of professionals and services exist and where one can find them. If it is necessary for individuals to choose between services for which they must pay and those which are available at no cost to the public, they have to know who is eligible for public care, where these different alternatives are located, and how one gains access to them.

Complete Health Care

Young people must be taught not only where to find the services, but something about the necessary content of routine health supervision and what should be done by various ages or stages of development. They should learn that certain problems require more than one visit for their complete care. They should be encouraged to keep health supervision and dental visits up to date and to follow through on problems which are found.

Appropriate Immunizations

Young people should understand and receive all the recommended childhood immunizations, and they should be particularly encouraged to maintain immunity against rubella becuase of its potential for damaging a baby when the mother is pregnant. Rubella immunization must be completed at least 3 months prior to the conception of a baby, since the virus lingers in the body and might damage the fetus.

Physical Examinations Before Pregnancy

Both males and females should have complete physical examinations before a pregnancy which they have planned is initiated. At this time, health problems can be treated and any genetic problems can be discussed. Testing may be done as indicated, and genetic counseling can be arranged.

Appropriate Prenatal Care by Risk Status

The mother's health status should influence the selection of the source of prenatal care. If indicated, referral may be done by the person who does the prepregnancy physical examination. Recommendation for amniocentesis after the pregnancy is started can be based on the genetic history and be part of genetic counseling. It should be understood that when amniocentesis is recommended, the possiblity of abortion may present a moral quandary or need for decision during the pregnancy. The earlier this can be worked through, the better.

Availability of Abortion

When a problem pregnancy warrants abortion, it is necessary for this service to be available for everyone. The group that historically has had problems obtaining safe abortions is the medically indigent group. The advantages of planned childbearing, particularly for this group which is particularly handicapped by excessive childbearing, are so great that barriers to abortion must be prevented.

Availablitiy of Hospital Care at Appropriate Level

Women who are characterized by certain risk factors at the time they undertake pregnancy need not only specialized prenatal care but also eventually maternity care at a hospital capable of providing an appropriate level of care at the time of delivery. Referral of the mother to this hospital and a specially prepared means of transportation when she goes into labor are necessary. Sometimes a high-risk pregnant woman requires hospitalization prior to her delivery date. Since high-risk women are more apt to be medically indigent than otherwise, the availability of public funding for this sort of care is essential. Not only must the mother be educated to understand why this type of care is important so that she will seek it and follow the necessary advice, but society must ensure that the servies are available and that there are no barriers to receiving them.

Levels of Care

The definition of levels of care in terms of hospital maternity medical care differs slightly from state to state but correspond in general to national standards that have been developed as part of the concept of regionalization of perinatal care.[38] Essentially, mothers at low risk for problems may deliver in primary-level licensed community facilities. Home deliveries are not recommended. It is expected that blood banks and radiological services are available in case of common difficulties. The secondary levels of care include the services of skilled technicians, trained obstetricians and gynecologists, and relatively expensive equipment which may be brought into play on behalf of a mother experiencing complications of labor and delivery. Tertiary maternity care includes more of the same facilities available at secondary-level centers, and in addition an even greater concentration of subspecialists and expensive equipment and laboratory services. Tertiary levels of care are usually located within university medical centers and serve a large population on a regional basis. Secondary levels of care relate in a definite way to smaller regional boundaries and a given set of community hospitals. All units are bound together by communication and continuing medical education linkages, as well as referral and transportation systems. It is not only essential for the professionals to understand the linkages and the capacities of the different parts of the system, but also for the families to understand why referral is recommended and necessary.

Education for Labor and Delivery

Childbirth education should be provided for both parents and "significant others" during the prenatal period. Control of breathing and learning the technique of focusing thoughts so as to reduce the amount of perceived pain are helpful to many laboring mothers. The father or significant other person can provide emotional support as well as some physical comfort to the mother during labor, provided that the person understands what to expect during the process and how to be most helpful. Instructors trained in Lamaze techniques are available in many communities, and other credentialed childbirth educators exist. Many private physicians as well as clinic settings include education for childbirth as one of their services. The content and timing of such education has been described in the literature.[39] Objectively the effects appear beneficial for fetal as well as maternal outcomes, but obstetricians believe further study is necessary to prove this.[40]

Education for Breast-feeding and Child Care

During late pregnancy, the mother-to-be develops a greater interest in the details of breast-feeding and child care. This is therefore an appropriate time to educate her and allow questions and discussions on these topics. Fathers and significant others can play important roles in the discussions, since their attitudes are bound to have an influence on the mother. From the point of view of the mother's health, breast-feeding may be described as natural and associated with more rapid return of the uterus to its normal size following delivery, pleasant physical sensations, and a special feeling of closeness and importance to the infant. The milk is of the highest nutritional value for the child, sterile, the right temperature, and always available, making child feeding optimally convenient. Not every woman will be able to breast-feed. Care should be taken not to arouse guilt in these mothers, but to support them in their own priorities. Sometimes insight and a little ingenuity, however, can help a hesitating mother overcome the barriers she perceives to successful breast-feeding.

External Social Supports

Many mothers will not need social supports beyond what is already available to them within their own family. Mothers with a supportive husband, relatives, or close friends; mothers with adequate education; and mothers with adequate income can manage without external arrangements. However, socially isolated mothers, those who are medically indigent, and those whose education and experience have not prepared them for the childbearing experience may benefit from one or more of the following:

PUBLIC HEALTH NURSE
   Nurses from local public health agencies usually include among their duties visits to high-risk newborns. They are able to assess the needs of the new mother and infant and provide educational services as indicated. They may detect problems and make referrals for medical or social services.

SUPPLEMENTAL FOODS
Mothers may be eligible for supplemental foods under the WIC (Women, Infants and Children) program designed to provide medically-at-risk mothers with better nutrition and to involve these mothers and their infants in ongoing health services. In some areas, food stamp programs help mothers obtain more food for the money available to them.

SOCIAL SERVICES
   Some mothers need income assistance. Other social services available in many communities include job training and day care services for infants. For mothers who have not completed their high school education, some communities may have special classes or may simply admit the mother back into high school. For many mothers, such social services may make the difference between becoming a drop-out, dependent on society, and a useful, productive member of society.

SUPPORT GROUPS
   Some mothers, burdened by the new experience of motherhood or the demands of several children, may find comfort and assistance from parent groups who meet and talk about how they cope with the child-rearing needs of their own children. Group facilitators assist members of the group to help each other. Mothers who are potential child abusers, mothers who use drugs or alcohol, and mothers with other handicaps can obtain definite benefits from the close social support such groups can provide.

OTHER HOME VISITORS
   In some areas, homemakers exist who are supported by public health or other public agencies. The function of the homemaker is to visit the home of a woman who is unable to manage the situation by herself, to both assist and train her to become a better manager. Help from the homemaker can be temporary or relatively long-term.

Follow-up After Pregnancy

After a pregnancy termination, whether the termination resulted in a fetal loss or a live birth, follow-up should consist of complete health care. A mother of childbearing age is always a potential future childbearer, and it is desirable to maintain her in optimal health in order to help her be the best possible parent that she can for her living children, as well as be the healthy bearer of future healthy children. In the interconceptional intervals, it is assumed that family planning services will be necessary. It is also possible during this interval to give a mother needed vaccines. All health needs should be attended to, including dental care.

Termination of Fertility

After a woman has attained her desired family size, sterilization should be available to her as an option. Currently in the United States, about one third of the couples in the childbearing age range have been sterilized.[41] Worldwide, this has become a very popular method of terminal birth control. Of course, other methods of birth control should also remain available for women who have all the children they want.

Health Care for the Father

In this chapter as in other similar statements, little mention has been made of the father. This is not to deny the importance of his role in childbearing (fertility itself is health-related) and the essential role his health plays in maintaining a healthy family. The father who is not in good health cannot be as effective a worker, cannot be as physically helpful to his mate, cannot be as emotionally supportive to her, cannot play as well the important role of adult male of the family, as healthy fathers can. The father whose health is not good adds to the mother's burden of responsibility. To some extent, the mother must take love and support from the father in order to have enough to give the children. She, despite changing male and female roles in our society and greater participation of fathers in child care, still carries the main burden as primary caretaker in most homes.

Thus the reduction of risk for childbearing from the perspective taken in this chapter does imply maintenance of the father in optimal health. Health care resources utilized by the mother and professionals providing social support for her should always check into the well-being of the father in order to make sure that he is not neglected. Part of the education which is given to children in preparing them for their future role as parents should emphasize the significance of the father's strength and role as a parent and partner. His baby will not be as healthy as it possibly could be unless he maintains himself in good health and models the appropriate life-style, health care, and nutritional behaviors which he and the mother want to hand down to their children in their children's best interests.

REFERENCES

1. U.S. Department of Health, Education, and Welfare Monthly Vital Statistics Report, *Annual Summary for the United States, 1978.* DHEW Publication No. 79-1120, 27, August 13, 1979, pp. 1–29.
2. McLean, Roderick, Mattison, Ernest T., and Cochrane, Nancy E.; "Maternal Mortality Study." *New York State Journal of Medicine* 79 (January 1979), pp. 39–52.
3. Pritchard, Jack A. and MacDonald, Paul C.; *Williams Obstetrics, 15th ed., New* York: Appleton-Century-Crofts, 1976, pp. 1–1138.

4. Morris, Naomi M. and Udry, J. Richard; "Daily Immunologic Pregnancy Testing of Initially Non-Pregnant Women," *American Journal of Obstetrics and Gynecology* 98 (August 15, 1967), pp. 1148-1150.
5. Hertig, A. T., Rock, J., Adams, E. C., and Menkin, M. D., "Thirty-four Fertilized Human Ova, Good, Bad and Indifferent, Recovered from 210 Women of Known Fertility. A study of Biologic Wastage in Early Human Pregnancy," *Pediatrics* 23 (1959), pp. 202-211.
6. Wegman, Myron E., "Annual Summary of Vital Statistics," *Pediatrics* 64 (December 1979), pp. 835-842.
7. Richmond, Julius B., "Healthy People—The Surgeon General's Report on Health Promotion and Disease Prevention." DHEW (PHS) Publication No. 79-55071, 1979.
8. Shannon, D. C., Kelly, D. H., and O'Connel,: "Abnormal Regulation of Ventilation in Infants at Risk for Sudden-Infant Death Syndrome," *New England Journal of Medicine* 297 (1977), p. 747.
9. Jones, K. L., Smith, D. W., Harvey, M. A. S., Hall, B. D., and Quan, L., "Older Paternal Age and Fresh Gene Mutation: Data on Additional Disorders," *Journal of Pediatrics* 86 (1975), p. 84.
10. Siegel, E., and Morris, N. M., "The Epidemiology of Human Reproductive Casualties, with Emphasis on the Role of Nutrition." In *Maternal Nutrition and the Course of Pregnancy*. Washington, D.C. National Academy of Sciences, 1970.
11. Baldwin, W., and Cain, V. S., "The Children of Teenage Parents." *Family Planning Perspectives* 12 (January–February 1980), p. 34.
12. Siegel, E., and Morris, N. M., "Family Planning: Its Health Rationale." *American Journal of Obstetrics and Gynecology* 118 (1974), p. 995.
13. Pitkin, R. M., "Nutrition in Pregnancy," *Public Health Currents* 17 (January–February 1977), p. 1.
14. Naeye, R. L., "Weight Gain and the Outcome of Pregnancy." *American Journal of Obstetrics and Gynecology* 135 (September 2, 1979), p. 3.
15. Naeye, R. L., "Effects of Maternal Cigerette Smoking on the Fetus and Placenta." *British Journal of Obstetrics and Gynecology* 85, 1978 pp. 732-737.
16. Naeye, R. L., "The Duration of Maternal Cigarette Smoking, Fetal and Placental Disorders." In *Early Human Development*, Elsevier/New York: North-Holland Biomedical Press, 1979, pp. 229-237.
17. Clarren, S. K. and Smith, D. W., "The Fetal Alcohol Syndrome," *New England Journal of Medicine* 298 (1978), pp. 1063-1067.
18. Fricker, H. S. and Segal, S., "Narcotic Addiction, Pregnancy, and the Newborn." *American Journal of Diseases of Children* 132 (April 1978), pp. 360-366.
19. Nahas, G. G., "Current Status of Marijuana Research." *Journal of American Medical Association* 242 (December 21, 1979), pp. 2775-2778.
20. Herbst, A. L., Poskanzer, D. C., Robboy, S. J., Friedlander, L., and Scully, R. E., "Prenatal Exposure to Stilbestrol." *New England Journal of Medicine* 292 (February 13, 1975), pp. 334-339.
21. Henderson, B. E., Benton, B., Cosgrove, M., Baptista, J., Aldrich, J., Townsend, D., Hart, W., Mack, T. M., "Urogenital Tract Abnormalities in Sons of Women Treated with Diethylstilbestrol." *Pediatrics* 58 (1976), p. 505.
22. Doering, P. L. and Stewart, R. B., "The Extent and Character of Drug Consumption During Pregnancy." *Journal of American Medical Association* 239 (1978), pp. 843-846.
23. Greene, J. W., "Diabetes Mellitus in Pregnancy." *Obstetrics and Gynecology* 46 (December 1975), pp. 724-728.
24. Lewis, S. B., Murray, W. K., Wallin, J. D., Coustan, D. R., Daane, T. A., Tredway, D. R., and Navins, J. P., "Improved Glucose Control in Nonhospitalized Pregnant Diabetic Patients," *Obstetrics and Gynecology* 48 (September 1976), pp. 260-267.

25. Niswander,K. R., and Gordon, M., *The Women and Their Pregnancies*. DHEW Pub. No. (NIH) 73-379, 1972.
26. Hobel, C. J., Youkeles, L., and Forsythe, A., "Prenatal and Intrapartum High-Risk Screening: II. Risk Factors Reassessed." *American Journal of Obstetrics and Gynecology* 135 (December 15, 1979), pp. 1051-1056.
27. Smith, D. W., "Teratogenicity of Anticonvulsive Medications,.. *American Journal of Diseases of Children* 131 (December 1977), pp. 1337-1339.
29. Standley, K., Soulee, B., and Copans, S. A., "Dimensions of Prenatal Anxiety and Their Influence of Pregnancy Outcome." *American Journal of Obstetrics and Gynecology* 135 (September 1, 1979), pp. 22-26.
30. Sever, J. L., "Perinatal Infections Affecting the Developing Fetus and Newborn." In *The Prevention of Mental Retardation Through Control of Infectious Diseases*. USPHS Publ. 1692, Washington, D.C.: U.S. Government Printing Office, 1966, p. 396.
31. Bakketeig, L. S., Hoffman, H. J., and Harley, E. E., "The Tendency to Repeat Gestational Age and Birth Weight in Successive Births." *American Journal of Obstetrics and Gynecology* 135 (December 15, 1979), pp. 1086-1103.
32. Naylor, A. F., and Myrianthopoulos, N. C., "The Relation of Ethnic and Selected Socioeconomic Factors to Human Birth Weight." *Annals of Human Genetics* 31 (1967), pp. 71-83.
33. Udry, J. R., Bauman, K. E., Morris, N. M., and Chase, C. L., "Social Class, Social Mobility and Prematurity: A Test of the Childhood Environment Hypothesis for Negro Women." *Journal of Health and Social Behavior* II (September 1970), pp. 190-195.
34. National Academy of Sciences, Institute of Medicine, *Contrasts in Health Status*, Vol. I: *Infant Death: An Analysis by Maternal Risk and Health Care*, Washington, D.C.: National Academy of Sciences, 1973.
35. Zax, M., Sameroff, A. J., and Farnum, J. E., "Childbirth Education, Maternal Attitudes, and Delivery." *American Journal of Obstetrics and Gynecology* 123 (September 15, 1975), pp. 185-190.
36. Department of Health Education, and Welfare, Public Health Service, Division of Vital Statistics, *Wanted and Unwanted Births Reported by Mothers 15-44 Years of Age: U.S. 1976, Advance Data*, 56 (January 24, 1980), pp. 1-10.
37. Zelnick, M. and Kantner, J. F.: "Contraceptive Patterns and Premarital Pregnancy Among Women Aged 15-19 in 1976." *Family Planning Perspectives* 10 (May-June 1978), pp. 135-142.
38. Committee on Perinatal Health, *Toward Improving the Outcome of Pregnancy*. White Plains, N.Y.: The National Foundation-March of Dimes, 1976.
39. Chertok, L., "Psychocomatic Methods of Preparation for Childbirth." *American Journal of Obstetrics and Gynecology* 98 (1967), pp. 698-707.
40. Hughey, M. J., McElin, T. W., and Young, T., "Maternal and Fetal Outcome of Lamaze-Prepared Patients." *Obstetrics and Gynecology* 51 (June 1978), pp. 643-647.
41. Department of Health Education, and Welfare, Public Health Service, Division of Vital Statistics, *Contraceptive Utilization in the United States: 1973 and 1976*, *Advance Data* 36 (August 18, 1978), pp. 1-12.

5 / Risk Reduction from Birth to Kindergarten Age

Naomi M. Morris, M.D., M.P.H.

In Chapter Four, the focus was on parental health and how to prepare young people for parenting through education, optimal physical fitness, health care, and planning prior to and during pregnancy. The focus of Chapter Five is on perinatal (around the time of birth) care for mother and infant, and on early child health and health supervision. Some of the measures of risk and factors which influence risks from birth to age 4 were mentioned in Chapter Four, since, as was pointed out, many of the factors influencing immediate pregnancy outcome continue to contribute to the individual's risk of mortality or morbidity throughout and beyond the first year of life.

RISKS FROM BIRTH THROUGH AGE 4

Infancy (Birth to Age 1 Year)

INFANT MORTALITY

For 1978, the provisional U.S. infant mortality rate per 1,000 live births is 13.6[1] For whites alone, the final rate for 1977 was 12.3 For all other races, it was 21.7, which is equivalent to the rate for whites alone, 12 years earlier.[2] Since for whites and all other mothers there has been a steady decrease in infant mortality since at least 1935, and since rates in many other developed countries are lower than those in the United States, it would appear that further decrease is possible in the United States.

Neonatal Mortality: The key to the reduction of neonatal mortality, which is such a significant portion of all infant mortality, is the prevention of low-birth-weight births. Premature deliveries may result from maternal complications of pregnancy such as placenta previa. Low birth weight may be associated with congenital anomalies or other problems of the fetus which result in poor growth. In either case, babies weighing less than 2,500 gm account for two thirds of neonatal mortality.[3] If immediate delivery is not necessary to protect the mother or fetus, it is desirable to keep the baby in the womb as long as possible. Different methods of inhibiting premature labor exist and are used with some success to delay births.

As noted earlier, the major causes of neonatal mortality include immaturity and "other diseases of early infancy," which basically include problems of adaptation to life outside the womb; congenital anomalies; and birth injuries or catastrophic insults around the time of delivery.

Postneonatal Mortality: Beyond the age of 1 month, the current most common cause of death is believed to be sudden infant death syndrome (SIDS).[4] This problem is seen slightly more often in low-birth-weight babies. Other relatively important causes in the postneonatal period are infection of the respiratory tract or the gastrointestinal tract, accidents, and child neglect and abuse.[4]

INFANT MORBIDITY

Failure to Thrive: Babies who "fail to thrive" during infancy may have physical or behavioral problems.[5] Physical problems include damage to the central nervous system, congenital defects, hidden infections, nutritional problems, or other incipient illnesses. The most common behavioral disorder is poor maternal-child interaction. This may be due to a failure of maternal attachment or inadequate pair bonding. The problem may primarily be in the mother or it may be due to a problem in the baby affecting the baby's responses to the mother. Ideally the behavior of each is rewarding to the other. In the absence of appropriate responses the other's attempts at interaction may diminish.

Maternal neglect is often first manifested by a baby which fails to thrive. Failing to thrive roughly encompasses poor weight gain and an apparent lack of appropriate social responsiveness. In cases of neglect the baby seems apathetic more often than fussy. There is no clear sign of illness. The baby may show indiscriminate attachments to adults other than the parents. A wide range of tests and examinations may be necessary to rule out organic disease. Hospitalization of the infant often seems to cure the problem. The baby perks up, eats well, gains weight, and develops appropriate social responses. Return of the child to the home may result in relapse.

Developmental Delay: Developmental delay may become obvious during the first year in children with severe mental retardation. Quiet babies may be deaf or may be retarded; babies whose motor development is slow may have muscle disease or may be exhibiting developmental delay. Severe developmental delay unassociated with birth trauma or congenital defect is unusual; although approximately 3 per cent of the child population is retarded, most children are in the mild or borderline range.[4] Small premature babies exhibit developmental delays approximately equivalent to the number of weeks too soon that they were born. This "normal" delay must be distinguished from serious neurological damage suffered by some prematures. It is not always possible to do this until later in childhood.

Infectious Disease: Pneumonia is a common complication of many infant infirmities, and one of the most frequent causes of hospitalization during the first year of life.

Gastrointestinal infections are common complications of poor feeding techniques; hospitalization because of dehydration is an infrequent result. Most GI tract infections during infancy are preventable and reflect the child's environment.

Infants under 4 to 6 weeks of age may harbor serious infections without showing typical signs of infection. They also are susceptible to infection by organisms not commonly responsible for disease in older children. Thus, a jaundiced newborn with no fever, the usual clue to important infection, may be suffering from a serious bacterial infection. A newborn may develop an ear infection (otitis media) due to an organism such as *Pseudomonas*, rather than to the *Hemophilus influenaz* or the *Streptococcus pneumoniae* which commonly infect toddlers. These differences make diagnosis and treatment of infectious disease in infants particularly challenging. Yet, infections more than other health problems have become amenable to prevention and therapy in the last 50 years, and much of the marked reduction in infant mortality during this time is due to control of infectious disease.

Ages 1 to 4 Years

MORTALITY FROM ONE TO FOUR YEARS OF AGE

The major causes of mortality from 1 to 4 years of age are accidents, congenital defects, and cancer.[2]

Accidents: Accidents include automobile injuries, ingestions of toxic substances, falls, fires, and drownings. With regard to automobile accidents, children in this age group are most often the passive victims of accidents occurring while they are passengers in automobiles.[6] They may also become the victims of street accidents because of running unpredictably into a motor vehicle's path.

The most frequent ingestion used to be that of aspirin, but since the new child-proof packaging has become widespread, aspirin poisoning and other ingestions of medications are seen much less often.[7] Household cleansing agents still pose a large danger to exploring toddlers.

Fatal falls are especially characteristic of children living in high rise dwellings in urban areas. Ordinary falls, such as from cribs, do not usually result in death. Serious head injuries said to be the result of ordinary falls must lead to investigation of possible child abuse.

Drownings are sometimes seen in rural areas where unprotected ponds and natural bodies of water exist. In urban areas, accidents sometimes occur in private swimming pools, making fencing and protection of such pools mandatory.

Congenital Defects: Serious defects in the central nervous system, the heart, or other organs continue to claim lives in this age period. The immediate problem is most often superimposed infection.

Cancer: Some cancers, such as neuroblastoma, are seen in the newborn. Others, such as leukemia, may first be manifested in toddlers or preschoolers. Surgery, radiation, and chemotherapy are currently able to prolong the lives of many children with neoplasms. Complications of these therapies, however, particularly infection, may cause unanticipated deaths.

MORBIDITY FROM ONE TO FOUR YEARS OF AGE

Less Than Optimal Physical and Mental Development: During these years, a child's failure to grow or develop normally often becomes obvious to the parents for the first time. Investigation for serious health problems follows medical recognition of unusually small size. Because of its correlation with adult obesity, early obesity is also cause for medical concern.

Deficits of mental development are more subtle than growth deficits, but children with delayed speech or clumsy motor behavior may come to light as parents make comparisons with other children and start thinking ahead to kindergarten. With regard to mental development, 20 per cent of the school population manifests poor performance,[4] many of the learning problems seen in school-age children are evident in the preschool period, and 80 per cent of learning disorders are said to be remediable.[4] Starting remediation early is important for success, before the child's behavior starts to reflect a low self-image.

Behavior Disturbances: Children with deviations of growth, mental development, or motor development often have behavior disturbances as a result of problems within the peer group and the family. Problems originating elsewhere within the family may also generate behavior disturbances in children who are otherwise normal. Behavior disturbances in the preschool group include resistance to bedtime, night terrors, inability to play with peers (too aggressive), inability to separate from the mother, rhythmic movements such as rocking and head banging, unusual reactions to toilet training, stubbornness, crying easily, temper outbursts, thumbsucking, nailbiting, high activity level, and reluctance to eat.[8]

Child Abuse and Neglect: Problems of development and behavior call for investigation of family relationships. Poor nutrition, evidence of inadequate physical care, and an apparent accident-proneness are also clues to disordered relationships with the parents. Sexual abuse of a child may occur in this age group. The effects of child abuse or neglect result in attention being focused on the child, sometimes concealing the basic problem. Neglect and abuse are more commonly seen in children who were prematurely born or have some handicap of physical or mental development.[9]

Infectious Disease: The common contagious diseases of early childhood like whooping cough and measles are uncommon today because of early immunization. Nevertheless, some children are not immunized and remain at risk, especially in low socioeconomic status groups.

The most common infections which toddlers and preschoolers experience are upper respiratory, with the usual complications of associated ear infections and sometimes bronchitis or pneumonia. Recurrent otitis media may cause fluctuating hearing loss with resultant effects on speech development. For this reason, prompt care of ear infections is very important.

In some parts of the south, gastrointestinal parasitic infestations still occur, but the worm loads are usually not great enough to cause serious illness. Anemia, often seen in nonwhite toddlers, is usually associated with dietary inadequacies, although recurrent infections and, infrequently, parasites may play roles.

Parasites from pet animals (*Toxocara canis* or *gatis*) infect toddlers, but serious complications are rare. Most parents feel the benefits outweigh the risks.

Lead Poisoning: Children in this age group living in poor housing are at highest risk for ingestion of old lead-containing house paint, leading to elevated lead levels in the blood. Recent research demonstrates that there really is no safe, acceptable lead level.[10] A lead burden in a toddler damages the central nervous system, as is shown later in terms of reduced learning achievement. As many as 40 per cent of children living in blighted urban areas carry significant lead burdens, although very few children have high enough serum levels to become acutely ill and thus come to medical attention.[11] With the major morbidity variable being cognitive development, lead poisoning is extremely important as a preventable factor leading to less than optimal development.

FACTORS WHICH INFLUENCE RISKS FROM BIRTH THROUGH AGE FOUR

Factors During the Prenatal and Delivery Period

PARENTAL FACTORS LISTED IN CHAPTER 4

All parental factors which are associated with premature births and congenital defects influence risks from birth through age 4. These factors include low socioeconomic status, low educational level, childbearing at the extremes of age, several births close together in a very young mother, a history of poor pregnancy outcome, chronic illness in the mother, complications during the pregnancy, and lack of prenatal care.

MATERNITY CARE AT APPROPRIATE LEVEL HOSPITAL

Mothers at high risk of poor pregnancy outcomes are more apt to have their special needs met in secondary and tertiary level hospitals where the equipment and level of technical expertise available are appropriate for the potential problems to be encountered, as suggested in Chapter Four. When a crisis develops, if the mother is in a location such as home or a community hospital where facilities do not exist, time is lost in transferring her to appropriate care. This time may make a great deal of difference for the fetus.

NEONATAL CARE IN AN APPROPRIATE LEVEL NURSERY

As with high-risk mothers, high-risk newborns are best served in nurseries where the level of expertise and technological sophistication can provide appropriate therapy if and when problems develop. The time lost in transferring a newborn to a tertiary level nursery when the child is acutely ill may make a difference between brain damage or optimal survival.

OTHER FEATURES OF NEONATAL CARE

Although the emphasis has been on the technological aspects of neonatal care for high-risk newborns, in fact, the early development of good mother-child relationships is extremely important if the baby survives. Therefore for any newborn, high risk or normal, efforts to bring the mother and child together as early as possible and for as much time as possible are features to be found in high-quality care.

It has been shown that giving babies to their mothers immediately after delivery and leaving them with the mother for at least the first hour after birth, when both mother and baby are alert, and then returning them to the mother for extra time during the the newborn period, facilitate the mother's caring behavior and her attempts to stimulate communication later. These features seem to be associated with better cognitive development in the baby than when the dyad spends less time together in the newborn period.[12]

When the baby stays in the mother's room, that is, "rooming-in," the mother is able to learn the baby's waking pattern and to feed the baby when the baby is ready to eat. She learns to recognize the child's indications of need. Babies kept in a newborn nursery and brought to the mother at regular hours cannot be fed according to their own natural rhythms. This may interfere with the mother's ability to breast-feed, inasmuch as the baby will not be wide awake and interested in sucking when it is in the mother's presence. A sleepy baby also does not stimulate much speech in the mother, nor can the mother stimulate the baby in other ways helpful to early development.

The home delivery movement is in part a response to the awareness that the early relationships between mother and baby, and baby and the rest of the family have lasting effects on all involved. Early bonding experiences among baby, mother, and father provide very satisfying emotional responses in the parents which are not duplicated when initiated at a later age.

Factors After Discharge from the Nursery

NUTRITION

The baby's nutritional status is always critical for its health and development. New reasons have recently been found to support breast-feeding.[13] Although formulas can be created from cows' milk which contain nutrients supporting what appears to be normal growth, there is no question but what the specific ingredients of human milk are most appropriate for human babies and cannot be completely duplicated. In addition, human milk contains factors which fight against the bacteria with which the baby is most apt to become colonized, that is, those which the mother is carrying. These specific factors help keep the child well. Of course, increasing the content of the diet as the infant gets older is important for maintaining adequate nutritional status. Supplements such as iron, vitamins, and fluoride are also important. Toddlers generally arouse maternal anxiety because of the small quantities they seem to eat. The parents' knowledge of nutrition and diet is challenged at this time to ensure adequate essential foods within the acceptable total intake. Inadequate preschool nutrition has been related to abnormal cognitive development.[14] Currently there is professional concern about the effects of the more restrictive vegetarian diets on children of preschool age.[15]

PARENTING: ENVIRONMENTAL STIMULI

Much of the child's intellectual development is dependent upon appropriate stimuli coming from the environment. These include behaviors of the parents toward the baby and in response to the baby's behaviors. In homes where the parents have less education, there is a difference in the ways in which the parents respond to the baby's attempts to communicate and in their behavior toward the baby.[16] It is possible that these early differences lead to significant differences later in the child's intellectual ability. Head Start, preschool programs, and other attempts to enrich the early environment of children seem to make a lasting difference on the child's ability to learn within a school setting.[4,17] It is possible that some children who presently appear to be border-line mentally retarded would have performed at a higher level had their earliest environment been enriched.

SAFETY: ACCIDENTS, EXPOSURES

The use of adequate restraining devices in automobiles and protection of the toddler from wandering into dangerous streets or places where the child might fall are various means of protecting the child from fatal accidents. There is no real substitute for continuous supervision of a young child. However, homes can be made less hazardous by educated attempts to remove common hazards from children's reach. This includes putting all cleaning solutions and medicines beyond the child's reach; erecting barriers in front of exposed heaters, high windows, and stairways; keeping pots and pans turned inwards on the stove and out of reach; fencing a yard or a swimming pool; and teaching the child to avoid areas where dangers lie. Hazards such as peeling paint in old homes need repair. Awareness of other potential exposures also can lead to protection of the child. Such exposures might include toxic chemicals which might be carried home from the job on the parents' clothing.

INFECTION

Immunizations protect against childhood diseases. The principles of prevention must be understood by parents. How diseases are spread from person to person, through air, water and foods, and by insects and the rodents upon which insects live must be appreciated. The role of personal cleanliness in avoiding skin disease must also be recognized.

The family must learn which illnesses need medical attention. They must learn to take care of minor illnesses in appropriate ways.

CONTINUING MEDICAL SUPERVISION

A child needs periodic medical examinations for several important reasons. Through early detection of developing problems and early treatment, complications can be minimized. Complete immunization is accomplished. The parents are prepared to understand the behaviors which will next develop in the child. This helps them to protect the child and not to expect more than the child can do, thus preventing frustration in both children and parents. More details may be reviewed in the literature.[18,19] Much of child health supervision can be carried out by public health nurses, pediatric nurse practitioners, or child health associates.

CONTINUING SOCIAL SUPPORTS

Family: Socially isolated mothers are seen to obtain less health care for their children and to have higher risks of problems in the children. Children develop best when both parents are in the home, or the mother is part of an extended family, or there is someone else in the home, an older adult who assists with child care.[20] Not only is the family a source of experience and emotional support, but it plays an obvious economic role.

Community Agencies and Public Services: For many mothers lacking family support or living in poverty, or where employment or education is less than adequate, community agencies play a very important role in helping the mother give the child what it needs. Assistance may be necessary for varying periods of time, but it has been demonstrated that intervention makes a meaningful difference. For example, in the case of the Early and Periodic Screening, Diagnosis and Treatment Program for Title 19 eligible children, although only 25 per cent of the eligible population has been reached, many children have received preventive and follow-up health services which, without outreach, their families probably would not have provided.[21]

Programs based on federal laws help provide income, medical care, day care for preschoolers, and job training for young parents.

Local health and social agencies provide casework services for specific types of problems and provide access to health care.

ACTIONS TO PROMOTE HEALTH, HEALTHY INFANTS AND PRESCHOOLERS

Promoting Parental Fitness for Childbearing

Promotion of parent fitness for childbearing, as in Chapter 4, will reduce the risk factors which cause poor pregnancy outcome and thus reduce the risk factors extending through the first few years of life.

Supporting Regionalization of Perinatal Care

Standards developed by committees of the American College of Obstetrics and Gynecology, the American Academy of Pediatrics, the American Academy of Family Physicians, and the American Medical Association, cover what is currently recommended for regionalization of perinatal care.[22] Three levels of care in each field are described with referral from the community level to the most specialized level for high-risk mothers and babies. These standards exist, but they have not been put into practice everywhere. Implications of the standards include the shutting down of certain small, poorly equipped obstetric and neonatal services, and the consolidation in other hospitals of these activities. Local physicians often resist such changes because they do not want to send their own patients to other areas or to other physicians for care. Ultimately, local physicians support regionalization when they see that the results for their patients warrant the changes, when they realize that their patients return to them after the crisis is over, and when they believe that the standard of practice in effect in their area mandates referrals.

Educating Service Providers

REGIONALIZATION

REFERRALS
Service providers require education to understand their role within the larger system. Referral networks within regionalized systems need to be clearly spelled out and formalized. Good referrals will plan for continuity of maternal and newborn care from the prenatal period through delivery and then back to the community for the postpartum period.

ENCOURAGEMENT OF MATERNAL-INFANT BONDING
The service providers should establish within the various delivery settings where they do not already exist arrangements which encourage maternal-infant bonding. Insofar as possible, the mother should be awake at, or soon after delivery, and should be able to hold her newborn during the first hour after birth. The father's presence is desirable. Following the stabilization period, the baby should be in the mother's room as much as possible. Trained personnel should help the mother become acquainted with her baby in the hospital setting.

HEALTH EDUCATION
While the mother and newborn are hospitalized, the mother should not only learn what her particular newborn is like, but also be taught child care, child behavior, infant nutrition, maternal nutrition, and the patterns of health supervision which are appropriate for the newborn and herself. While the mother is learning about the care of the baby, it is helpful if the baby's father or the maternal grandmother or any significant other person is included in the educational process. This way, the same ideas are fostered in all who might provide care for the baby, which may help to avoid later arguments over what is best.

Educating the Public

CONCERNING BONDING
In order to understand the changes which have been made in hospital settings and the new trends for "significant others" to be present during labor and delivery, the public needs to be educated concerning maternal-infant attachment and the bonding process. This will help people in the mother's environment as well as the mother.

CONCERNING FEEDING
Mothers in general are at the mercy of the marketplace. When it comes to formulas and baby food, much advertising is directed at young parents. Also, the last generation fed babies in a totally different way from the present generation. Each generation tends to think their way is superior. The latest scientific notions concerning appropriate timing and character of feedings should be shared with the public. The peer group and the extended family may then support the parents in what they do, rather than create

conflicts. At least everyone will understand the doctor's advice better and be better able to evaluate commercial products.

CONCERNING REGIONALIZATION
Regionalization of services imposes certain hardships on families. When a mother or a baby must be hospitalized in a tertiary center, for many families this means that they will be at some distance from their home. Parents need to understand what regionalization is trying to accomplish, and why it might be important for them. If parents do not understand the purpose of referral to a distant place, they are less likely to accept the recommendation, and more likely to be upset by the whole process. For the smoothest possible utilization of regionalized services, everyone involved must understand what it is all about.

CONCERNING CONTINUING CARE FOR THE FAMILY
The public must appreciate what can be accomplished through continuing comprehensive health supervision for the family in order to desire continuing care.

CONCERNING HEALTH AND HEALTH CARE
Health education of the public requires continuous messages in the mass media.

Providing Periodic Child Health Supervision

Periodic child health supervision is described in standards developed by the American Academy of Pediatrics.[23] The timing and the content of visits have been worked out in detail. Both timing and content vary with the age of the child. Since it is not always possible for a child to appear at the exact age described in the schedule, there is some leeway for visits. However, the schedule developed represents an ideal pattern for a healthy child.

IMMUNIZATIONS
Routine immunizations are started in the first year and completed in the second with recommended boosters occurring at entry to grade school and then approximately every 10 years. Diphtheria, whooping cough, tetanus, poliomyelitis, rubella, rubeola, and mumps are diseases for which immunization is currently recommended. Diphtheria, whooping cough, tetanus, polio, and measles (rubeola) are illnesses which formerly were responsible for a sizable amount of mortality and morbidity in children through age 4.

EXAMINATIONS
Complete physical examinations and dental examinations are recommended as part of periodic child health supervision. Thorough examinations make possible the detection of small problems which can be dealt with before they become worse. Chronic problems such as congenital defects or acquired chronic illnesses may also need to be followed periodically so that needed care can be obtained.

ANTICIPATORY GUIDANCE
Since development usually occurs in approximately the same sequence, care givers can let parents know ahead of time what to expect. This helps the parents cope with

changing behaviors and other forms of development without interpreting the changes as something they cannot understand and with which they cannot cope.

Anticipatory guidance might include:

1. Discussion of accident prevention, related to the age of the child and typical behavior for that age.
2. Behavior as noted above.
3. Feeding in terms of selection of foods and quantity of foods that the child could be expected to eat at the present time. Assistance with diet may be of particular value for vegetarian parents.
4. Counseling in answer to the parent's questions. The American Academy of Pediatrics recommends the use of questionnaires which help the parents to list their present concerns about the child.[23] However the information is elicited, it is important to allow the parents the opportunity to raise their own questions at each contact.

REFERRALS

The routine care giver, detecting certain kinds of problems, can refer the child for more examination or counseling in depth by a specialist in the area. It might be that a dietitian could be of more help developing a preschool vegetarian diet. It might be that persistent otitis media needs evaluation by an audiologist or an ear, nose, and throat specialist. It might be that a child apparently slow in developing speech would benefit from a complete educational evaluation, including evaluation by a developmental psychologist, a speech and language specialist, an occupational and/or physical therapist, and a vision and hearing screener. For children whose parents cannot pay for expensive care, referral to a public agency such as the state Crippled Children's Services may be indicated. Under P.L. 94-142 the local school system may provide a complete educational evaluation at no cost to the parent. Special preschool education may also be available from this source.

For many reasons, day care or preschool experiences may be useful for a normal or a handicapped child. The care giver needs to be familiar with resources in the community for these services and must be able to discuss with the parent what to look for in seeking such a service. The care giver can also help the parent anticipate the child's adjustment to such a setting.

Providing Continuing Maternal and Paternal Health Supervision

BIRTH CONTROL—TIMING OF THE NEXT BIRTH

Following childbirth, it is important for the mother to have a good method of birth control in order to delay the next birth for a reasonable period of time. The timing of the next birth can be discussed with both parents. The mother should have her own physician, who helps with her gynecological care. Nevertheless, this subject can be brought up by the pediatrician or the person providing health care for the child.

GENERAL HEALTH

The interconceptional period is an appropriate time to make certain that all the mother's and the father's health needs are being met. If necessary, the person taking care of the child should ask whether the mother and the father are looking after their own health and assist them in obtaining appointments if this seems useful. As noted earlier, the health status of the child can be facilitated by ensuring good health in both parents. Any health problem in the family detracts from the energies available to stimulate and care for the child.

FAMILY RELATIONSHIPS, MENTAL HEALTH

The caretaker for the child always needs to inquire about harmony within the family. Evidence of problems, whether behavior disorders appear first in the child or come out through questioning of the parent, always needs attention in order to foster the child's well-being. Referrals for mental health support of the parents may be looked upon as preventive therapy in relation to the child's well-being.

REFERRAL FOR SOCIAL NEEDS

The child's care giver, because of sensitivity to the needs of the parents, may find it important to refer the parents for help with education, financial assistance, family problems, job training, or group social support or therapies, such as Alcoholics Anonymous or Parents Anonymous. The child's total environment must be considered in the assessment of parental needs for assistance. The child under the age of 5 is particularly vulnerable to problems within the home, inasmuch as outside adults as yet have no continuing responsibility. The health care provider therefore has a particular responsibility during this time before the child is in school to consider broadly all the influences impacting on family life and to attempt to be helpful. The health sector registers newborns and should take the responsibility for tracking the child at least until the child is in school.

REFERENCES

1. Wegman, Myron E., "Annual Summary of Vital Statistics—1978." *Pediatrics* 64 (December 1979) pp. 835–842.
2. Department of Health, Education, and Welfare, Public Health Service, National Center for Health Statistics, *Facts of Life and Death*, DHEW Publication No. (PHS) 79-1222, November 1978.
3. Niswander, K. R., and Gordon, M., *The Women and Their Pregnancies*, DHEW Pub. No. (NIH) 73-379, 1972.
4. Richmond, Julius B., *Healthy People—The Surgeon General's Report on Health Promotion and Disease Prevention*. DHEW (PHS) Pub. No. 79-55071, 1979.
5. Wright, James C., "Growth Failure: Short Stature and Failure to Thrive," In *Ambulatory Pediatrics II*, Morris Green and Robert J. Haggerty, eds. Philadelphia: W. B. Saunders Co., 1977, pp. 354–360.
6. Baker, Susan P., "Motor Vehicle Occupant Deaths in Young Children." *Pediatrics* 64 (December 1979), pp. 860–861.
7. Scherz, Robert G., "Impact of Safety Packaging on Accidental Poisoning." *Pediatrics* 63 (May 1979), pp. 816–817.
8. Haggerty, Robert J., Roghmann, Klaus J., and Pless, Ivan B., *Child Health and the Community*. New York: John Wiley and Sons, 1975, p. 97.
9. Klein, M. and Stern, L., "Low Birthweight and the Battered Child Syndrome." *American Journal of Diseases of Children* 122 (1971), p. 15.
10. Needleman, Herbert L., et al., "Deficits in Psychologic and Classroom Performance of Children with Elevated Dentine Lead Levels. New England Journal of Medicine 300 (March 29, 1979), pp. 698–695.
11. Lin-Fu, Jane S., "Lead Exposure Among Children—A Reassessment." New England Journal of Medicine 300 (March 29, 1979), pp. 731–732.
12. Kennell, John, Voos, Diana, and Klaus, Marshall, "Parent-Infant Bonding." In

Child Abuse and Neglect: The Family and the Community. Rey E. Helfer and C. Henry Kempe, eds. Cambridge, Mass.: Ballinger, 1976, pp. 25–54.
13. Roy, C. C. et al., "The Rediscovery of Breast Feeding." *Canadian Medical Association Journal* 119 (July 22, 1978), pp. 109–112.
14. Winick, M., "Malnutrition and Brain Development." *Journal of Pediatrics* 74 (1969), p. 667.
15. Dwyer, J. T. et al., "Preschoolers on Alternate Life-Style Diets: Associations Between Size and Dietary Indexes with Diets Limited in Types of Animal Food." *Journal of the American Dietetic Association* 72 (1978), pp. 264–270.
16. Schaefer, E. S., "Parents as Educators: Evidence from Cross-Sectional, Longitudinal, and Intervention Research," *Young Children.* 27 (1972), pp. 227–239.
17. Darlington, Richard B. et al., "Preschool Programs and Later School Competence of Children from Low-Income Families." *Science* 208 (April 11, 1980), pp. 202–204.
18. Morris, Naomi M., "Pediatric Health Promotion Through Risk Reduction." *Family and Community Health* 3 (May 1980), pp. 63–76.
19. Alpert, Joel J., "Infancy and Early Childhood." In *Ambulatory Pediatrics II*, Morris Green and Robert J. Haggerty, eds., Philadelphia: W. B. Saunders Co., 1977, pp. 384–401.
20. Baldwin, Wendy and Cain, Virginia S., "The Children of Teenage Parents." *Family Planning Perspectives* 12 (January–February 1980), pp. 34–43.
21. Department of Health, Education, and Welfare, Health Care Financing Administration, "EPSDT; *Overview*," (HCFA) 77-24524, Washington, D.C.: The Medicaid Bureau, Office of Child Health.
22. Committee on Perinatal Health, *Toward Improving the Outcome of Pregnancy*. White Plains, N.Y.: The National Foundation–March of Dimes, 1976.
23. Committee on Standards of Child Health Care, *Standards of Child Health Care*, 3rd ed. Evanston, Ill.: American Academy of Pediatrics, 1977.

6 / Risk Reduction in the Middle Childhood Years

Naomi M. Morris, M.D., M.P.H.

The middle childhood years encompass school-aged, prepubertal children. Literature and statistics to be cited do not refer to a uniform age period. Mortality risks experienced at this time are the lowest for any period during life, 34.8 per 100,000 population for the 5 to 9 age group, and 37.6 per 100,000 for the 10 to 14 age group, in 1976.[1] Morbidity risks, on the other hand, are high, with infections and accidents very common events. Children missed 4.7 (high income) to 6.6 (low-income) days of school in 1976 for acute illness.[1] Injuries were the most common reason for hospitalization.[1] School failure is probably the most important morbidity. Some risk reduction during this period is dependent on the behavior of the individual child. Previously, risk reduction was accomplished solely through the behavior of parents and society.

RISKS TO BE AVOIDED IN THE MIDDLE CHILDHOOD YEARS

Mortality

ACCIDENTS
In 1976, accidents accounted for approximately 17 deaths per 100,000 individuals ages 5 to 14. Accidents thus constituted approximately half of all mortality in this age group. Of accidents to children over 1 year of age, those associated with automobiles were about 20 per cent, drowning about 8 per cent; and fires about 6 per cent.[2] There is a large sex differential in mortality from accidents in school-age children: boys' rates are consistently much higher than girls', the difference peaking during adolescence.[1]

CANCER
Cancer took five lives per 100,000 children, ages 5 to 14, in 1976.[2,3] The most common cancers are leukemia and central nervous system tumors.

CONGENITAL DEFECTS
The mortality rate from congenital defects in 1976 was two per 100,000 children, age 5 to 14.[3] The most commonly fatal congenital defects are within the heart.

OTHER
Other important causes of mortality in the 5-to-14-year age group in 1976 were homicide, influenza and pneumonia, heart disease, cerebrovascular disease, and suicide.[3] Some of the homicide cases were the results of child abuse. Suicide has been increasing in children 10 to 14 years of age, and has only recently appeared in the top ten causes of death for children.[4] It has been recognized in children 5 to 9.[5]

It is noteworthy that the only category in this list related to infectious disease is the one which is entitled "influenza and pneumonia." Many of these deaths occur in

85

children suffering from underlying problems, such as congenital defects, problems of the immune system, or neoplasms for which they are receiving chemotherapy.

Morbidity

CHILDHOOD INFECTIOUS DISEASES

On the average, young children have 6 to 7 upper respiratory infections per year, most of them mild.[6] Of the common childhood diseases, only chicken pox occurs with its historic frequency (188,396 cases in 1977). Most (whooping cough, 2,177 cases in 1977; diphtheria, 84; polio, 18; measles, 57,345; rubella, 20,395; mumps, 21,436) have been greatly reduced in frequency because of routine immunization.[7]

Scarlet fever must be added to the list of common childhood diseases infrequently seen. It has been reduced, not through vaccination, but through the earlier recognition and prompt treatment of streptococcal infections with penicillin or other antibiotics.

In recent years, cases of atypical rubeola have occurred in some young adolescents who had received killed measles vaccine as infants.[8] Also there are children who received earlier types of rubella vaccine who recently have been found to have inadequate antirubella titers.[9] It therefore may be necessary to reimmunize selected individuals in order to protect them against rubeola and rubella. Overall, however, the incidence of childhood communicable diseases has been reduced tremendously over the experience of 40 years ago.

Scarlet fever must be added to the list of common childhood disesases infrequently seen. It has been reduced, not through vaccination, but through the earlier recognition and prompt treatment of streptococcal infections with penicillin or other antibiotics.

In recent years, cases of atypical rubeola have occurred in some young adolescents who had received killed measles vaccine as infants.[8] Also there are children who received earlier types of rubella vaccine who recently have been found to have inadequate antirubella titers.[9] It therefore may be necessary to reimmunize selected individuals in order to protect them against rubeola and rubella. Overall, however, the incidence of childhood communicable diseases has been reduced tremendously over the experience of 40 years ago.

VISION DEFICITS

In terms of medical problems needing correction, vision deficits are one of the most common. Approximately 17 per cent of children 6 to 11 have a binocular visual acuity of 20/40 or less (Snellen ratio) without correction.[3]

HEARING DEFICITS

Approximately 3 per cent of children have hearing deficits, many due to repeated and chronic otitis media.[2] Most of the deficits are mild, but they may interfere with the child's classroom experience.

SPEECH DEFECTS OR PROBLEMS TALKING

Approximately 6 per cent of children 6 to 11 have speech defects or problems talking, according to interviews with parents during the Health Examination Survey.[3] The major handicapping condition among school children in 1974–75 was speech impairment.[10]

ACCIDENTS

Accidents are the most common cause for hospitalization of school-age children. Twenty-five per cent of hospitalized children on any given day are there because of injury. Accidents are frequently associated with recreational activities and equipment. For children 6 to 11, bicycle, swings, and skateboards are responsible for the majority of emergency room visits.[1,2]

HOSPITALIZATIONS

Common causes of hospitalization for children under age 15 include, in addition to injuries, pneumonia and upper respiratory infections, gastroenteritis, and appendicitis. Regarding the rate of discharges from hospitals, for children under age 15 by the leading surgical procedures, the leading operation for both boys and girls in the United States in 1975 and 1976 was tonsillectomy with or without adenoidectomy. The rate for boys was 8.5 and for girls 8.6 per 1,000 children. The next most frequent surgical procedure in the hospital for children of both sexes was operation to the tympanic membrane. The rate for boys was 4.5 and for girls 3.4 per thousand children. For boys, repair of inguinal hernia, reduction of a fracture, and appendectomy were the next most common procedures, respectively. For girls, the order was appendectomy, reduction of a fracture, and dilatation of the urethra.[1] Although the rate has been halved in the last 15 years, most pediatricians feel that tonsillectomy and adenoidectomy are performed far too often, reflecting historical conviction rather than present science.

DEVIATIONS OF GROWTH AND DEVELOPMENT

Growth: Overeating is the most prevalent nutritional problem today. About one third of currently obese adults were overweight children.[2] Children such as these readily stand out from their peers in school, and may suffer psychological as well as physical consequences of their obesity.

Excessively short children are also noticeable. Some are genetically small. Family disorganization and serious problems in the mother may account for the rarely seen undernourished child.[11]

Marked deviations of growth in school-age children deserve attention. Underlying problems may be chronic and difficult to change, but in middle childhood there is still hope for normalizing growth when nutrition has been faulty.

Development: With the reduction in incidence of childhood infectious diseases, a group of old problems has assumed new relative prominence. These have been labeled "the new morbidities." Among these are problems in school. About 20 per cent of children have reading or learning disabilities. School failure and school drop out are frequent results. For children with reading or certain learning disabilities, intervention can enable 80 per cent to place in the normal range for their age.[2]

Approximately 3 per cent of the school-age population have been classified as mentally retarded, but of these, 90 per cent are in the mild or borderline range. It is likely that many of these children come from backgrounds which have provided inadequate stimulation or opportunity for learning. With appropriate educational assistance starting at an early age, fewer such children may fall into the retarded category in the future.

Behavior Disturbances: Some school failure is due to disturbed behavior within the school setting. Causes for inappropriate behavior may be social or psychological in origin.

CHILD ABUSE

It is estimated that there are 200,000 to 4,000,000 cases per year of child abuse in the United States.[2] Child abuse is grossly underreported in most areas. Not only physical abuse—punishment and beatings—affect children in the middle childhood years; during this period sexual abuse of children is increasing, to peak in adolescence. Sexual abuse constitutes about 10 per cent of all cases of reported child abuse.[12]

The consequences for individuals who have been abused as children include abuse of their own future children when they become parents. For children who have been sexually abused, normal adult relationships are often affected. The child devalues himself or herself and may turn early to delinquent behavior.[12,13]

DENTAL CARIES

By age 11, on the average, a child will have decay in three permanent teeth. By age 17, eight to nine permanent teeth will either be missing, have decay, or contain a filling.[2] In recent years, knowledge of the effects of sticky sweets and the value of fluoride in the diet has contributed to a reduction in the amount of dental caries seen in children.

FACTORS WHICH PREDISPOSE TO THESE RISKS

Psychological Development

In middle childhood the individual spends more and more time out of the home. Teachers and peers become more important. The child has new models with whom to identify. Guidance from the home may be rejected as the child becomes more independent. This may lead to communication problems and parent-child conflict unless the parent understands and supports the need for independence within expanding boundaries. With regard to peer groups, this age group is very fond of clubs and societies of their own making. Loyalty to the group makes a child willing to follow suggestions of peer leaders, even when better judgment might dictate otherwise.

Favorite Activities

The school-age child is becoming more daring and adventurous, with a need for strenuous physical activity. He or she may play in hazardous places unless facilities for supervised adequate recreation are provided. Need for approval from the peer group may lead to daring or hazardous feats during games or utilizing recreational equipment. Some activities for which protective equipment is advisable are undertaken without such equipment.

More than half of all injuries leading to restricted activity or medical attention are incurred in or adjacent to the home.[1] Hazardous play is therefore not always too distant for parental evaluation and modification.

Certain Risk Factors in the Parents

Risk factors in the parents which predisposed children to cancer, congenital defects, mental retardation, or premature birth in earlier periods continue to contribute to the child's risks in middle childhood. The existence of the conditions affect the child's health, development, and education. Children with such problems should have been identified and tracked from their preschool period with planning for appropriate assistance and education.

Family Environment and Life-Style

Many characteristics of family life-style and the environment provided the child contribute to the risks experienced by school-age children. The family may fail to obtain appropriate health supervision for the child, which may result in failure to obtain care for health problems, available vaccines, dental services, dietary guidance and guidance in teaching the child principles of safety. Poverty and low levels of parental education may lead to poor living conditions and a lack of intellectual stimulation. Lack of strong family support systems and social isolation, immature or impulsive parents, parental abuse of alcohol or drugs, and marital discord, or single-parent households also add to pediatric risks for this age group.[1] A community may have social support systems available, but some families for various reasons may not take advantage of the existing services.

ACTIONS TO PROMOTE HEALTH IN MIDDLE CHILDHOOD

Through the Parents

PARENTAL RISK FACTORS
Reduce parental risk factors before conception and during pregnancy, the child's infancy, and preschool years as suggested in earlier chapters.

FAMILY PLANNING
Assist the parents with birth control for child-spacing to enable adequate attention to the development and well-being of each child.

PARENT'S LIFESTYLE
Assist the parents to achieve a healthy life-style through parental education concerning the use of cigarettes, drugs, alcohol, proper nutrition, and exercise. Parental education on these points may be initiated wherever the parents have contact with health or social services, including the child's health care provider or social agencies. Education may also be directed at entire communities through the mass media. Schools may send information home to parents or may contribute to parental education through the Parent-Teachers Association meetings.

SPECIAL NEEDS OF PARENTS
Parents merit referral for help with such things as alcohol abuse, marital problems, or signs of a potential for child abuse. Many communities have mental health services available or lay-organized groups such as Alcoholics Anonymous or Parents Anonymous, which can provide support to troubled parents. Indirectly, these services protect children.

ANTICIPATORY GUIDANCE
Parents can utilize continuous education on the subject of child-rearing from the period before they have their first child throughout the child's period of dependency.

Anticipatory guidance for the parents concerning behavior, diet, and development in general is a routine part of child health supervision. Relationships of the child to siblings, grandparents, schoolteachers, and peers should be subjects of the discussions between care providers and parents. The parents can use the information to better understand the behavior they see in the child. This protects the child from the consequences of inappropriate expectations on the part of the parents.

A very important part of the parents' education concerns the child's sexual development. During middle childhood, boys and girls usually go their separate ways. Yet each has ideas about what families are like and how they are formed. In a separate section of their minds, they are becoming more and more familiar with their bodies and physical sensations in the genital area. Children do not put physical sex and their romantic ideas together until puberty. However, prior to that time, they need to be "immunized" by adequate information in order to prevent mistakes later. Middle childhood is a very important time for sex education.

The parent can be the best sex educator of the child, providing the parent has adequate vocabulary and an understanding of child behavior in the social sphere surrounding the child. Health care providers and schools should contribute to parental education, so that the parent in turn can little by little provide the information the child needs. The parents' role modeling and information create a context within which the child can weigh and measure information and behavior perceived from outside sources.

The parents are role models not only for family life, but for all the aspects of healthy life-style, including nutrition, exercise, and the use of cigarettes, drugs, and alcohol. Education aimed at the parents should not only have as a goal the improvement of the parents' life-style, but specific guidelines for adequate nutrition, and so on for the child. The parents can help the child learn to like a well-balanced diet. Attractive and delicious home cooking is part of a child's heritage which he or she never really loses, although at the time he or she may seem unappreciative. Parents must be educated to realize that although they may try to impose rules on the child which incorporate what is best for the child, these rules will not be totally persuasive unless they follow all the applicable ones themselves.

Through the Child

COMPREHENSIVE HEALTH EDUCATION IN SCHOOL

Nutrition: School feeding programs can contribute to the child's appreciation of a balanced diet, much as home cooking does. In addition, theoretical reasons for diet composition can be taught as part of the school curriculum.

Alcohol and Drugs: The effects of substances on the body can be taught as part of the school curriculum. Older children can participate in discussions which incorporate value judgments and decision making.

"Know Your Body": The "Know Your Body" (KYB) program is an experimental curriculum which has been incorporated into several school systems.[14] Students learn about risk factors and their own risks by participating in physical examinations, blood tests, and classroom exercises focused on how to reduce risks. This program is described in detail elsewhere in this book. Modified versions of the KYB Program are being tried in many schools.This specific type of health education appears well adapted to the school-age child's level of cognitive development, concrete operationalized thought, characteristic of the child between 7 years of age and advanced adolescence. Concepts dealt with only in the abstract may not be considered applicable to the self in this age group.[15]

Puberty and Adolescence: Children must be taught the physiology of puberty and adolescence. In addition, they want to know something about the *meaning* of growing up. Behaviors and values need to be aired among the peer group with adult guidance.

The anatomy and physiology of reproduction are basic information. Birth control and family planning can be examined as necessities in the process of rational family formation and individual development. The most explicit lessons should be saved for children beginning to show signs of biological puberty.

Decision Making: Older children respond well to seminarlike discussions which enable them to make their own decisions on behaviors where values play a role. Sexuality as well as substance abuse is an area around which such discussions often focus.

Accident Prevention: Young children must be taught the safe use of matches, stoves, electrical sockets, and knives, and other dangerous objects. They need practice in handling such objects, and opportunities for this under seupervision may reduce the fascination such things hold for private experimentation, or at least make private use safer. Young children also need guidance in learning to cross streets with heavy traffic and play near busy streets, particularly in urban areas where other play areas do not exist. They must become conscientious users of seat belts when passengers in autobiles.

Lessons for older children appropriately focus on sports and recreational activities. Role modeling is very important for the motivation of school children to employ safety-oriented equipment and behavior, but the theory behind the use of such equipment and behavior can also be taught in a curriculum employing books, pictures, and movies. The equipment would include safety equipment for team sports, padding and helmets for children utilizing bicycles and skateboards. Children need to be taught swimming skills from as early an age as possible. They need to be taught respect for firearms. Drivers' education usually is provided in high school, but younger children need to learn traffic laws, since they apply to pedestrians and bicycle riders.

The school has an important role to play in dealing with all these subjects. In addition to providing education on these topics through the school system, communities can support public education on these subjects through the mass media and through local recreational programs.

COMPREHENSIVE HEALTH CARE

Comprehensive health care, which should have begun before birth, must continue through the school years. Health care providers must be especially sensitive to behavioral and educational problems.

School Health Services: Many school systems require that immunizations be completed before a child is admitted. The majority of children come with records of immunization from their private source of health care. If immunizations have not been completed, sometimes arrangements are made for them to be provided at school or by the local health department.

At periodic intervals, schools may provide vision and hearing screening. Children may be weighed and measured. There may be a dental health program including dental examination. At times, cleaning the teeth, application of fluoride or fluoride rinse programs, and dental education are also provided. Psychological testing and referrals for mental health services may be provided. Follow-up to make certain all identified problems are under care has been an important role of school health services.

Outside the School: Periodic examination with all the usual elements of comprehensive health care are suggested by the American Academy of Pediatrics to occur every year or two for the school-age child.[16] During these visits, more and more direct communication with the child is possible, as he or she grows up. Children who are showing the first signs of pubertal changes are ready for specific professional counseling concerning adolescence and reproduction.

When children can use special evaluation or services, the routine source of periodic health supervision should assume the responsibility of making such referrals and following up to see that appropriate actions are taken.

SUPPORT SERVICES IN THE COMMUNITY

The reduction of risks to the school-age child cannot be done by the parents, the health providers, and the schools alone. The community and federal, state, and local governments can create important environmental changes or opportunities. These include the special educational programs which meet the needs of children with specific physical or learning handicaps. In the '70s Public Law 94-142 legislated appropriate education for all school-age children with supporting services as needed.[17] Intervention during the school years is expected to reduce the permanent handicapping which results from behavioral disturbances, mental retardation, hearing, vision or speech impairment, or other health impairments. Twelve per cent of children 5 to 17 were eligible for service under P.L. 94-142.[18] Minimal requirements for educational opportunities for the handicapped were stated in the federal law, P.L. 94-142, but some states were able to add more services for more children, reaching into the younger-than-5 age group particularly. In 1981 with federal funding withdrawn some states may not choose to support as many services for children with special needs, but models for community systems have been developed.

On a community level, fluoridation of water is useful for reducing dental caries. Youth organizations provide opportunities for supervised and constructive play and physical development. Supervised recreational settings contribute to safety during activities enjoyed by school-age children.

Standard setting and enforcement are important governmental functions. Since some injuries are related to specific sports or to contact with certain devices, the government can enforce standards and encourage improved product design and engineering. Local governments can enforce compliance with safety rules and regulations such as where bicycles can be ridden.

The monitoring of infectious disease at the state and federal levels assists communities to know against what illness in particular measures must be taken at any given time. The monitoring of immunization levels of children led to the recent federal drive to bring levels up when it was discovered that the overall number of children completely immunized had fallen to a dangerously low level.

Monitoring of the environment in terms of air pollution, water pollution, and industrial wastes is also important, as school-age children range further than younger children and, as growing individuals, are still among the most vulnerable members of the population.

Environmental monitoring might include what appears on television and through other mass media. School-age children are very aware of current events and are trying very hard to grow up and act like adults. If their perception of adult behavior incorporates violence, cigarette smoking, alcohol consumption, drug use, and promiscuous sexuality, one can be certain that these are the behaviors that will be imitated. To protect the children, one can either change adult behavior or put in place the means to reduce the consequences of the behavior when it is begun in childhood. Both alternatives require a high level of community commitment and responsibility.

REFERENCES

1. Department of Health, Education, and Welfare, Public Health Services, *Health, United States, 1978.* DHEW Publication No. (PHS) 78-1232, December 1978.
2. Department of Health, Education, and Welfare, Public Health Services, *Healthy People: The Surgeon General's Report on Health Promotion and Disease Prevention.* DHEW (PHS) Publication No. 79-55071, 1979.
3. Department of Health, Education, and Welfare, Public Health Services, *Facts of Life and Death.* DHEW Publication No. (PHS) 79-1222, November 1978.
4. Vaughan, III, Victor C., and McKay, R. James, "The Field of Pediatrics." In Vaughan and McKay, eds. *Nelson Textbook of Pediatrics,* 10th ed., Philadelphia: W. B. Saunders Co., p. 4.
5. Tishler, Carl L., "Intentional Self-Destructive Behavior in Children Under Age Ten." *Clinical Pediatrics* 19 (July 1980), pp. 451–453.
6. Dingle, J. H., Badger, G. F., and Jordan, W. S., *Illness in the Home.* Cleveland: Cleveland Press of Western Reserve University, 1964.
7. Department of Health, Education, and Welfare, Public Health Services, Center for Disease Control, *Reported Morbidity and Mortality in the United States, Annual Summary 1977,* 26 (September 1978), pp. 2–4.
8. Department of Health, Education, and Welfare, Public Health Services, Center for Disease Control, *Morbidity and Mortality Weekly Report* 27 (November 3, 1978), pp. 427–437.
9. Balfour, Henry H., "Rubella Reimmunization Now." American Journal of Diseases of Children 133: 1231–1233, Dec., 1979.
10. U.S. Bureau of the Census, *Statistical Abstracts of the United States, 1977,* 98th ed., Washington, D.C.: U.S. Government Printing Office, 1977.
11. Kerr, Mary Ann D., Bogues, Jacqueline Landman, and Kerr, Douglas S., "Psychosocial Functioning of Mothers of Malnourished Children." *Pediatrics* 62 (1978), pp. 778–784.
12. Schechter, Marshall D. and Roberge, Leo, "Sexual Exploitation." In *Child Abuse and Neglect, the Family and the Community,* Ray E. Helfer and C. Henry Kempe, eds., Cambridge: Ballinger, 1976, p. 129.
13. Kempe, C. Henry, "Sexual Abuse, Another Hidden Pediatric Problem: The 1977 C. Anderson Aldrich Lecture." *Pediatrics* 62 (September 1978), pp. 382–389.
14. Williams, Christine L., Arnold, Charles B., and Wynder, Ernst L., "Primary Prevention of Chronic Disease Beginning in Childhood, The Know Your Body Program: Design of Study." *Preventive Medicine* 6 (1977), pp. 344–357.
15. Lowrey, G. H., "Behavior and Personality." In *Growth and Development of Children.* Chicago: Yearbook Medical Publishers, 1978, pp. 133–203.
16. Committee on Standards of Child Health Care, *Standards of Child Health Care,* 3rd ed. Evanston, Ill.: American Academy of Pediatrics, 1977.
17. The Education for All Handicapped Children Act of 1975, P.L. 94-142, 20 U.S.C. 1401 et seq. *Federal Register* 42: 163 (August 23, 1977), pp. 42474–42518.
18. Palfrey, Judith S., Mervis, Richard C., and Butler, John A., "New Directions in the Evaluation and Education of Handicapped Children." *New England Journal of Medicine* 298 (April 13, 1978), pp. 819–824.

7 / Risk Reduction in the Adolescent Years

Naomi M. Morris, M.D., M.P.H.

Adolescents are young people who are no longer children but not yet adults. The beginning and ending of the adolescent years are variable among individuals. The beginning of adolescence is generally related to biological puberty. Boys enter puberty at an older average chronological age than girls; no other generalization can be made except that most of the people usually conceptualized as adolescent are between the ages of 10 and 19. Statistics collected for different purposes use different dividing lines. To make comparisons among groups it is important to pay attention to the age groups cited in any statistics concerning adolescents.

Younger adolescents differ from older adolescents in many biological and psychological ways. Risks shift abruptly as new behaviors are initiated, for example, as teenagers switch from being automobile passengers to becoming automobile drivers, as they compete in contact sports, or as they become sexually active.

Some risks, such as mortality from congenital anomalies, are left over from earlier periods of life. Some risks relate particularly to the teenage period of development. Some risks are important mainly because of their implication for future well-being. As in infancy, during adolescence rapid change makes the individual vulnerable; it also gives particular significance to patterns of problem-solving and developing habits. Not only preparation for childbearing and family formation are at stake. Risk reduction in adolescence truly sets the stage for adult life.

RISKS IN THE ADOLESCENT AGE GROUP

Mortality

In 1976 the death rate for children 10 to 14 years of age was 34.6 per 100,000. For the age group 15 to 19, it was 97.1. For the age group 20 to 24, it was 131.3 per 100,000.[1]

The difference between the male and female experience increases with age. In the 10-to-14-year age group, for males the death rate is 44; for females the rate is 25.0. In the age group 15 to 19, for males the rate is 139.9; for females the rate is 53.2. In the age group 20 to 24, for males the rate is 198.4; for females the rate is 64.4. Subsequently, the ratio shifts back, although male mortality rates always exceed female mortality rates.

For children 12 to 15, diseases and conditions play a more prominent role in mortality than in later adolescence when accidents and violence account for a steeply rising rate of male deaths.[2] In 1976, 37.5 per cent of deaths in 12 to 15 year-olds were due to diseases and conditions, almost one third of which were neoplasms; in 16 and 17-year-olds, only 23.2 per cent of deaths were due to diseases and conditions. The remainder in each case is attributed to accidents and violence. The motor vehicle death rate specifically climbed from 28.3 in 12 to 15-year-olds to 43.2 per cent in 16 to 17-year olds.

AUTOMOBILE-RELATED ACCIDENTS

Alcohol is implicated in many automobile-related fatalities.[3] About half of fatally hurt drivers are found to have blood alcohol concentrations at or above the legally defined level of intoxication. Lower levels in teenagers, the elderly, and others sensitive to alcohol might increase the likelihood of an accident. Young people driving under the influence of marijuana or other drugs also place themselves at greater risk.

Eighty per cent of Americans do not use lap and shoulder belts.[3] Young people are known to harbor different attitudes about risk than older people. Excessive speed is more apt to be a factor in the vehicular fatalities involving teenagers 15 to 19 years old than in those involving older drivers.

Thirty per cent of Americans killed in motorcycle accidents in 1977 were under 20 years of age.[3] Motorcyclists have a seven-times greater chance of fatal injury per mile driven than automobile drivers.

OTHER ACCIDENTS

Drowning and fires are other causes of fatal accidents. Alcohol is often associated with boat-related accidents and drownings. Handguns, snowmobiles, minibikes, and private aircraft contribute to other possibly preventible fatalities.

HOMICIDE

Murder accounts for over 10 per cent of all deaths among the 15 to 24 age group, just under 7 per cent for whites but almost 30 per cent for blacks.[3] The American homicide rate is much greater than those of most other developed nations. In 60 per cent of murders in this country, victim and offender are related or acquainted. Sixty to 80 per cent of homicides are the result of personal disagreements and conflict, while robbery, sexual assault, and other circumstances are blamed for the remainder. As with other fatal injuries, homicide reflects the poor, weekends and nights, and alcohol abuse.[3]

SUICIDE

Suicide is the third leading cause of death in the 15 to 24 age group. More than 10 per cent of deaths in this age group in 1977 were due to suicide.[3] In contrast to homicide, suicide is more common among whites.[3,4,5] The rate in the 1970s is higher than it was in the fifties and sixties.[3] The incidence has been increasing in the 10-to-14-year age group as well as in older adolescents.[5] An increasing rate of suicide has been seen among young people in other industrialized nations.[3]

CANCER

Cancer is the fourth prominent cause of mortality during the adolescent years.[3] This is apparently not due to an increasing incidence, but to control of deaths from infectious disease, some of which used to be particularly threatening during the teenage years (e.g., tuberculosis).

Morbidity

Illness rates, the use of medical services, and hospitalizations are low for adolescents.[2] Kovar reports that in 1975–76, there were 361 hospitalization days for every 1,000 children 12 to 17 years of age. For boys 35 per cent and for girls 13 per cent of the days spent in the hospital were because of injuries. For girls 12 to 17 years of age, 18 per cent of the days in the hospital were because of childbirth. Among boys 12 to 15, there were 89 days of hospitalization per 1,000 per year for injuries, and among boys ages 16 to 17, there were 164 days per year. Among girls ages 12 to 15, there were 35 days of hospitalization per 1,000 per year for deliveries, and among girls ages 16 to 17, there were 162 days per year. Adolescents had, on the average, 2.4 acute conditions per year, missing 4.8 days from school. Adolescents 12 to 17 years of age made 1.6 visits to office-based physicians per year in 1975–76.

When asked, adolescents list their problems as nervousness, dental, acne, anxiety over health, scholastic difficulties, sex, and religion. Drugs and alcohol appear very low on self-ranked lists of problems.[4,6–8]

From an epidemiological standpoint, most of the problems listed by the adolescents are important, and only a few need be added.

CHILDHOOD DISEASES

The attack rate for measles (rubeola) is presently (1977 to 1979) highest in the 10-to-14-year age group, at the rate of 42. 8 cases per 100,000 population.[9] In 1977 more than 20 per cent of reported cases occurred in the 15 to 19 age group, with over 60 per cent of cases in individuals over 10.[10] Rubella has an even greater concentration during adolescence. In 1977, 70 per cent of cases occurred in those 15 and older.[11] The attack rate was highest in the 15 to 19 year age group, at 47 per 100,000.[12] In 1978 this rate was lowered slightly, and the attack rate in the 20 to 24 year group went up.[12]

ELEVATED BLOOD PRESSURE

A very small percentage of adolescents have overtly abnormal elevations of blood pressure. However, by definition, values over the 95th percentile for age are suspect, even though they may not exceed the usual borderlines defined for adult hypertension.[13] Data suggest that individuals with values on the upper end of the range will continue to occupy this position in relation to the rest of the population. Therefore, as they age, they will be the first to become hypertensive, and therefore constitute a high-risk group. However, adolescents are known to have labile blood pressure values, responsive to the situation of the moment. It is not clear whether brief and recurrent elevations have any significance for a future sustained hypertension. Since the issue is not settled, it appears worthwhile to identify adolescents who exhibit elevated values, in order to follow them carefully. Stamler et al. suggest following children with sustained blood pressures over the 75th percentile for age and sex, especially when there is a family history of hypertension or the child is overweight.[14] For children 12 and over, the 95th percentile value falls at levels considered high for adults, approximately 140 systolic over 90 diastolic. For 12-year-olds the 75th percentile value is 125/80.

MALNUTRITION

Obesity: Approximately 15 to 20 per cent of high school children are more than 20 per cent over the mean weight for their height, one definition used for obesity.[15] The prognosis for permanent weight reduction in adolescents is not good. Obese adolescents tend to become obese adults.[16] Nevertheless, behavior modification techniques and support groups can help some individuals.[17]

Common Dietary Deficiencies: In adolescents, the most common dietary deficiencies are iron, calcium, and zinc, and vitamins A, B_6, C, and folacin.[17] Simple iron-deficiency anemia is seen in 5 to 15 per cent of male and female adolescents, particularly blacks. Forty per cent of Spanish-American teenagers and 10 per cent of white as well as black teenagers have been found to have low plasma vitamin A levels; and in low-income families, plasma folicin has been found in 9 per cent of boys and 5 per cent of girls. Other below-standard intakes have not been reflected in laboratory measurements.

Special Needs Associated with Growth: The increase in body weight in adolescence, particularly in males, calls for great increases in consumption of calories and protein. With the exception of poverty-level females, teenagers in the United States generally consume more than the recommended amount of protein. Their caloric intake is slightly under the recommended dietary allowances (RDA).[18]

Special Needs Associated with Pregnancy: For those adolescents who become pregnant, there are nutritional needs not only to support adolescent growth but also to provide nutrients for the developing fetus. This means specifically increased intake of iron and calcium as well as some extra calories, particularly in the second half of pregnancy. Nutritional requirements are calculated by adding the recommended increment for pregnancy in older women to the recommended dietary allowance appropriate for the adolescent's age.[19]

Vegetarian Diets: Many adolescents in the last decade have become vegetarian for ecological or religious reasons. Those diets which omit only meat but include eggs, milk, and sometimes fish provide adequate nutrients. The individual must learn the food content of different foods and how to combine them, but no problems ordinarily result. Vegetarian diets which omit eggs, milk, and milk products become difficult to balance without vitamin and mineral supplementation. The addition of dietary supplements may avoid deficiency diseases. The most strict vegetarian diets, consisting only of simple grains, are inadequate, and result in dietary deficiencies.[17]

Other Dietary Considerations: Many adolescents, especially girls, are dissatisfied with their body image. Girls are particularly apt to attempt to lose weight. In some girls dieting of extreme degree may be part of a condition called anorexia nervosa. Endocrine changes may be associated with anorexia nervosa. The onset of menses may be delayed in girls who have not menstruated. Other girls, already beyond menarche, may cease having menstrual periods. Beneath a critical weight or proportion of body fat for each height, menstruation will not occur. The exact mechanism is not totally understood, but there is a relationship between weight and the integrity of the reproductive system.[20] Anorexia nervosa is at the extreme end of a spectrum of dietary patterns aimed at weight loss and requires medical care.

The diet selected by adolescents is guided by considerations other than its nutritional content in many cases. When weight loss is desired, various crash diets or food fads may be pursued. Adolescents with no concern for body weight may select their diet as mood and opportunity dictate. Notoriously fond of fast foods, adolescents who need high calorie intakes will not necessarily do poorly with selections such as hamburgers and milkshakes. Problems may arise from excessive use of candies, cakes, cookies, soft drinks, and other foodstuffs containing high concentrations of sugar and fats with little else. Satisfaction from such high-density food materials may preclude adequate intake of fruits, vegetables, and grains.

DENTAL HEALTH

Caries: Partly due to the ingestion of frequent high sugar snacks and partly due to neglect, caries appear in increased numbers during adolescence. Based on dental examinations of a sample of the civilian noninstitutionalized population of the United States from 1971 to 1974, 53.6 per cent of children 12 to 17 were found to need decayed tooth repair, 13.4 per cent needed gingivitis treatment, and 27.5 per cent needed dental cleaning.[21] By age 17, eight or nine permanent teeth have decayed, been filled, or are missing.[3]

Orthodontia: The best time for correcting abnormalities of bite or appearance is during the period of rapid growth. In the survey mentioned above, 7.1 per cent of children 12 to 17 were judged in need of orthodontic care because of severe malocclusion.[21]

ACNE

Acne in some degree is an almost universal problem of adolescence. Skin hygiene and local therapy control most cases. Dietary changes usually are not recommended. A few cases of cystic acne with obvious infection respond to more aggressive therapy, including the use of tetracycline orally. Long-term antibiotic therapy is no longer as popular as it once was. Systemic therapy particularly with tetracycline is contraindicated during pregnancy; tetracycline damages fetal tooth development.

MENTAL HEALTH

"Out-of-Control" Behavior: For every case of death by suicide, it has been estimated that there are up to 200 unsuccessful attempts.[22] As noted earlier, there has been a growing suicide rate in the adolescent population of the United States and other industrialized countries. This signal of distress points up the impact on adolescents of the pressures in society today. Suicide is not the only sign of an adolescent in pain. Other "out-of-control" behaviors include vandalism, shoplifting, running away, substance abuse, and promiscuous sexual behavior.[23]

Younger as well as older adolescents are involved in these behaviors, indicating a stress level beyond their ability to cope. Peaks of low self-esteem and poor self-image are known to characterize children at entry to junior high school.[24] The new environment with its academic challenges and its teen culture can be very difficult for children trying at the same time to adapt to the bodily changes of early puberty. For some children the path is downhill from this point. Parental expectations for academic achievement and vocational selection can impose a heavy burden on top of a critical load. Parental expectations and courses offered may not fit the adolescent's abilities or interests.

Data from various sources concerning the multiple anxieties of adolescence support the adolescent's own complaints that "nervousness," school difficulties, and "anxiety over health" are important problems during the teenage years.[6-8]

Learning Problems: Learning problems can influence behavior and mental health. A high percentage of children attempting suicide have records of school failure, truancy, and discipline problems. Psychologic tests show "minimal brain dysfunction" more often in such children than in a control group.[25]

Only recently has the educational system been required by law to provide appropriate education for *all* children. This includes children who have educational handicaps which prevent them from succeeding in the ordinary school curriculum. The evaluation of such preschool and grade-school age children and curricula appropriate for them are newly developed. Evaluations and curricula for handicapped adolescents are not yet at all well-developed.[26]

Substance Abuse: Adolescents place substance abuse low on the list of problems which they perceive as important. Nevertheless, because of the known consequences of substance abuse, the following statistics are of interest: among all adolescents ages 12 to 17, 53 per cent have tried alcohol, 47 per cent have tried tobacco, and 28 per cent have tried marijuana. In 1978, it was estimated that 29 per cent of high school seniors smoked cigarettes daily, while 6 per cent used alcohol and 9 per cent used marijuana daily. Trends seem to indicate that alcohol and cigarette use may be decreasing in older alolescents and marijuana use is increasing.[2]

PROBLEMS RELATED TO SEXUAL BEHAVIOR

Sexually Transmitted Diseases: Sexually transmitted diseases are rare among adolescents younger than 15. They are common among the 16 and 17-year-olds.[2]

In 1976, 3 of 1,000 younger adolescents and 20 of 1,000 older ones acquired gonorrhea. The case rate for 15 to 19-year-olds in 1975 was 12.9 per 1,000, which is three times the rate of 20 years earlier. Gonorrhea is more common among female adolescents than among males of comparable age, in contrast with adult men and women. Gonorrhea is a serious illness for girls, in that pelvic inflammatory disease occurs in 17 per cent of all women who have gonorrhea, and sterility may result in 15 to 40 per cent of cases of pelvic inflammatory disease, even when adequate treatment is received.[2]

Syphilis and other major types of venereal disease are less common but chlamydial, trichomonas, and yeast infections are seen with increasing frequency in teenagers. The health consequences of *Chlamydia trachomatis* infections are not negligible, either for males or females, and risk may extend to the fetus when pregnancy occurs.[27]

The herpes virus, which infects the genital tract and poses a serious threat to an infant at delivery, is suspected of a role in the etiology of cervical cancer also. The epidemiology of cancer of the cervix is like that of a sexually transmitted disease.

Adolescent Pregnancies: In 1976, there were 1.2 live births per 1,000 women 10 to 14 years of age, 34.6 live births per 1,000 women 15 to 17, and 81.3 live births per 1,000 women 18 to 19. The birth rate of 15 to 17-year-old girls, as in all older age groups, has been falling since 1972. The rate for 10 to 14-year-olds has been steady. There were approximately 12,000 births to girls under 15 in 1976.[2] The latter are still children themselves, not really ready for pregnancy. The physical risk to the infant is increased, and the mother is psychologically, economically, and educationally unprepared for parenthood.

Statistics concerning what happens to children born to young teenagers show that they have a relatively deprived and handicapped future. In large part, the prognosis is due to the circumstances surrounding the adolescent. Adolescents who have such early births generally come from poor socioeconomic backgrounds.[28]

The age of a young woman at the birth of her first child affects her ultimate educational attainment. The chance of a young teenager completing high school is small.[2] Teenage mothers also tend to have more children. They subsequently have a greater risk of poverty and welfare dependency.[2]

Not all teenagers who become pregnant carry the child to term. More adolescents under age 15 obtained legal abortions than had live births in 1976.[2] In the age group 15 to 17 the ratio of abortions to liveborn children was about two to three. The declining birthrate in the 15-to-17-year-old group is partly due to increased numbers of abortions, as well as to an increase in the use of contraception. About one third of legal abortions each year have been for women under the age of 20.[2]

FACTORS WHICH PREDISPOSE TO THESE RISKS

Bracketed in the period of transition between childhood and adulthood, adolescents are vulnerable physically, psychologically, and socially.

Physical Vulnerability

RAPID GROWTH

During the period of rapid growth, there is a need for adequate sleep and nutrition. Nutrition provides the building blocks for growth, and during sleep as yet incompletely understood endocrine patterns provide internal environments unique to the adolescent period and probably growth-related. In addition to dietary deficiencies, certain defects become prominent during the period of rapid growth. Among these are scoliosis, susceptibility to damage to the growing end of bones (e.g., Osgood-Schlatter's disease; Legg-Perthes disease), and dental problems as related earlier. The problems of chronic illnesses, such as congenital heart disease or cystic fibrosis, may be exaggerated as a consequence of the growth process, or may cause stunting of growth. Most common, simple dietary excess leading to obesity predisposes the adolescent to hypertension and negative self-image.

CERTAIN ILLNESSES

Diabetes and thyroid disease are two endocrine disturbances which may appear for the first time during adolescence. Diabetes of earlier onset may become more troublesome at this time, partly because of the self-discipline needed to control the disease.

Perhaps because of the adolescent's tendency to exercise vigorously, sleep less than needed, and obtain less than optimal nutrition, as well as to enter new environments, the adolescent is susceptible to certain infectious diseases. Historically, adolescence was a common time for the onset of tuberculosis. Presently, infectious mononucleosis is frequently recognized in this age group, hepatitis consequent to the use of unsterile equipment in drug abuse is a serious problem, and epidemics of influenza, streptococcal infection, and meningococcal infection are frequently seen in young military populations or other groups formed by adolescents.

Other problems originating during adolescence include alcoholism, duodenal ulcer, hypercholesterolemia, labile hypertension, irritable colon syndrome, and migraine headaches.[4]

Psychological Vulnerability

PSYCHOLOGICAL DEVELOPMENT

The psychological tasks of adolescence include becoming independent from the parents, learning to like oneself, becoming admired by the peer group, establishing a heterosexual relationship, and defining the direction for vocational activity. The adolescent experiences a return of conflicts concerning aggressiveness, and awareness of sexual energy. The adolescent fears loss of control because he or she is aware of changes in mood and anxieties within himself or herself. Sometimes, this is exaggerated into a fear of insanity. The adolescent is unaware that these concerns are universal. The psychological tasks may create anxiety as the social context in which the problems must be solved may create various problems, as will be discussed in the following sections.

The adolescent's attempts to impress his or her peer group and to act adult lead to many behaviors which are interpreted by adults as rebellious and inappropriate. Symbols of adulthood in our society include smoking, the use of alcohol, and, for girls, pregnancy and motherhood. Depending on the social setting, behaviors related to these outcomes are or are not reinforced. Competition for status within the peer group also explains certain aggressive and impulsive behaviors as well as concern over personal appearance.

SECONDARY EFFECTS OF GROWTH

The adolescent is aware of the changes in the shape of his or her body. These changes require adaptation and a new self-image. Anxiety over breast size in girls and height and muscle development in boys may lead to behaviors which are designed to have some beneficial effect, or may lead to states of depression. The boy who is a late maturer, too short, or both is at a disadvantage in our society. The girl who matures very early may be extremely self-conscious and withdrawn. Early and late maturers experience the adolescent period differently.[29]

Cognitive changes are not necessarily in phase with growth. Learning ability seems to spurt along with height,[30] but judgment may lag behind bodily changes which invite sexual behavior, use of alcohol, aggressive responses, and so on. A person may obtain a driver's license before his or her judgment is mature. Pregnancies similarly can occur before mature judgment can play a role in preventing an unwanted pregnancy or planning the timing of a desired one.

Social Vulnerability

SEXUAL ACTIVITY

Heterosexual behavior has an obvious biological base, but it is a social necessity, not a biological one. The mass media teach children in our society that sexual behavior is part of adulthood. Sexual activity is also made to appear desirable and rewarding. During this century, increasing proportions of unmarried adolescent girls have had intercourse, and they have had their first experience at a younger age.[31] (There are no national data for boys.) Even during the 1970s, large changes in female experience have been documented. In 1971, 27 per cent and in 1976, 41 per cent of unmarried 17-year-old women reported that they had had sexual intercourse at least once. The proportion of sexually active 15-year-olds increased from 14 per cent in 1971 to 18 per cent in 1976.[32] There are differences by ethnic groups; larger proportions of blacks at each age are sexually experienced than whites. The increase in recent years has been greater for whites, and the gaps between the groups are narrowing.

Superficially, what appears to be happening is a reduction of the double standard, so that girls are free to experiment with sexuality much as boys have been. Not every woman sees this as a step forward, since the risks for females are still greater than the risks for males, and reduction of the double standard gives women more freedom to act like men, but possibly less freedom to follow their own inclinations.[33] Discussions among adolescent groups reveal that those who prefer to abstain from sexual relationships until a later time need support because of peer group pressures in the opposite direction.

One problem related to early sexual behavior is the need for birth control by individuals who barely recognize that their behavior is equivalent to adult sexual behavior. Adolescent sexuality is an area about which most adults and most school systems prefer not to talk. Society on the one hand encourages the behavior by its modeling and messages, but on the other hand fails to recognize it and protect young adolescents from its consequences. The instruction and services necessary for responsible heterosexual behavior are not made readily accessible to young adolescents. The children have some of the required knowledge, but are not assisted in applying the knowledge to their own experience with concrete discussions of sexual behavior. Risks relating to sexual behavior therefore remain a relatively abstract concept relevant to adults. To these young people whose stage of cognitive development may still be at the cognitive development may still be at the concrete level, such risks do not seem applicable to themselves and their own behavior, since they do not see themselves as adults to whom the norms concerning pregnancy and birth control apply.[34]

VOCATIONAL CONSIDERATIONS

In line with a new commitment to equal opportunities for females, that is, reduction of the double standard in vocational opportunities, girls are now encouraged to prepare themselves for the competitive world of work the same as boys. This situation is both a welcome one and a difficult one for females, since most females continue to desire marriage and children at some time in the future and may recognize that in the real world, working women shoulder the bulk of responsibility for household management regardless. This recognition may cause compromise in goal-setting. Some females are experiencing increased pressure for educational or vocational achievement because of societal trends, perhaps resulting in anxieties over grades and admission to graduate studies, which formerly were reserved for males. In addition, some girls without career orientations appear defensive about their life plans. There is some unease about accepting the older feminine role.

Vocational decisions by either sex are complicated by the fact that society is changing very rapidly at the present time, and occupations adaptive for present needs may not exist 20 or 30 years from now. Occupations held by parents may not be appropriate for those planning to live in the future world, so parents cannot model vocational roles. There is no question but that skills will be necessary for future employment; an unskilled person cannot count on finding much work in our increasingly technological society. Needless to add, education or training for the handicapped becomes even more complex and important given this situation.

Adolescents who have not yet acquired job skills are nevertheless ready to be consumers and need incomes to support their consumer demands. Clothes, food snacks, transportation, and recreation require expenditures by adolescents. Parents with adequate resources can provide allowances to cover these needs, yet in support of a work ethic it seems desirable for youth to find work. Work is not even available for all those adults who need it, let alone adolescents who have not completed their schooling or who by virtue of their living arrangements are apparently still the dependents of responsible adults. The needs of minority-group adolescents for work are particularly pressing.

THE IDEALS OF YOUTH

In many ways, the adolescent has been encouraged to develop ideals for the way he or she thinks life and society should be, but more and more, through observation and studies of the real world, the awareness develops that things are really not that way. The adolescent is disillusioned and at the same time forced to define his or her role within a real world which is imperfect.

Further, solutions to problems presented by the mass media appear to be instant. Even though time frames may be defined as long, problems are often solved within a half-hour or so. This does not strengthen the ability to defer gratification, so necessary for solutions to real problems and achievement of difficult goals.

Not only with regard to prolonged periods of education in order to acquire skills for employment, but also with regard to heterosexual relationships, the adolescent is often unwilling to wait. Informal housekeeping is being attempted by many adolescents, particularly college students. Some sociologists see advantages to "trial marriages," at least in terms of the pair getting to know each other and making a more reasoned judgment as to whether they wish to spend life together. As long as children do not bless the couple, there may be logic to this reasoning. Prolonged sexual relationships seem preferable to promiscuity.

One other problem has been identified in relationship to the ideals of youth, and this is the cynical effect of too much too soon. Excessive material advantage, early, may influence a person's motivation to work. Substance abuse and vandalism by adolescents from comfortable homes have been in part attributed to the parent's excessive generosity with material things. This may conceal stinginess with regard to the parents' attention, however. It is probably better not to blame affluence per se for negative adolescent behaviors.

THE GENERATION GAP

History records that every generation has had some problems communicating with the next one. Features of society, particularly those relating to change, inevitably make it necessary for the child to adapt to what is coming. The parent finds it easier to remember the environment of his or her youth. Each, therefore, approaches the present with different assumptions. The rapid rate of change characterizing the twentieth century may have exaggerated this problem.

Adolescents in immigrant groups descending on the United States experience the generation gap to an even greater degree. Foreign adolescents reject their parental standards and traits in the process of adaptation to their new environment. The orientation of native-born Americans to outsiders at times adds greatly to the burden of social vulnerability borne by adolescents who have ethnic backgrounds different from the majority.

ACTIONS TO PROMOTE HEALTH IN ADOLESCENTS

Periodic Medical Examinations

The American Academy of Pediatrics has defined standards for the pattern and content of periodic medical examinations for all children according to their age group.[35]

IMMUNIZATION

A booster for diphtheria and tetanus is needed at approximately age 15. Special efforts should be made to determine the immune status of girls concerning rubella. Ideally, rubella immunization should be provided for girls who do not have satisfactory antibody titers against the disease before they become sexually active. In any event, rubella vaccination may be completed providing the girl will not become pregnant for the following 3 months. The status of immunity to other childhood diseases should also be reviewed.

SCREENING

Various screening services may be performed prior to school entry at the junior high level or at school. These include hearing, vision, dental health, height and weight, skin, and tuberculin testing. In some schools screening for elevated blood pressure and scoliosis are also provided.

HEALTH EDUCATION AND COUNSELING

The most important element of periodic health examination for adolescents is actually health education and counseling. The health care provider at this time is able to discuss with the adolescent the adolescent's status with regard to growth and development. The examiner can talk about puberty and relate the adolescent's stage of secondary sexual characteristics to his or her overall potential development. Sexual behavior, including contraception, can be discussed. The adolescent's particular interest in sports and exercise can be investigated. The adolescent's diet can be reviewed and commented upon. Any concerns which the adolescent expresses concerning self, family, school performance, future vocation, use of alcohol, drugs and tobacco can be discussed. The use of seat belts and safety equipment during recreational activities can be encouraged.

Dental Care

Dental screening is important, and all adolescents should continue to be seen at approximately 6-month intervals. Those who need restoration and orthodontic care should be encouraged to obtain whatever is necessary. This advice can be given directly to the adolescent as well as communicated to the parent.

Community-Based Counseling and Services

The particular needs of adolescents suggest that a variety of special clinics or services can contribute to the adolescent's health and well-being.[4] A "hot line" for seeking help during crises is popular in many communities. Mental health clinics sponsored by state or local agencies can help teenagers and their families. Teen clinics which provide comprehensive services shaped particularly to the needs of teenagers seem better than sources of care where teenagers have to mingle either with younger children or with older adults. Family planning clinics have served many adolescent patients. Planned Parenthood and local and state public health agencies frequently provide services for adolescents. Student health services in colleges have been slow to take up contraceptive services, but many have now done so. In high schools, it has been difficult to incorporate the actual prescription of birth control methods, although more and more school nurses are able to refer students for this assistance. Venereal disease clinics are usually sponsored by local public departments. Adolescents represent a large proportion of the people needing care for sexually transmitted diseases. This service should be provided in any clinic providing medical services to teenagers. In all settings, the wishes of the adolescent for confidentiality and even anonymity should be respected, although involvement of parents when treatment is needed for younger adolescents should be encouraged.

Help for Parents

Education concerning the tasks of adolescence should be provided parents by the adolescent's health care provider and by the schools. Parents cannot automatically understand the adolescent's viewpoint. Parents in midlife are often experiencing crises of their own. Special groups dealing with typical parental problems may help the parents to cope. The PTA may also assist parents in the child-rearing tasks relating to their adolescents through support and educational activities. The parent's physicians or other therapists can play a role in helping them through their children's adolescence, by being sensitive to the special characteristics of family relationships during this time of life.

Driver Education

The schools provide education for safe automobile driving and motorcycle safety. This education is extremely important and should be supported in every community.

Sports Education

Most schools, from the junior high school level up, sponsor competitive team sports. Actually, sports should be taught not only the 5 per cent of children who are athletically talented, but all children in the system. Youth should be encouraged to participate in activities that will provide them exercise and pleasure, and they should learn to use the appropriate safety gear.

Family Life Education

Family life education should be taught in the schools, starting from the earliest level, as discussed in Chapter Four. In addition, as adolescents go through junior high school and high school, courses such as human ecology, sociology, psychology, and biology should contribute to their understanding of human life. Seminar discussions of decision making concerning various behaviors are valuable adjuncts.

School Services

Many school systems provide health and social services within the school setting. If these are not available in school, there should nevertheless be systems for screening out children in need of services and making referrals for these services, with follow-up to make sure that the services are obtained. Among the particular services which are useful for adolescents are those relating to general health, family planning or birth control, sexually transmitted diseases, prenatal care, and mental health counseling.

In some high schools, day care centers for the adolescent's children have been established. Within these centers, the mothers and other adolescents can learn about child development and child care. Having a place to leave her child is also helpful to the adolescent mother who is completing her high school education.

Healthy Living

The school system in its curriculum should include the theory behind behaviors recommended for healthy living. This includes nutrition, exercise, smoking, and the use of drugs and alcohol. In some schools an innovative program known as the "Know

Your Body" program, which focuses on specific risk reduction, has been introduced.[36] This program is discussed elsewhere in this book. Its particular appeal to young people is its concrete approach. Each child learns his or her own blood pressure, and learns to measure it in others. The children find out their cholesterol levels. They look at their weight in relationship to height, and they record details of their diets. Over a period of time, changes in their specific risk factors can be related to their specific behaviors. Discussions within the classroom help each child in decision making for healthy behaviors.

In schools where the principles of healthy living are reinforced by such things as a balanced diet in the school lunch room and the absence of junk foods or cigarettes in machines, there is an unspoken commitment to improving the children's life-style. This is an important reinforcement and requires teachers' cooperation, since they may be tempted to behave in ways different from what they teach.

Other Community Support Services

RECREATION

It has been mentioned that exercise and sports for lifetime health promotion need to be provided for all adolescents, not just for those interested in competitive sports. In addition to what is available in the school, it is desirable for communities to have organized programs and space in which to carry them out, including parks, bicycle paths, and swimming facilities, with supervision for young people.

VOCATIONAL TRAINING

In addition to traditional schools, communities should provide alternative educational pathways or vocational training for students who do not fit into the standard program. The Department of Labor may provide Job Corps experiences which provide income and training for future work. Another helpful program has been the CETA program which also provides income during on-the-job training for certain types of work. The future of this program is clouded at this time due to federal funding cutbacks.

SHELTERS

Many children and sometimes adults leave home with various problems and have nowhere to go. Communities can support shelters for runaways, for abused children and mothers, for pregnant girls, and for substance abusers, with service to help the individuals get through a period of crisis and develop realistic plans for the future.

SPECIAL PROGRAMS

Communities can sponsor special programs which involve youth who otherwise might lack guidance and direction. These programs might be like the Boy Scouts, conventional youth organizations; or they might be special municipal programs organized by police departments or social service agencies.

The commitment of communities to providing services for adolescents is an extension of a national commitment to the future of our country. Pediatric risk reduction must be broadly conceptualized to include not only health care providers, but also social service, educational, and community groups working together for the survival and optimal development of young people. Hopefully today's adolescents will continue this commitment on behalf of tomorrow's children.

REFERENCES

1. Department of Health, Education, and Welfare, Public Health Services, *Health, United States, 1978.* DHEW Publication No. (PHS) 78-1232, December 1978.
2. Kovar, Mary Grace, "Some Indicators of Health-Related Behavior Among Adolescents in the United States." *Public Health Reports* 94 (March–April 1979), pp. 109–118.
3. Richmond, Julius B., *Healthy People–The Surgeon General's Report on Health Promotion and Disease Prevention.* DHEW (PHS) Publication No. 79-55071, 1979.
4. Millar, Hillary E. C., *Approaches to Adolescent Health Care in the 1970's.* DHEW Publication No. (HSA) 75-5014, 1975.
5. Holinger, Paul C., "Violent Deaths Among the Young: Recent Trends in Suicide, Homicide, and Accidents." *American Journal of Psychaiatry* 136 (September 1979), p. 9.
6. Brunswick, Ann, "Health Needs of the Adolescent: How the Adolescent Sees Them." *American Journal of Public Health* 59 (1969), p. 1730.
7. Sternlieb, Jack J, and Munan, Louis, "A Survey of Health Problems, Practices, and Needs of Youth." *Pediatrics* 49 (February 1972), pp. 177–186.
8. Parcel, Guy S., Nader, Philip R., and Meyer, Michael P., "Adolescent Concerns, Problems, and Patterns of Utilization in a Triethnic Urban Population." *Pediatrics* 60 (August 1977), pp. 157–164.
9. *CDC Morbidity and Mortality Weekly Report* 28 (August 31, 1979), pp. 410–411.
10. *CDC Morbidity and Mortality Weekly Report* 27 (November 3, 1978), pp. 427–436.
11. *CDC Morbidity and Mortality Weekly Report* 27 (November 17, 1978), pp. 451–459
12. *CDC Morbidity and Mortality Weekly Report* 28 (August 17, 1979), pp. 374–375.
13. "Report of the Task Force on Blood Pressure Control in Children." *Pediatrics* 59 (Supplement), pp. 797–820.
14. Stamler, Jeremiah et al., "Blood Pressure in Children." *CIBA-GEIGY,* (1980).
15. Lowrey, George H.; *Growth and Development of Children,* 7th ed. Chicago: Year Book Medical Publishers, 1978, pp. 438–442.
16. Charney, E. et al., "Childhood Antecedents of Adult Obesity." *New England Journal of Medicine* 295 (1976), p. 6.
17. Marino, Deborah Dunlap and King, Janet, "Nutritional Concerns During Adolescence." In *Pediatric Clinics of North America,* Vol. 27. Philadelphia: W. B. Saunders Co., February 1980, pp. 125–139.
18. Department of Health, Education, and Welfare, *Advance Data,* Vol. 6. DHEW Publication No. (HRA) 77-1250, March 30, 1977, pp. 1–15.
19. Food and Nutrition Board (National Research Council), *Recommended Dietary Allowances,* (9th ed.) Washington, D.C.: National Academy of Sciences, 1979.
20. Frisch, R.E. and McArthur, J. W., "Menstrual Cycles: Fatness as a Determinant of Minimum Weight for Height Necessary for Their Maintenance or Onset." *Science* 185 (1974), pp. 949–951.
21. Department of Health, Education, and Welfare, *Data from the National Health Survey: Basic Data on Dental Examination Findings of Persons 1–74 Years, United States, 1971–1974.* DHEW Publication No. (PHS) 79-1662, May 1979.
22. Marks, A., "Management of the Suicidal Adolescent on a Nonpsychiatric Adolescent Unit," *Journal of Pediatrics* 95 (1979), p. 305.
23. Friedman, Stanford B. and Sarles, Richard M., "Out-of-Control Behavior in Adolescents." In *Pediatric Clinics of North America,* Vol. 27. Philadelphia: W.B. Saunders Co., February 1980, pp. 97–107.
24. Hamburg, Beatrix A., "Early Adolescence: A Specific and Stressful Stage of the Life Cycle." In *Coping and Adaptation,* G. Coelho, D. Hamburg, and J. Adams, eds. New York: Basic Books, 1974, pp. 101–124.

25. Rohn, R. D. et al, "Adolescents Who Attempt Suicide." *Journal of Pediatrics* 90 (1977), pp. 636–638.
26. Scranton, T. and Downs, M., "Elementary and Secondary Learning Disability Programs in the U.S.: A Survey." *Journal of Learning Disabilities* 8 (1975), pp. 394–399.
27. Klein, Jerry R., "Update: Adolescent Gynecology." In *Pediatric Clinics of North America*, Vol. 27. Philadelphia: W.B. Saunders Co., February 1980, pp. 141–152.
28. Baldwin, Wendy and Cain, Virginia S., "The Children of Teenage Parents." *Family Planning Perspectives* 12 (January–February 1980), pp. 34–43.
29. Gross, Ruth T. and Duke, Paula M., "The Effect of Early Versus Late Physical Maturation on Adolescent Behavior." In *Pediatric Clinics of North America*, Vol. 27. Philadelphia: W. B. Saunders Co., February 1980, pp. 71–77.
30. Lindgren, G., "Peak Velocities in Height and Mental Performance: A Longitudinal Study of Schoolchildren Aged 10–14 Years." *Annals of Human Biology* 6 (1979), pp. 559–584.
31. Udry, J. Richard, Bauman, Karl E., and Morris, Naomi M., "Changes in Premarital Coital Experience of Recent Decade-of-Birth Cohorts of Urban American Women" *Journal of Marriage and the Family* 37 (November 1975), pp. 783–787.
32. Zelnick, M. and Kantner, J. F., "Sexual and Contraceptive Experience of Young Unmarried Women in the United States 1971 and 1976." *Family Planning Perspectives* 9 (March-April 1977), pp. 55–71.
33. Hite, Shere, *The Hite Report.* New York: Dell, 1976, p.457.
34. Nadelson, Carol C., Notman, Malkah T., and Gillon, Jean W., "Sexual Knowledge and Attitudes of Adolescents: Relationship to Contraceptive Use." *Obstetrics and Gynecology* 55 (March 1980), pp. 340–345.
35. Committee on Standards of Child Health Care, *Standards of Child Health Care*, 3rd ed. Evanston, Ill: American Academy of Pediatrics, 1977.
36. Williams, Christine L. Arnold, Charles B. and Wynder, Ernst L., "Primary Prevention of Chronic Disease Beginning in Childhood, The Know Your Body Program Design of Study." *Preventive Medicine* 6 (1977), pp. 344–357.

8 / Mental Health Risk Reduction for Children

Jules R. Bemporad, M.D. / William Beardslee, M.D. / Felton Earles, M.D.

It is often difficult to determine with any great validity what the true risk factors are for children in the area of psychological health. This lack of certainty results from the child being an underdeveloped organism with marked abilities for adaptation that can later compensate for early traumas or deprivations. Our concept of childhood is one of rapid change and development during which the individual displays flexibility and a capacity for reorganization. Causative factors are not linear in the sense that a certain experience at, say, age 2 will have a certain result at age 9, or that an acquired characteristic, good or ill, remains unchanged throughout ontogeny. Rather, the effects of experience at any stage are thought to be reworked and modified as the child goes through the developmental process. Normal growth is seen as a progression through stages in which accomplishment in each stage depends partially on the successful mastery of the developmental tasks of the previous stage and in turn prepares the individual for the following developmental stage. Therefore, the effects of any risk factor are complex and modified by a multiplicity of influences. Nevertheless, as will be discussed later, certain risk factors have been identified as having fairly lasting pathogenic effects if therapeutic, or at least compensatory, intervention is not offered. Before proceeding to a discussion of these factors, however, a general presentation of current opinion regarding the gauging of psychopathology in childhood, and even how childhood psychopathology may be conceptualized, appears warranted.

Diagnosis of psychological health or illness in childhood is often not an easy matter. The well-worn criteria that the clinician normally uses to assess psychopathology in adults are not suitable for usage with children. For example, subjective discomfort is commonly taken as an indication of severity in estimating the psychopathology of adults, but children become extremely distraught over nonpathogenic experiences while seeming to ignore what appear to be severe symptoms to an observer. Another frequently used criterion of adult pathology, the inability to function consistently in work or in relationships, cannot be used in assessing children who are normally prone to fluctuations of functioning and lability in most of their endeavors.

Further difficulties arise when we see children manifest symptoms as part of their coping with conflicts which arise from the developmental process itself. Such symptoms are not only considered "normal" but their absence may indicate problems in development. Among these "normal" symptoms could be listed the stranger anxiety of the infant, the transient fears of the preschooler, and the obsessions of the latency-age child. These manifestations of conflict diminish and disappear as the child masters the problems posed by his or her expanding awareness as well as the increasing demands of the environment.

These difficulties in assessment have caused a good deal of consternation among clinicians who must decide which symptoms merit intervention lest they cause problems in later life and which symptoms can be left to be resolved by the child as he or she continues to mature. One valuable approach to this whole problem of assessment has been proposed by Anna Freud and her co-workers in London. Basically, Freud suggests that any symptom merits serious consideration if it is blocking the normal development of the child. The severity of any manifest pathology is to be appreciated by how it impedes the expected developmental process. Anna Freud describes how play, freedom of fantasy life, school performance and stability of relationships, and social adaptiveness have all been proposed as the major parameter by which to gauge the mental health of children. Yet none of these successfully grasped the "vital aspects" of psychological health in the sense that the adult's ability to love and work were indications of absence of pathology. She concludes that there is only one factor in childhood whose impairment can be used as an accurate index of the absence of significant pathology and that is "the child's capacity to move forward in progressive steps until maturation, development in all areas of personality, and adaptation to the social community have been completed. Mental upsets can be taken as a matter of course so long as these vital processes are left intact"[1].

Therefore, according to this approach, risk factors would be those conditions that either impede the developmental process or cause it to become markedly deviant. Consequently, each developmental stage could be seen as having specific risks that are characteristic of the child's particular developmental tasks at that level, although some profound traumas, such as growing up with a severly disturbed parent, would retain their pathogenicity throughout development. While such a system of stage-related risk factors would be ideal in conceptualizing the possible problems that affect development, we still lack sufficient knowledge of the various developmental stages, the needs of the child at each stage and the abilities for later remediation to propose such a neat scheme with any confidence. At our current state of knowledge, such factors can be delineated only as arising from inborn, familial, or extrafamilial origins (as will be detailed in the next section). In addition, it may be added that any of these risk factors, if prolonged, give rise, either through psychological pain or the formation of pathological characteristics, to a further impediment to growth: the child's own personality. Thus, any risk factor, whether it be exposure to a chaotic family, the loss of a parent, or growing up in a poor neighborhood, eventually will express itself in the child carrying within himself or herself ideas, feelings, and expectations that eventually will produce either pathology or functioning that is much below potential in adult life. It is, in fact, in the effort to prevent this "internalization" of external difficulties that it is important to identify risk factors and to attempt to effect prompt remediation before they achieve permanence in the structure of the personality.

TYPES OF RISK FACTORS

Knowledge of factors that either cause or are associated with psychological disturbances in children has come from a variety of areas. The largest source of information has been simple clinical experience with children who had suffered some sort of trauma during development. One of the earliest studies of this type is Rene Spitz's[2] well-known work with infants who were separated from their mothers at 6 months of age. Spitz not only pointed out that these infants went through a depressive type of reaction but that later in life they were developmentally retarded. Later, other authors[3] noted that children who had suffered maternal separation or loss often became delinquent in adolescence. These studies relied largely on clinical observations and have been criticized as too subjective and lacking in experimental rigor.

In the past few decades, more systematic studies on risk factors have been attempted.

These have been epidemiological studies which sampled large numbers of children in order to determine the factors that were associated with psychological difficulties.

Other systematic studies were those which selectively chose "children at risk" and examined how such children were functioning at various stages of development. Children were defined as being "at risk" for various reasons: some had a severely disturbed parent while others were organically damaged, born prematurely, grew up in socially deprived settings, or went to inferior schools. These studies have shed much light on the causes of psychopathology in childhood and have also given rise to a whole new field of inquiry: the study of coping. This interest arose from the finding that some at-risk children did very well, contrary to expectations. This observation obviously drew the interest of investigators who wished to learn how these children were able to "cope" with adverse circumstances, so that their beneficial experience could be generalized to less-fortunate children. Although it is too early to make any definite statements about what allows certain children to overcome risk factors, some indications will be presented in the next section.

Before proceeding with a description of risk factors, it should be noted that it is rare to find only one factor acting alone. It is more common to find families in which risk factors are clustered and thus risk reduction is more difficult. For example, economic difficulties (risk factor one) often lead to marital discord (risk factor two) and to exposure to a pathogenic social setting (risk factor three) and so on. The appreciation of this accumulation of risk factors is important for, as Rutter[4] has shown, the effect of risk factors is not simply additive. Rutter's data from epidemiological studies on the Isle of Wight and in London identified six family variables, all of which were strongly associated with psychiatric disturbances in the child. These variables were (1) severe marital discord; (2) low social status; (3) overcrowding in the family unit; (4) parental criminality; (5) maternal psychiatric illness; and (6) admission of the child into care outside the home, for example, foster homes. Children who experienced only one of these risk factors seemed to be functioning as well as children who had none. However, children experiencing two of these risk factors were four times as likely to demonstrate pathology. With three factors, the likelihood of disturbance increased many-fold. Therefore, the presence of more than one risk factor strongly increases the odds of disturbance and should prompt particular attention from clinicians.

With this brief introduction, we will attempt to enumerate the types of risk factors and the conditions in which they have been implicated. These factors are also presented in Table 1 and for convenience have been organized into inborn, intrafamilial, and extrafamilial types.

TABLE 1.   Types of Risk Factors

I. Constitutional Risk
   A. Genetic
   B. Nongenetic

II. Intrafamilial Risk
   A. Mental status of parents
   B. Quality of parents' marriage
   C. Parent-child and sibling-sibling relationships

III. Extrafamilial Risk
   A. Quality of physical environment
   B. Quality of schooling
   C. Historical change (excessive life events)

INBORN GENETIC RISK

With an increasing degree of certainty, although still far from proven, genetic factors have been documented in the major psychoses, [5] autism,[6] some types of learning disabilities,[7] and personality disorders.[8] Traditionally, these studies were dependent on finding sufficient pairs of identical and nonidentical twins to calculate indexes of inheritability. The studies using the Denmark Psychiatric Register of Kety, Rosenthal, and Wender[9] represent the most convincing data that the schizophrenias are, in part, genetically determined, although even these data have been criticized[10] on the basis of overinclusive diagnostic criteria.

This approach is complemented by family and pedigree studies of families containing one or more persons with a defined psychiatric disorder.[11] Using methods of population genetics and quantitative biology, conceptual models have been developed to test genetic theories of causation,[12] although ultimate confirmation of the genetic origins of psychiatric disorders will depend on demonstrations at the neuronal and molecular levels of analysis.

The clinical relevance of this research is still far from clear. Considerable attention is being given to the identification of a physiological vulnerability or set of vulnerabilities to develop a psychosis among children at genetic risk.[13,14] The influence of environmental factors in an illness with such a long incubation period as schizophrenia or manic-depressive disorder greatly complicates simple extrapolations from genotype to phenotype. The most that can be said at this point is that the probability of having a psychotic disorder given one or two parents with a similar disorder ranges from about 10 to 40 percent.[9] Identification of children at risk for future disorder, based on behavioral or physiological grounds, is still an academic exercise, and will probably remain so for several years to come. The ultimate importance of this research, aside from demonstrating causative factors, will be to find strategies of creating a specific environment which can compensate and, perhaps, nullify the genetic predisposition to illness. It is hoped that the complexity and adaptability of the human nervous system can be utilized to overcome inborn predispositions in an optimal environment.

NONGENETIC, CONSTITUTIONAL RISK

A second category of risk factors is of nongenetic constitutional origin and has a much longer history of clinical relevance. This group of factors invariably involves some degree of known or inferred insult to the developing nervous system. In general, damage inflicted by any one of a variety of endogenous or exogenous insults are inversely related to age; the younger the organism, the more profound the damage. The range of insults includes chromosomal damage; neuronal and glial (cellular) damage incurred at times of differentiation, proliferation, and migration; and functional disorder of cell masses in the central nervous system (CNS).[15] For each type of damage, a different causal mechanism exists. For example, maternal malnutrition may contribute both anatomical and functional insults to the developing nervous system. Unfortunately, emphasis has been devoted primarily to the degree of intellectual impairment resulting from this category of risk factors.

Emotional factors are commonly thought to represent secondary phenomena when coexisting with intellectual retardation or learning disabilities. This trend reflects a bias generated by the existence of better standardized methods for measuring intelligence and by the social and administrative needs which result from a system of universal education. Nevertheless, the reverse might be true; emotional and motivational deficits may be primary, and intellectual factors (except as severe levels of retardation) may be secondary.

It has been argued that tempermental characteristics have a constitutional origin.[16] If this is true, the existence of certain temperamental traits observable in infancy (distractibility, regularity of biological rhythms, high intensity, and so on) may represent behavioral and emotional predispositions toward the development of psychiatric disorder.[17] As another example of a risk factor in this category, there is presumptive evidence that the coexistence of several minor physical anomalies in infants and young children asre associated with high activity levels in boys.[18] Clearly, early behavioral manifestations establish expectable parental responses which may in themselves produce distorted patterns of relationship ultimately giving rise to emotional, learning, and language problems. For example, Thomas, Chess, and Birch[16] have been able to delineate three temperament types which appear stable throughout development. They called these types the difficult child, the easy child, and the slow-to-warm-up child. These authors found that so-called difficult children were much more vulnerable to behavior disorders in later childhood. They also emphasize that the specific match between a child's basic temperament and parental style is a potent factor in a child's emotional development. As a result, parents should acknowledge and learn to accept (and optimally deal with) each child's specific temperament style.

INTRAFAMILIAL AND EXTRAFAMILIAL RISK

In child psychiatric research, most attention has been given to risk factors stemming from the psychosocial environment, and this is justifiably an area of emphasis, since it represents phenomena that are more amenable to change than constitutional factors. As reflected in Table 1, such risk factors may be conceptually grouped as either intrafamilial or extrafamilial.

Extensive reviews already exist documenting the potential impact that this variety of factors may have on children's emotional and intellectual development. Robins,[19] for example, found that disharmonious homes, sociopathic parents, and inconsistent discipline was associated with continuation of childhood delinquent behavior into adult life. Epidemiological studies conclude that the presence of mentally ill parents and marital strain appear to be the most closely linked to childhood psychiatric disorder.[4]

It is more difficult to draw casual inferences about the influences of extrafamilial factors. These types of psychosocial risk factors may also exert their influences differentially with age. As examples, the presence of marital discord may be more harmful to children of preschool age than older children, particularly with regard to the origins of conduct disorders;[20,21] societal, institutional, and cultural influences may have their maximal influence in early adolescence.[22] In addition, the geographic setting may exert an effect. For example, Lavik[23] found that low social class increased the rate of psychiatric disorder in Norwegian adolescents but that youngsters in Oslo were more affected than those living in rural areas. Finally, these complex combinations of risk factors can be observed from epidemiological studies of child abuse. Baldwin[24] found that low-income status (an environmental characteristic) increases the rate of abuse but that young parents, large family size, and psychiatric instability are also contributing factors. Others have found that children with difficult temperaments are more likely to be abused. Therefore, there is a combination of societal, familial, and individual characteristics which interact to create a severe risk factor for child abuse. It would be difficult, if not impossible, to separate each of these effects as particularly causative with any assurance.

CAUSATIVE MODELS OF RISK

Since it seldom, if ever, happens that a psychiatric disorder is caused by a single factor, the task of research becomes that of explaining how several different risk factors operate interdependently in producing outcomes of clinical importance. At the present level of methodological refinement, this is a complex pursuit; the accurate measurement of a single factor is often troublesome enough, let alone that of several factors. When it is recognized that concepts of risk must be placed within a developmental framework and that knowledge is ultimately a result of tracking children with established risk over time, the extensive labor necessary for such studies becomes apparent.

Models of causation commonly exist beyond the coping capacity of practical and ethically safe research designs and existing methods. These models range from simple interactional models to sophisticated double-threshold models originating from quantitative biology.[25] A problem in contemporary research is to coordinate the conceptual development of models with testable hypotheses, making use of presently available methods. Epidemiologic approaches are in the most strategic position to carry forth this mission, since valid and reliable data can be generated in sufficient scope from general populations to test causative and predictive models.

In the course of an epidemiologic study to determine the prevalence and causes of behavior problems in preschool children, Earls et al.[26] have developed and tested a parsimonious three-variable risk model composed of a temperamental characteristic, the parent's marital satisfaction, and the interaction of these two factors. The model is illustrated in Figure 1, which demonstrates that beyond a certain threshold on a continuum from satisfactory to unsatisfactory marriages, the added influence of a "difficult" temperament increases the probability of a behavior problem in the child.

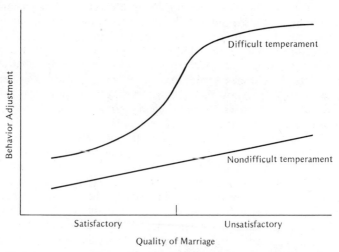

FIGURE 8-1.   **Two factor model illustrating the relationship of quality of marriage and temperament to behavior adjustment.**

The importance of placing risk factors in a developmental time framework has been emphasized by Sameroff,[27] and he uses the term *transaction* to represent the influence of multiple risk factors at different ages. Behavioral symptoms also need to be interpreted within a developmental framework; for example, enuresis in a 3-year-old carries quite a different clinical meaning from the same symptom in a 10-year-old. As well, invariant aspects of development, such as sex, must be represented in causal models. Although the sex ratio is more balanced in studies of preschool children[28] and during middle adolescence,[29] it is widely recognized that prior to puberty, boys are vastly overrepresented in clinical samples of emotionally and intellectually handicapped children.

Although complex models will eventually be required to help explain complex behavioral outcomes, given our present level of sophistication, the illustration in Figure 2 is helpful in clarifying interpretations regarding development of psychiatric disorder in the first few years of life. The period from birth to 3 years is called a phase of induction—a phase during which a physiological risk (e. g., prematurity) or an environmental one (e.g., a mentally ill mother) sets the stage for later difficulty. The period from 3 to 7 years is a phase of symptom formation. Behavior problems arising during this period may be validly observed, but the differentiation between those which are transient and those which are indicators of a persisting problem may be difficult to ascertain. Beyond the age of 7, the presence of behavioral symptoms should be more carefully considered to represent an established and, therefore, treatable disorder.

Two other related issues remain to be discussed: the efficacy of screening for risk factors and ethical considerations arising from what action should be taken once a constellation of risk factors has been identified. A principal strategy of epidemiologic research is the two-stage field survey in which a population is first screened for possible cases of a certain disorder; then those persons exhibiting positive tests are recalled for a more thorough diagnosis. In detecting asymptomatic or subclinical physical disorders, such as hypertension or tuberculosis, the purpose of screening is to apply a highly sensitive measure which guarantees that all possible cases will be detected without regard for the number of false-positive cases misidentified. In psychiatric studies, a different situation exists, primarily for ethical reasons. When screening for risk or presence of psychiatric illness, it is undesirable to misclassify persons as potential cases (false-positives) when they are normals. The ethical problem of identifying a normal child as potentially deviant, and then subjecting that child and family to a more intrusive examination, can greatly undermine the integrity and consequently, the importance of research. This is no easy matter to resolve. It first requires a clear hypothesis or body of evidence on the salience of the risk factor or factors being examined. Second, highly specific tests (those that carry a high probability of accurately identifying normals) are

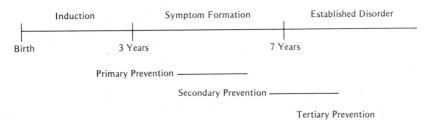

FIGURE 8-2.   Three phases in the genesis of common childhood psychiatric disorders.

needed. Third, the benefits that accompany identification of risk factors should be carefully described and supported by the research work. Often the benefits of such research are as difficult to define as the operation of risk factors.

This brief discussion should indicate how complex "risk" research is in the area of mental health. The reduction of risk factors, one critical strategy in the primary prevention of psychiatric disorder, does not necessarily depend on the final existence of scientific proof that factors X and Y are causally linked to outcome Z. As an example, the United States is currently witnessing an unexpected decline in mortality from cardiovascular disease at a time when scientific evidence on the influence of a host of risk factors in conflictual.[30] The fall in mortality rates may be linked to a reduction in one or more risk factors, such as removing saturated fats from the American diet, because it seemed practical and safe, but not because proof existed linking saturated fats or any other single factor to heart disease.

In the case of psychiatric illness, the combination of genetic counseling, good prenatal care, anticipatory guidance, particularly to parents of children with "difficult" temperaments, and stable caretaking environments might substantially reduce overall rates of disorder and actually eliminate some types of disorders. An important function of research, then, is the definition and description of the range of possibilities for prevention. It therefore rests on the ingenuity of teachers, therapists, architects, policy makers, and ordinary citizens to prevent psychiatric disorders.

COPING MECHANISMS: PROTECTIVE FACTORS IN CHILDREN AT RISK

Having acknowledged the complexity and the interaction of psychological risk factors, some further comments may be added about children who have coped with adverse environments in order to clarify protective factors. There is a paucity of literature on these protective factors and most of our current information derives from studies of children at risk, which found that, contrary to expectations, certain children were functioning well at the time of examination. However, encouraging as this finding may be, there is no absolute assurance that this sample will continue optimal functioning in adult life. In the studies reported to date, most of the children examined were preadolescent and were rated on four rather general parameters: relationships outside the family, relationships within the family, social and academic activities, and sense of self (or self-esteem). These four parameters do not define coping per se but are to be taken as outward evidence of some still undefinable inner resource that allows a child to overcome adverse situations.

Rutter[31] attempted to define some factors which facilitated coping as a result of his epidemiological studies. His group found that children with an adaptable temperament were less prone to be scapegoated by psychiatrically ill parents than were children with difficult temperaments, and thus were spared some of the abuse and insults ot the sense of self. Another possibly innate protective factor described by Rutter's group is high intelligence. This ability would allow the child to gain esteem from extrafamilial pursuits such as school work and preserve or consolidate a positive sense of self.

Environmental protective factors mentioned by Rutter center on the child being able to form a close relationship with a psychologically healthy unit. In some cases of families with parental psychopathology, this relationship was with the healthy parent, while in others the child related to someone outside the nuclear family. Wynne,[32] who has studied the children of schizophrenic parents, also noted the beneficial effects of a bond with a healthy parent. In another context, Cochran and Brassard[33] describe the importance of a family's social network on providing the child with opportunities for rewarding participation outside the family. Finally, Rutter found that parental supervision and structure appear to prevent the development of delinquency. Rutter and his co-workers[34] have also recently documented the major important effects that schools have on children's development, and their potentially harmful or protective effect.

Another researcher who has described protective factors in children at risk is E. J. Anthony,[35] whose work has focused on children raised by a psychotic parent. Anthony observed that the children who appeared to overcome this severe risk factor had resisted becoming engulfed in the parent's illness and developed an objective and somewhat detached view of the parental psychopathology. Anthony also mentioned that these children often received support from the nonpsychotic parent and at times exhibited special creative talents. He speculates that the creation of a detached attitude, while sparing the child from the psychotic contagion of the parent, may carry over into other relationships and to later restrictions on the self.

Kaufman et al.[36] have also reported on children of severly psychiatrically ill mothers and, like Anthony, have discovered a few children who are functioning quite normally. These "super kids," as Kaufamn and his associates call them, had close relationships outside the home and considerable creative talents (as also described by Anthony in his study). In addition, it was found that the "super kids" had an affectionate relationship with the mother who also provided intellectual stimulation despite her mental illness. Finally, Kaufman et al. stress the importance of close and satisfying peer relationships as a protective factor.

In summarizing this brief literature on children who managed to turn out well in highly stressful situations, certain recurrent themes become apparent. One is the history of a close relationship with a healthy adult or peer, either within or outside the family group. It may be speculated that this relationship allows the child to adopt a healthier model and also to gain a more realistic view of the world than is presented at home. However, this relationship may also give the child the needed response to form an adequate and positive sense of self. The second recurrent factor, that of exceptional creative talent or high intelligence, also allows the child to gain needed self-esteem and to secure gratification outside the pathogenic home environment.

These studies are extremely instructive since they show that every child needs to feel adequate, loved, and respected as an entity in himself or herself. Ultimately, these environmental responses create a healthy regard for self which the child carries into adult life and hopefully will provide protection from later pathology.

REFERENCES

1. Freud, A., *Normality and Pathology in Childhood*, New York: International Universities Press, 1965.
2. Spitz, R., "Anaclitic Depression." *Psychoanalytic Study of the Child* 2 (1946), pp. 313–342.
3. Bowlby, J., *Forty-four Juvenile Thieves*, London: N.P., 1946.
4. Rutter, M., et al, "Attainment and Adjustment in Two Geographical Areas. III. Some Factors Accounting for Area Differences." *British Journal of Psychiatry* 126 (1975), pp. 520–533.
5. Matthysee, S. and Kidd, K. K., "Estimating the Genetic Contribution to Schizophrenia." *American Journal of Psychiatry* 133 (1976), pp. 185–191.

6. Folstein, S. and Rutter, M., "Infantile Autism: A Genetic Study of 21 Twin Pairs." *Journal of Child Psychology and Psychiatry* 18 (1977), pp. 297–321.

7. Owen, F. W., "Dyslexia—Genetic Aspects." In *Dyslexia: An Appraisal of Current Knowledge*, A. L. Benton and D. Pearl, eds. London: Oxford University Press, 1978.

8. Cloninger, C. R. and Guze, S. B., "Psychiatric Illness in the Families of Female Criminals: A Study of 288 First Degree Relatives." *British Journal of Psychiatry* 122 (1973), pp. 697–703.

9. Kety, S. et al, "The Types and Prevalence of Mental Illness in the Biological and Adoptive Families of Adopted Schizophrenics." In *The Transmission of Schizophrenia*, D. Rosenthal and S. Kety, eds. Oxford: Pergamon Press, 1968.

10. Benjamin, L. S., "A Reconsideration of the Kety and Associates Study of Genetic Factors in the Transmission of Schizophrenia." *American Journal of Psychiatry* 133 (1976), pp. 1129–1133.

11. Winokur, G. et al., "The Iowa 500. II. A Blind Family History Comparison of Mania, Depression and Schizophrenia." *Archives of General Psychiatry* 27 (1972), pp. 462–464.

12. Reich, T., Cloninger, C. R., and Guze, S., "The Multifactorial Model of Disease Transmissions. 1. Description of the Model and Its Use in Psychiatry." *British Journal of Psychiatry* 127 (1975), pp. 1–10.

13. Fish, B., "Neurobiologic Antecedents of Schizophrenia in Children: Evidence for an Inherited, Congenital Neurointegrative Defect." *Archives of General Psychiatry* 34 (1977), pp. 1297–1306.

14. Venables, P., "Progress in Psychophysiology: Some Applications in a Field of Abnormal Psychology." In *Progress in Psychophysiology*, P. Venables and M. J. Christie, eds. New York: John Wiley, 1975.

15. Dobbing, J., "Vulnerable Periods in Developing Brain." In A. N. Davidson and J. Dobbing, eds. London: Blackwell, 1968.

16. Thomas, A., Chess, S., and Birch, H. G., *Temperament and Behavior Disorders in Children*. New York: New York University Press, 1969.

17. Sostek, A. M. and Anders, T. F., "Relationships Among the Brazelton Neonatal Scale, Bayley Infant Scales and Early Temperament." *Child Development* 48 (1977), pp. 320–323.

18. Waldrop, M. et al., "Newborn Minor Physical Anomalies Predict Short Attention Span, Peer Aggression, and Impulsivity at Age Three." *Science* 199 (1978), pp. 563–565.

19. Robins, L., "Sturdy Childhood Predictors of Adults' Antisocial Behavior: Replications from Longitudinal Studies." *Psychological Medicine* 8 (1978), pp. 611–622.

20. Wallerstein, J. S. and Kelly, J. B., "The Effects of Parental Divorce: Experiences of the Preschool Child." *Journal of the American Academy of Child Psychiatry* 14 (1975), pp. 600–616.

21. Wallerstein, J. S. and Kelly, J. B., "The Effects of Parental Divorce Experiences of the Child in Later Latency." *American Journal of Orthopsychiatry* 46:2 (1976) pp. 256–269.

22. Earls, F., "Social Reconstruction of Adolescence." *Perspectives in Biology and Medicine* 22 (1978), pp. 65–82.

23. Lavik, N., "Urban-Rural Differences in Rates of Disorder." In *Epidemiological Approaches in Child Psychiatry*, P. J. Graham, ed. New York: Academic Press, 1977.

24. Baldwin, J., "Child Abuse: Epidemiology and Prevention." In *Epidemiological Approaches in Child Psychiatry*, P. J. Graham, ed. New York: Academic Press, 1977.

25. Reich, T., James, J. W., and Morris, C. A., "The Use of Multiple Thresholds in Determining the Mode of Transmission of Semi-Continuous Traits." *Annals of Human Genetics* 29 (1965), pp. 51–71.

26. Earls, F., "Epidemiological Child Psychiatry: An American Perspective." In *Psychopathology of Children and Youth*: A Cross-Cultural Perspective, E. Purcell, ed. New York: forthcoming. Josiah Macy, Jr., Foundation, pp. 3–27.

27. Sameroff, A. J. and Chandler, M. J., "Reproductive Risk and the Continuum of Caretaking Casualty." In *Review of Child Development Research*. F. Horowitz, M. Hetherington, and S. Scarr-Salapatek, eds. Chicago: University of Chicago Press, 1975.
28. Earls, F., "The Prevalence of Behavior Problems in Three-Year Old Children: A Cross-National Replication." *Archives of General Psychiatry* 37 (1980), pp. 1153–1157.
29. Graham, P. and Rutter, M., "Psychiatric Disorder in the Young Adolescent: A Follow-up Study." *Proceedings of the Royal Society of Medicine* 66 (1973) pp. 1226–1229.
30. Garraway, W. M. et al., "The Declining Incidence of Stroke." *New Engalnd Journal of Medicine* 300 (1979), pp. 449–452.
31. Rutter, M., "Invulnerability, Or Why Some Children Are Not Damaged" In *New Directions in Children's Mental Health*. C. J. Shamsie, ed. New York: Spectrum, 1979.
32. Wynne, L. C., "Risk-Reducing Factors in Schizophrenia." *Psychiatric Opinion* 16:2 (1977).
33. Cochran, M. M. and Brassard, J. A., "Child Development and Personal Social Networks." *Child Development* 50 (1979), pp. 601–616.
34. Rutter, M., Maughan, B., Mortimore, P., and Ouston, J., *Fifteen Thousand Hours, Secondary Schools and Their Impact on Children*, Cambridge: Harvard University Press, 1979.
35. Anthony, E. J., "Thy Syndrome of the Psychologically Invulnerable Child." In *The Child in His Family, Children at Risk*, E. J. Anthony and C. Kospernik, eds. New York: John Wiley, 1974.
36. Kaufman, C., Grunebaum, H., Cohler, B. and Gamer, E., "Superkids: Competent Children of Psychotic Mothers." *American Journal of Psychiatry* 136 (1979).

9 / Promoting Mental Health and Reducing Risk for Mental Illness

Paul C. Mohl, M.D.

The first thing that must be said about mental health promotion is that it is extremely difficult. Reviews of the field have generally been very pessimistic.[1-3] The reason for this is that two of the major risk factors for mental illness, coping deficits and environmental stress, are extremely difficult to change, and a third, genetic loading, is impossible to alter. Mental health professionals were not always so pessimistic. In the 1940s and 1950s there was hope that psychoanalytic insights and techniques would help everyone to cope more effectively, to achieve greater life satisfaction, and to raise a new nonneurotic generation. But it was psychoanalysis which ultimately taught us that coping patterns, once established in childhood, take years of hard work to alter. In the early 1960s there was hope that mental health consultation would result in early case detection, more therapeutic social systems, and effective psychotherapy delivered widely by supervised paraprofessionals. However, in the 1970s community mental health centers have become overwhelmed by the need for outpatient maintenance of chronic psychiatric patients. In the late 1960s and early 1970s various encounter group interventions were proposed as vehicles for promoting mental health. Much of the flurry of activity (marriage encounter, marathons, Esalen-type retreats) is now seen as so much narcissistic self-indulgence.[4] Given this history, one must be cautious in evaluating the current darling of mental health promotion: stress management.

These movements were not total failures. Psychoanalysis remains fundamental to all psychotherapy. Community consultation gave us crisis intervention, still a central element in preventive psychiatry. Encounter groups gave us a permanent appreciation of the importance of social support in modulating stress. Also, group therapy has become an essential psychiatric treatment. Thus, it is likely that the relaxation techniques used in current stress management programs will have an enduring place in mental health promotion.

THE MENTAL ILLNESSES AND THEIR RISK FACTORS

When considering risk factors, it must be remembered that we are speaking of conditions that range from mild transient situational disturbances to chronic schizophrenia, a lifelong disabling condition. Recently, an entirely new diagnostic schema has been published by the American Psychiatric Association.[5] It includes in the range to 200 separate psychiatric disorders. For our purposes we may consider *five broad categories of mental illnesses and their risk factors.*

The organic mental disorders involve actual physiologic lesions of the brain causing intellectual and cognitive impairment. The economic cost is high in both lost productivity and cost of care. The risk factors are the same as for physical illness of other organ systems and are generally unaffected by the interventions described in this chapter. The schizophrenic disorders are chronic, recurrent psychoses involving delusions, hallucinations, paranoid ideation, and other bizarre disturbances of thinking and perception. They usually result in severe incapacity in work and social life. Thus, the cost is extremely high in lost productivity. It has been estimated that schizophrenia accounts for 100 million hospital days annually in the United States and an economic cost of $20 billion.[6] The risk factors are a matter of controversy with strong evidence implicating genetic and biochemical factors, solid evidence for early infant learning, and some evidence for sociological effects. Life stress commonly precipitates an acute psychotic decompensation.

The major affective disorders involve severe disturbances of mood, depression or euphoria, sometimes of psychotic proportions including delusions, hallucinations, suicide attempts, and grandiose behavior. The economic cost is moderate since most of these patients are productive members of society between episodes of the disease. On the other hand, these patients are nearly totally unproductive, frequently requiring hospitalization during an acute episode. Risk factors include clear genetic vulnerability, early childhood losses, and acute environmental stress (commonly a loss of some sort).

The treatment and prevention of *the major psychoses* (schizophrenia and major affective disorders) will probably always be the responsibility of psychiatrists since medication, hospitalization, and long-term follow-ups are required. Recent preliminary research suggests that biochemical and family screening may be useful but extensive further work is necessary.[7,8] The important role for hospital and community health administrators, and for prevention-minded family physicians and nurses is in early identification and referral of these patients.

The fourth major category of mental illness is *the substance use disorders*. Most patients who abuse alcohol or illicit drugs also have some other mental illness which expresses itself in the form of substance abuse. Additional risk factors include cultural background, possible genetic components, social disintegration, and stress. The economic cost is incalculable, especially if one considers the medical care required for the sequelae of substance abuse (liver disease, heart disease, hypertension, and so on) and the cost of criminal behavior associated with drugs and alcohol. The social cost of substance abuse is also devastating, with family disintegration and financial ruin common. The prevention of substance abuse generally lies in the reduction of the risks of other mental disorders. Once substance abuse occurs, treatment requires a comprehensive, expensive, usually medically based program. However, early recognition and referral can markedly reduce the social and economic costs.

The final category of mental disorders is also the most common: *disorders of adaptation* which include anxiety, impulse, transient adjustment, personality, psychosexual, somatoform, dissociative, and minor affective disorders. Studies have indicated that the prevalence of psychiatric symptoms in the general population is 25 per cent.[9] Most are disorders of adaptation in which a wide variety of chronic, sometimes mild, symptoms (headache, depression, obsessions, anxiety, irritability, hypochondriacal concerns, unexplained physical complaints, maladaptive behavior patterns, unusual sexual practices, and so forth) result from a failure to cope with stresses of day-to-day living. The cost is measured in failure to achieve full potential productivity, not in hospital costs. But there is recent evidence that there is increased susceptibility to physical illnesses in these individuals.[10,11] The risk factors are coping deficits, which generally exist from early childhood, and environmental demands and stresses. *It is this category of mental illness to which the average, apparently healthy person is most susceptible and toward which risk-reducing interventions should be directed.*

The interventions currently available, which are both economically feasible and effective are, crisis intervention, stress management, group support, and mental health consultation. Prior experience has shown that educational campaigns directed to altering coping mechanisms are ineffective. Also, more research is necessary before bio-chemical screening or genetic counseling could become viable interventions.

MENTAL HEALTH CONSULTATION

This intervention is very simple in description but complex in action. A trained profes-sional, usually a psychologist or psychiatrist, is made available to an organization for a few scheduled hours each week. How such an individual may be used is highly variable, ranging from didactic training programs to group and individual support. It seems that a major use of such consultation would be to aid in early identification and referral. By presenting problem situations to the consultant, troubled individuals who might never seek help or who might deteriorate substantially before receiving assistance may be identified and referred. A second use of such consultation would be in identifying the stressful elements and alternatives in trouble spots. A third use is in supervising individuals to whom others go, seeking counsel, thus maximizing their helpfulness.

Suppose one were looking at a large organization (community or company) and had a mental health professional available 5 hours each week. How should one use him or her? There are several possibilities, High-stress areas will generally send up some kind of "noise." This may take the form of higher rates of crime in one area of town, a sense of political ferment in other areas, or high job turnover or absenteeism in partic-ular sections of a business. The consultant should be available to such areas. If there are more areas than there is consultant time, it must be remembered that steady con-sistent impact in selected areas is more effective than diluted involvement in many areas. There are also certain areas which send up little "noise" but which are, nonethe-less, at high risk for mental illness. These include various programs which rehabilitate people who have suffered in some way: sheltered workshops, job retraining programs, orphanages, and so on. If these kinds of programs do not meet the psychological needs of their participants the risks are very high. Brief consultation can be very effective.

Once having identified the areas involved, with whom should the consultant consult? There are several principles. It must be someone who has direct contact with the target population; it must be someone who has the power to change some things; it must be someone who wants to help. If the consultant is perceived as an emissary from the authorities to catch errors, the consultation will be a waste of time. Thus, the presenta-tion and introduction of the consultant is crucial. Specific individuals to consider offering consultation to include judges, policemen, shop stewards, supervisors, person-nel officers, project and program managers, teachers, guidance counselors, ministers, community organizers, and general physicians.

An example of the kind of impact that consultants may have is in the legal system. Judges, district attorney, and police officers have a difficult time distinguishing crim-inal behavior from acting out (in which maladaptive behavior is used to express internal conflicts). The legal system generally has only two responses to misbehavior: do nothing or punish. Mental health consultation can help create other options (such as refer to the emergency room) and sort out the most appropriate one. Police are often called upon to intervene in family problems which are not criminal (drunkenness, quarrels, and so on). Their response may affect the future course of the family toward more disintegration or towards more stability. These are simple examples of the way a mental health consultant may be used. Further information is available in the writings of Gerald Caplan[12,13] who first developed programs in community consultation.

CRISIS INTERVENTION

This chapter distinguishes between stress, which tends to be chronic, insidious, and covert, and crises, which are acute, temporary, and usually obvious. A crisis is generally defined as a major transitional moment in a person's life. Thus, it is more restricted than stress. During a crisis, and individual's usual coping mechanisms are overwhelmed. Normally unconscious material is available to awareness, and interpersonal relationships are in flux. The outcome of the crisis may be personal growth, regression, or increasing rigidity of prior coping patterns. It is a high risk–high gain situation. Skilled rapid intervention may prevent later mental illness and may result in the development of better coping skills. The stimuli to crisis situations may be expectable, major life events (births, deaths, marriage, job change), or unexpected catastrophes (natural disasters, economic reverses, war, and others).

One central element in crisis intervention is availability and accessability. Crises are brief, lasting minutes to hours, only occasionally lasting more than a few days. During that brief time the outcome is highly unpredictable, ranging from suicide to damaging life decisions (quitting a job, divorce, impulsive moves) to reintegration to significant personal growth. Thus, an effective crisis intervention program must be established so that it is easily available with minimum complexity for the person in crisis to negotiate. The three most common programs have been: placement of psychiatrists in emergency rooms (an uncommon practice before the 1960s), crisis and suicide hotlines, and 24-hour walk-in clinics. Adequate publicity is necessary to ensure accessibility. A walk-in clinic of which the community is unaware will not be very effective. Extensive advertising and community support are important.

Another element in accessibility is the perception of the resource by the target population. Commonly, the target population of these programs is a group which ordinarily avoids seeking professional counseling. Thus, great efforts are sometimes made to dissociate the programs from usual medical or other establishment institutions. Individuals who would never dream of seeing a psychiatrist might be willing to seek help at a "Family Problem Center," "Human Growth Center," or "Free Clinic." One of the problems of these programs is that with all of the publicity they receive they have become points of contact for seriously disturbed, sometimes chronic psychiatric patients. Thus, despite the nonestablishment presentation, thorough backup, training, and consultation by skilled mental health professionals is essential. More detailed organizational descriptions of some of the most successful crisis intervention programs, including the original Los Angeles Suicide Prevention Center, are available in McGee's admirable summary.[14]

The effective elements in crisis intervention are as difficult to define as for any psychotherapy. Nonetheless, we shall try. The four elements seem to be support, ventilation, advice, and interpretation. The central aspect of support is the personal contact. One of the worst aspects of a crisis is the loneliness of it. Crises commonly involve real, threatened, symbolic, or fantasized loss. Thus, crises are often acute grieving processes. The importance of replacing the acute loss with personal contact is a widely acknowledged human need. A new sense of hope is engendered and the person's natural healing processes are mobilized. Alcoholics Anonymous makes particularly good use of this element, providing each member with a partner who is on-call 24 hours a day to be with the individual feeling an overpowering urge to drink.

Once contact and support are offered, ventilation of feelings should be encouraged. Persons in crisis are usually experiencing several intense, often conflicting feelings.

These feelings are often not viewed as acceptable nor socially appropriate (e.g., rage at a loved one). The feelings most commonly experienced are: rage, terror, and sadness. It is very important to give permission to experience and express these feelings. The ventilation of these emotions often allows discharge of the pent-up tension, thus relieving the acuteness of the crisis, allowing the individual to approach the situation more reflectively and rationally. Direct advice on the crisis is rarely indicated or effective in crisis intervention; however, information about resources available to the person, advice to avoid major life decisions while in acute emotional turmoil, and information about the grieving or crisis resolution process are all helpful. Persons in crisis often need to have the obvious suggested (e. g., "talk to a lawyer"). Also, advice such as "allow yourself to experience and work through your anger" can help patients resist their natural inclination to suppress painful feelings.

Interpretation is simply clarification for the patient of the feelings and conflicts he or she is experiencing. Labeling feelings accurately can, by itself, give a sense of understanding and mastery to the person in crisis. Once the issues are clarified, courses of action and choices are frequently clearer. Effective interpretation, however, is extremely difficult requiring a good basic grounding in psychotherapeutics and extensive supervised experience in listening. This is another reason why crisis intervention programs require heavy involvement of trained professionals. The price of an ill-timed or insensitive interpretation can be high.

A little-employed aspect of crisis intervention, but one with great potential, is the model used in the first well-publicized effort at crisis intervention. I refer here to the Coconut Grove Fire in Boston in 1942. A substantial number of psychiatrists were mobilized and moved to a large group of individuals in crisis.[15,16] They intervened with the acutely traumatized individuals and their families, including emergency room interviews, hospital unit follow-up, and home visits. They found that by assisting the grieving process in bereaved family members psychiatric symptoms were markedly reduced 1 year later. They also found that adaptation problems in traumatized individuals were reduced. The Israeli military has employed this model of handling combat neuroses and debriefing after particularly traumatic battle situations.

GROUP SUPPORT

Support groups serve two functions in reducing risk for mental illness. There is a substantial body of data suggesting that social support modulates the noxious effects of stress.[17] Second, the move from small tightly knit communities to large, poorly organized living groups is a substantial stress in itself and, thus, a risk factor for mental illness. In the extreme, social deterioration and dislocation are considered major etiologic factors in many mental illnesses.[18] To put it bluntly, the way we live causes mental illness. Most people, even though they are aware of the risks of our mobile, disorganized life-styles, would not prefer to revert to tightly knit social units which are often rather restrictive. Thus, a variety of artificial social support systems have been used to fill the void.

The groups may be organized in a variety of ways. They may be task-oriented or support-oriented. They may be time-limited or open-ended. They may have open memberships or closed memberships. There are many other dimensions upon which groups may be defined. For our purposes we may consider four major types of groups: postillness, work environment, retreats, and life circumstance groups.

Postillness groups, while very specialized, are particularly important in mental health promotion. Illness represents a major life crisis. Chronic illness becomes a chronic stress. The individual's and family's coping capacities are frequently stretched to the limit. These groups provide a focus for socialization at a time when patients and family members are inclined to become withdrawn and isolated. They provide support at a time when persons commonly feel embarassed and ashamed. They provide advice and information for dealing with the illness. Sometimes the groups define themselves frankly as offering support for afflicted patients and families. In other instances this aspect is more covert and the overt agenda is some other task (fund-raising, politicking, and so on) related to the disease. Time-limited support and educational groups have also been offered to patients prior to discharge from the hospital.[19] The most famous of these groups is Alcoholics Anonymous (Al Anon for family members). Others include ostomy groups (for people who have had colostomies or iliostomies), cancer groups ("I Can Cope," "Make Today Count"), arthritis groups, and mental retardation groups (for parents coping with afflicted children). Information on these groups is available through the national organizations concerned with the particular disease.

Work environment groups attempt to build support and cohesion within the work group while reducing and resolving conflict. This reduces work-related stresses, improves job satisfaction, and increases productivity. These groups may be crisis-related, meeting only as needed, or ongoing, meeting regularly to deal with a chronically stressful task. They usually focus on fostering open communication and expression of feelings so that conflicts and stresses may be identified and dealt with. This is very threatening at first and, thus, these groups should usually be conducted by a trained outsider. They have been used effectively in many work settings including hospitals,[20] the military,[21] and business.[22] As with mental health consultation, the target settings can be identified by the "noise" produced in response to the stress and conflict. One of the most difficult tasks is enlisting the interest of the target population. Sometimes, presenting these activities as training programs eases the acceptance problem. It is best to use a total outsider with no responsibilities to anyone within the organization in order to gain the trust of the target population. The outside group facilitator should have no job other than to help the particular work unity deal better with its stresses. A community health agency might consider having a list of mental health professionals interested in this kind of work available to businesses and other local institutions. This would function exactly as does the agency's list of available consultants. This type of intervention can be very effective for business and employees but will likely not be spontaneously considered by them.

Retreat groups usually are intense, time-limited experiences with open memberships. A group of individuals, usually strangers, leave their usual environment to spend a weekend or a week in an isoloated area together. Most of the time is spent in intense emotional interaction under the leadership of a trained professional. The stated object is growth: personal, spiritual, or marital. The model for these groups is the Esalen Institute, Big Sur, California. These groups are commonly organized by churches around a spiritual theme. They have also been used to support marital growth (marriage enrichment). They are also used as training exercises for future psychotherapists. Regardless of the stated agenda, these groups have in common the goal of promoting honest interaction between people. Most participants report the experience to be rejuvenating and enriching, A renewed sense of social bonding is found. There have also been a few reports of serious negative effects for some people from the intense encounters,[23] which makes the presence of a trained professional very important.

The life circumstance groups are similar to the postillness groups. The common bond, however, is some shared, stressful situation. These groups are organized around the recognized need for support in coping with certain difficult problems. The regular weekly or monthly meetings frequently have programs on a wide variety of topics, but the avowed purpose is the creation of a support system for those who ordinarily have none. Among the high-risk groups which have been successfully supported are senior citizens (American Association of Retired Persons), single parents (Solo Parents, Parents Without Partners), the obese (Take Off Pounds Sensibly, Weight Watchers), and women (consciousness-raising groups).

STRESS MANAGEMENT

This is the newest intervention of mental health promotion. Among the most exciting developments in medicine recently has been the growing evidence that implicates stress in the etiology of many mental and physical illnesses. Paralleling this has been a new knowledge on the ability of humans to control their own physiology. This came at a time when there was growing realization that learned coping mechanisms and environmental stresses are extremely difficult to change. The result was an attempt to teach people to control their physiological responses to stress: stress management.

The notion that stress is related to disease is an old one, dating back to the Greeks, but its modern incarnation began in the 1930s when Hans Selye[24] began exploring some of the implications of Walter Cannon's fight or flight formulation of automatic nervous system activity. What, Selye wondered, would happen if fight and flight from a threatening stimulus were blocked? His experiments led to the formulation of a general adaptation syndrome, composed of discrete stages, involving specific prolonged physiological responses, and resulting in exhaustion and death. His notion of stress was a state of chronic physiological arousal resulting from the presentation of a noxious stimulus under circumstances in which the usual fight or flight response was not possible.

Our understanding of the nature of stress and its physiology has become more complex in the intervening years, but the basic hypothesis that chronic noxious environments produce behavioral effects and physiological changes which, if sustained, lead to tissue damage, has been repeatedly confirmed. A high incidence of life changes (positive or negative) has been correlated with virtually every mental or physical illness (including accidental injury);[25] bereavement has been associated with increased mortality;[26] hard-driving, competitive behavior has been correlated with heart disease;[27] chronic subclinical depression has been associated with cancer;[28] repression of emotions has been associated with hypertension;[29] to mention a few. Thus, the effects of stress go far beyond the increased risk of mental illness. One of the most disturbing aspects of these otherwise exciting discoveries is the pervasiveness of the kind of stress and behavior linked to illnesses. It is extremely difficult to achieve success in our society without being mobile, competitive, and perspicacious with one's emotions. Major life changes, including significant loss, are universal. In short, our entire life-style is hazardous to our health.

In the late 1960s it was established that physiological responses could be consciously controlled. This led to the virtual explosion of biofeedback techniques, exciting research in meditation, and renewed interest in hypnosis. In the mid-1970s Herbert Benson[30] proposed that there is a physiologically distinct relaxation response. Relaxation had, until then, always been defined as an absence of arousal (Cannon's fight/flight response). Benson reasoned that, if one could train individuals to produce the relaxation response (slowed heart rate and respiration, decreased blood pressure, reduced adrenal output, increased electroencephalogram alpha waves) rather than the arousal response, the noxious effects of stress might be alleviated without making major life-style, environmental, or personality alterations. This idea remains an incompletely confirmed hypothesis although it has formed the basis for using a variety of stress management techniques in and out of the medical setting. Stress management programs outside of traditional settings have proliferated as did encounter group programs in the late 1960s.

Shortly after Benson's work, Pelletier[31] expanded upon these ideas and provided the outlines of current stress management programs. They usually have as their core a specific technique for evoking the relaxation response. Pelletier describes the techniques of autogenic training, Jacobson relaxation, transcendental meditation, and a form of yoga. To these may be added biofeedback training and training in autohypnosis. Common to all of these techniques is the instruction by a benevolent authority figure, a period of guided practice in a secure, quiet, peaceful location, and the requirement for extensive, continuing daily practice.

Practitioners of these techniques often report dramatic subjective experiences: changes in self-perception, improved ability to handle stressful situations, and inner feelings of serenity and peace (being at one with the universe). Research has demonstrated significant physiologic changes during the practice of these techniques in most people and sustained physiologic changes in some. Despite the probability that there is a faddish element to these programs, there is a high likelihood that there will be enduring value to these techniques as a part of risk reduction in mental illness. Stress management programs are also particularly efficient. The techniques can be taught in fairly large groups in a relatively few number of sessions (three to ten), and the practice time requirement is about 15 to 20 minutes two or three times daily. This is the kind of program that can be offered relatively inexpensively to a large number of people without requiring that they "seek help."

When organizing a stress management program there are generally two major goals: information on stress and its effects, and training in particular techniques for modulating the physiologic responses. Most people are not aware of the many forms stress takes nor of the severe sequelae. Neither do they understand its pervasiveness nor its constant demands on their coping mechanisms. Usually some didactic presentations are important in achieving this goal. Didactic presentations are not enough, however, and homework assignments involving greater attention to one's own life stresses are helpful. An important aspect of this is the sharing of these discoveries in a group setting. This helps the individual learn to use group support in dealing with stress. The group discussion also dispels the individual's fear that only he or she struggles with stresses, that other people cope smoothly and comfortably. The learning of the specific techniques involves periods of instruction and practice followed by group discussions of the difficulties involved. In order to provide adequate practice between sessions, they should be spaced weekly or biweekly. Each session should be 1 to 2 hours long. The sessions are best conducted in a small group of 10 to 12 persons, however, a large group may be used if there are sufficient personnel available to lead smaller discussion groups. In the latter case, the small discussion groups should have consistent membership and leadership. The program should be conducted in a comfortable, somewhat secluded area. Large auditoriums or bare, noisy meeting areas generally are not conducive to learning contemplative relaxation techniques. Audiovisual aids are generally not useful except for audiotapes which may be helpful in instruction in Jacobson relaxation or self-hypnosis techniques. Followup reinforcement meetings one month, three months, and 6 months after completion of the basic program may increase the utilization of the techniques learned. The followup sessions can be used as open-ended discussions to see who has continued using the techniques, who has not, and how successful they have been.

A basic stress management program will include education about stress, stress awareness exercises, one relaxation technique (progressive muscle relaxation, self-hypnosis, meditation, autogenics, biofeedback, or guided imagery), and one active coping technique (refuting irrational ideas, thought stopping, assertiveness training, time management, or coping skills reinforcement). All of these techniques are clearly described in a new handbook of stress management techniques which can be used as an instruction manual.[32] Below is a sample ten session stress management program:

Session 1: Didactic presentation on stress, its relationship to illness and life changes, followed by discussion group on the stresses.
> Homework: complete Life Change questionnaire and maintain daily stress diary.

Session 2: Discussion of participant's life changes and daily stresses followed by didactic presentation on bodily signs of stress.
> Homework: maintain diary of events and bodily sensations.

Session 3: Discussion of bodily sensation diaries followed by instruction and practice in relaxation technique.
> Homework: twice daily practice of relaxation technique.

Session 4: Discussion of effect and difficulties with relaxation technique—further instruction.
> Homework: continued practice.

Session 5: Brief discussion of effects and difficulties with relaxation. Initital presentation of active coping technique.
> Homework: continued relaxation technique practice, diary of coping used.

Session 6: Small group discussion of and instruction in coping technique.
> Homework: continued practice of both techniques.

Session 7, 8, 9: Discussion of use of coping technique, obstacles, successes, failures, further instruction.
> Homework: continued practice of both techniques.

Session 10: Review and reinforcement of information and techniques, suggestions for additional resources if wanted, arrangements for follow-up.

Evaluation of such a program is best accomplished by using any of the short stress symptom checklists available. They are best administered before session 1, at session 10, and on two later occasions. A more sophisticated evaluation program might use a control group and follow-up of performance, medical, and personnel records.

ADDITIONAL SAMPLE PROGRAMS

The community mental health movement began in the early 1960s and resulted in a wide proliferation of mental health centers and programs. Thus, it would be impossible to review all risk-reduction programs. Further, almost all are really partprograms. That is, I have found no report of any program which attempted to apply a wide variety of interventions to an entire institution or community. In most cases either a particular intervention or a particular target group was selected and intensive effort applied in that direction. Insofar as many different programs exist in any community, this seems to be the result of independent actions, not the result of careful needs assessment and planning. Many of these partprograms are described in the three major journals of this area: *Hospital and Community Psychiatry, Journal of Community Psychology*, and the *Community Mental Health Journal*. Readers who wish to become familiar with the wide variety of programs available may review these periodicals. Articles on needs assessment and identifying target populations are also published in them.

There are or have been, however, several programs worth considering in some detail. The first is the Haight-Ashbury Free Clinic, founded by David E. Smith, M.D. Here there was an identifiable population, at high risk for a variety of problems, unlikely to make use of medical care through the usual medical channels. The population was, of course, the "flower children" of the 1960s. The stresses were social dislocation, isolation, unstable interpersonal relations, extensive drug use, promiscuous sexual practices, and impoverishment. Smith established a storefront clinic in the Haight-Ashbury section where all the activity was occurring. He established an unmedical clinic. The physicians, nurses, and carefully trained paraprofessionals appeared, for all the world, like flower children themselves. Anyone was welcome, for any reason; no questions asked; no records kept; no names even required. The resource was advertised in the underground newspapers, on the street, and at rock concerts. The Free Clinic became a place where people on bad trips could be taken, where people who were lonely or depressed could come, where people with no place to go could feel secure. It participated in establishing overdose treatment tents at some of the concerts. Smith also did his political homework with the established powers in San Francisco. Despite early anxieties, they were, in the long run, pleased to have a responsible institution dealing with the problem.[33]

The Haight-Ashbury Free Clinic had a definable population area and task before it. A very different problem presented itself to health planners in San Antonio when they wanted to establish programs for the aged. Among the goals were the reduction of interpersonal isolation, malnutrition, and cognitive understimulation, all risks for depression and organic mental disorders in the elderly. The problem was identifying the elderly dispersed throughout a city of a million in neighborhoods which tended to be self-contained and resistant to extensive boundary crossings. Another problem involved the existence of small neighborhood and private programs distant from sources of support, anxious to expand their programs, yet resistant to outside influence.

Two governmental organizations, the City Department of Human Resources and the Alamo Area Council of Governments, evolved into kinds of crossroads for information and support. They made contact with the existing organizations and assisted the development of new ones, funneling information, assisting grant applications, providing contacts and program development advice. These two agencies also maintained contact with appropriate federal agencies and with the governor's commission on aging, keeping abreast of resource and new programming developments. The result has been the blossoming of three kinds of programs countywide but on a neighborhood-by-neighborhood basis. Twenty-five to 30 congregate feeding sites have been established throughout the city along with a citywide Meals-on-Wheels program. These sites are operated by neighborhood organizations which have used the situation to develop adjunctive socialization programs. El Centro del Barrio has attempted to foster relationships between members which will extend beyond the nutrition center so that the older people may assist each other. Project Free is especially proud of its multiracial, multiethnic, and multilingual programming.

More directly aimed at socialization are the programs of the San Antonio Chapters of the American Association of Retired Persons (AARP). There are 21 chapters scattered across the city; each meets monthly, usually in a local church, providing a variety of entertainment, socialization, and educational programs. Most chapters also organize a socialization network, maintaining daily telephone and occasional personal contact with those unable to initiate such on their own. The AARP collaborates with the Retired Teachers Association and with San Antonio College to maintain the San Antonio Institute of Lifetime Learning, Inc. A recent catalog listed no fewer than 77 separate classes lasting 8 to 16 weeks for the fall semester. The classes ranged from painting to Spanish to health to dancing to literature to estate management, and others.

The Boston State Hospital faced a still different kind of situation when it was handed Dorchester as its catchment area for community activities.[34] It faced a manifestly disorganized community, divided against itself along racial lines, suspicious of outsiders, yet without any clear definition of needs. Their first activity was to recruit and train a few members of the community who were then sent out to canvass the felt needs of the neighborhood by means of interviews. The almost universal concern with their children's education led to the formation of a comprehensive school consultation program and an after-school cultural enrichment program. Observations from these activities led to the identification of particularly disrupted families which were referred to a newly established family treatment center. Trained members of the community were highly visible in these endeavors. Later, as the nature of the community became better known to the psychiatrists, four high-risk groups were identified: unwed mothers, biracial marriages, alcohol abusers, and teenage and young-adult misdemeanor offenders. Therapy and educational groups were set up for the first two populations. A comprehensive alcohol treatment program was established. A collaborative program with judges and probation officers was developed in which a training school was used for young convicts not yet committed to a criminal life-style. Until then, the only recourse was prison.

Liaison psychiatry is not ordinarily thought of as part of the preventive psychiatry field, yet James Strain, who developed the most extensive program in the country, clearly defines it in terms of Caplan's concepts.[35] Liaison psychiatry programs may serve as useful models of risk reduction in areas such as hospitals, businesses, and health maintenance organizations. The foregoing examples have come from programs looking at large communities. A hospital is a large institution composed of patients, who are usually in crisis, and caretakers who are under chronic stress. Strain has advocated the "island of excellence" model for developing a systemwide program. Thus, the liaison psychiatrist would select a single area (most often determined by the receptivity of the area) and design a comprehensive series of interventions for it. In a coronary care unit this might include relaxation training for patients, crisis intervention for nurses and family members, an educational group for patients and spouses, and didactic work with physicians. On an oncology unit the program would be somewhat different: support groups for everyone, training the nurses in the teaching of stress management ot the patients, and routine consultation to the physicians. Some liaison psychiatry programs have not pursued the "island of excellence" model but have seized on one particular kind of intervention, offering it hospital-wide. In one hospital, weekly support groups for nurses have been widely offered. At other places, stress management programs have been made available to all staff and patients. These are frequently presented as inservice training programs in order to obviate any resistance to the programs due to labeling oneself or one's unit as "needing support."

GOALS FOR THE FUTURE

By now my own ideas about an ideal mental illness risk reduction program have probably come through: persons in acute stress need crisis intervention, persons under chronic stress need group support and stress management techniques, persons under intermittent stress (almost everyone) need stress management, and persons and institutions which create and/or respond to stress need mental health consultation. I am aware of no community nor institution which has attempted to establish such a comprehensive program, much less reported on it. A further goal for the future is solid evaluative research, especially on the true efficacy of stress management programs. More work with mobile crisis intervention teams should also be attempted. Events such as fires, accidents, murders, plant closings, or other major community upheavals represent serious crises in people's lives.

There appear to be fadlike cycles in the targeting of individuals for mental health promotion. In the last twenty years the focus has shifted from the suicidal to the disadvantaged, to women, to the elderly. Perhaps the next focus will be on the chronically ill. An interesting program might consist of support groups for *all* who suffer from chronic illness (diabetes, congestive heart failure, stroke, etc.) with initial contacts developed in hospitals and physicians' offices.

Perhaps the most important goal for the future is better basic research on the risk factors themselves. Stress is a very elusive concept, which defies definition. Further, one man's stress is another man's pleasure. Research has also shown that positive life · changes may be as toxic as negative ones. Selye has attempted to deal with this dilemma by distinguishing eustress from distress. Careful research on what stresses are toxic for which people would greatly assist in· defining high-risk populations and high-risk situations.

CONCLUSIONS

This chapter has reviewed the known risk factors in mental illness, the available techniques for risk reduction, and a few specific programs in the area. It has not included detailed reviews of needs assessment techniques, nor means for identifying high-risk populations. These have been implied in the examples offered and the interventions discussed. Several chapters in the *American Handbook of Psychiatry* provide useful information on the detailed organizational issues involved in a variety of settings.[36,37,38] The reader is also referred to the community mental health journals which publish many articles in these areas. A variety of state and federal agencies publish compendia of various programs, as well.

We return, however, to our original observation that mental health promotion is very difficult. The risk factors have not yet been defined sufficiently to allow the development of highly specific programs such as smoking prevention or exercise in heart disease risk reduction. Further, insofar as some risk factors are known, they are extremely difficult or expensive to change. What can be done at this point is to modulate the impact of stresses and crises thus preventing them from interacting with preexisting genetic or developmental vulnerabilities to produce overt, incapacitating symptomatology.

REFERENCES

1. Zusman, J. "Primary Prevention." In *Comprehensive Textbook of Psychiatry*, Vol. 2, 2nd Ed. A. M. Freedman, H. I. Kaplan, and B. J. Sadock, eds. Baltimore: Williams and Wilkins Co., 1975, pp. 2326–2332.
2. Davis, J. A., *Education for Positive Mental Health: A Review of Existing Research and Recommendations for Future Studies.* Chicago: Aldine Publishing Co., 1965.
3. Panzetta, A. F., *Community Mental Health: Myth and Reality.* Philadelphia: Lea & Febiger, 1971.
4. Lasch, C., *The Culture of Narcissism*, New York: W. W. Norton, 1979.
5. *Diagnostic and Statistical Manual of Mental Disorders*, 3rd ed. Washington, D.C.: American Psychiatric Association, 1980.
6. Eisenberg, L. and Parron, D., "Strategies for the Prevention of Mental Disorders," In *Healthy People: Background Papers for the Surgeon General's Report on Health Promotion and Disease Prevention.* Washington, D.C.: U.S. Department of Health, Education, and Welfare, 1979.
7. Buchsbaum, M. S., Coursey, R. D., and Murphy, D. L., "The Biochemical High Risk Paradigm: Behavioral and Familial Correlates of Low Platelet Monamine Oxidase Acitvity. *Science* 194 (1976), pp. 339–341.
8. Erlenmeyer-Kimling, L., "Genetic Approaches to the Study of Schizophrenia." *Birth Defects* 14 (May 1978), pp. 59–74.
9. Srole, L., Langner, T. S., Opler, M. L., and Rennie, T. A. C., *Mental Health in the Metropolis.* New York: McGraw-Hill, 1962.
10. Vaillant, G. E., "The Natural History of Male Psychological Health: IV. What Kinds of Men Do Not Get Psychosomatic Illnesses." In *Psychosomatic Medicine* 40 (October 1978), pp. 420–436.
11. Betz, B. J. and Thomas, C. B., "Individual Temperament as a Predictor of Health or Premature Disease." *John Hopkins Medical Journal* 144 (March 1979), pp. 81–89.
12. Caplan, G., *Principles of Preventive Psychiatry.* New York: Basic Books, 1964.
13. Caplan, G., *The Theory and Practice of Mental Health Consultation.* New York: Basic Books, 1968.
14. McGee, R. K., *Crisis Intervention in the Community.* Baltimore: University Park Press, 1974.
15. Cobb, S. and Lindemann, E., "Neuropsychiatric Observations After the Coconut Grove Fire." *Annals of Surgery* 117 (1943), p. 814.
16. Lindemann, E., "Symptomatology and Management of Acute Grief." *American Journal of Psychiatry* 101 (January 1944), p. 141.
17. Cobb, S., "Social Support as a Moderator of Life Stress." *American Journal of Psychosomatic Medicine* 38 (September 1976), pp. 300–314.
18. Fromm, E., *The Anatomy of Destructiveness* New York: Holt, Rinehart and Winston, 1973.
19. Rahe, R. H., Ward, H. W., and Hayes, V., "Brief Group Therapy in Myocardial Infarction Rehabilitation: Three to Four Year Follow-Up of a Controlled Trial." *Psychosomatic Medicine* 41 (May 1979), pp. 229–242.
20. Mohl, P. C., "Group Process Interpretations in Liaison Psychiatry Nurse Groups." *General Hospital Psychiatry* 2 (July 1980), pp. 104–111.
21. Glass, A. J., "Military Psychiatry and Changing Systems of Mental Health Care." *Journal of Psychiatric Research* 8 (1971), p. 299.
22. McLean, A., "Occupational (Industrial) Psychiatry." In *Comprehensive Textbook of Psychiatry*, Vol 2, 2nd Ed. Freedman, A. M., Kaplan, H. I., and Sadock, B. J., eds. Baltimore: Williams & Wilkins Co., 1975, pp. 2368–2375.
23. Lieberman, M. A., Yalom, I. D., and Miles, M. B., *Encounter Groups: First Facts.* New York: Basic Books, 1973.

24. Selye, H., *Stress in Health and Disease*. Boston: Butterworth, 1976.
25. Gunderson, E. K. E. and Rahe, R. H., eds., *Life Stress and Illness*. Springfield, Ill.: Charles Thomas, 1974.
26. Jacobs, S. and Ostfeld, A., "An Epidemiological Review of the Mortality of Bereavement." *Psychosomatic Medicine* 39 (September 1977), pp. 344–357.
27. Friedman, M. and Rosenman, R. H., "Association of Specific Overt Behavior Pattern with Blood and Cardiovascular Findings." *Journal of the American Medical Association* 169 (1959), pp. 1286–1296.
28. Bahnson, C. B., "Second Conference on the Psychophysiological Aspects of Cancer." *Annals of the New York Academy of Science* 164 (1969), pp. 307–634.
29. Weiner, H., Singer, M. T., and Reiser, M. F., "Cardiovascular Responses and Their Psychological Correlates." *Psychosomatic Medicine* 24 (1962), pp. 447–498.
30. Benson, H. *The Relaxation Response*. New York: Morrow, 1975.
31. Pelletier, K. R., *Mind as Healer, Mind as Stayer: A Holistic Approach to Preventing Stress Disorders*. New York: Delacorte Press, 1977.
32. Davis, M., Eschelman, E. R., McKay, M., *The Relaxation and Stress Reduction Workbook*. Richmond, Calif.: New Harbinger Publications, 1980.
33. Smith, D. E., and Luce, J., *Love Needs Care: A History of San Francisco's Haight-Ashbury Free Clinic and Its Pioneer Role in Treating Drug Abuse Problems*. Boston Little, Brown, 1971.
34. Becker, A., Wylan, L., and McCourt, D., "Primary Prevention—Whose Responsibility?" *American Journal of Psychiatry* 128 (1971), pp. 412–417.
35. Strain, J. J. and Grossman, S., *Psychological Care of the Medically Ill*. New York: Appleton-Century-Crofts, 1975.
36. Cohen, Raquel, R., "Community Organizational Aspects of Establishing and Maintaining a Local Program." In *American Handbook of Psychiatry*, Vol. 2, 2nd Ed., G. Caplan (Vol. 2 ed.) S. Arieti, ed. New York: Basic Books, 1974, pp. 649–661.
37. Brickman, R., "Organization of a Community Mental Health Program in a Metropolis." In *American Handbook of Psychiatry*, Vol. 2, 2nd ed. G. Caplan, (Vol. 2 ed.) S. Arieti, ed. New York, Basic Books, 1974, pp. 662–672.
38. Dillon, J. "Community Mental Health in a Rural Region." In G. Caplan (Vol. 2 ed.) *American Handbook of Psychiatry*, Vol. 2, 2nd ed., S. Arieti, ed. New York, Basic Books, 1974, pp. 673–685.

10 / Stress Reduction for Business and Industrial Employees

R. G. Troxler, M.D. / Tommie G. Cayton, Ph.D.

The decision on whether or not to embark on a stress management program for business and industrial employees is not an easy one to make. One must first consider the advantages and the disadvantages. The costs in employee time away from the job, in hiring specially trained personnel (or contracting for the training), and the effort involved in convincing top management to accept stress-reduction programs are definite disadvantages.

There is, however, a growing awareness among the leaders of business and industry of the potential benefits of a stress management program. Cooper and Marshall have pointed out that the organizational symptoms of job stress are low productivity, absenteeism, and high staff turnovers.[1]

In 1979 Rosch reported in the *Journal of the American Medical Association* that "stress related conditions are responsible for 10 to 20 billion dollars annually in loss of industrial productivity."[2] Jere Yates, in the American Management Association's publication on managing stress, feels that the productivity losses are closer to $60 billion.[3] It would appear that, in loss of productivity alone, generally the advantages outweigh the disadvantages.

The question remains as to whether or not an individual company should institute a stress management program. The standard medical approach to determining if a disease (job stress) is present is to check for the pattern of symptoms (effects of job stress) specific for that disease. Besides low productivity, absenteeism, and high turnovers, Cooper and Marshall[1] have stated that the effects of job stress also include poor physical health such as increased pulse rate, high blood pressure, high cholesterol levels, smoking, ulcers, and cardiovascular disease and poor mental health such as low motivation, lowered self-esteem, job dissatisfaction, job-related tension and escapist drinking.

Industrial health care workers concerned about job stress should survey the health records of company employees and determine if the prevalence of the effects of job stress are higher in their particular company than in the general business community. If the rate is higher, it would seem prudent to consider a stress management program.

Levi points out that alcohol abuse, a symptom of job stress, is one of the biggest social and medical problems of the world.[4] Alcohol abuse plays a major role in traffic accidents, leads to bad relations with supervisors and fellow workers, results in decreased productivity and an increase in absenteeism. The causation is multifactorial but job stress and family stress play important roles.

This interaction complicates any study on the relationship between job stress and disease. But on the other hand, it increases the opportunity for the industrial health care worker to develop a program with the potential to help the worker with stress both inside and outside of the work situation.

Since the effects of job stress are elevations of risk factors associated with heart disease and mental disease, the potential benefits of a successful stress management program may be useful in the prevention of two of the most common maladies of our society. Finally, the data derived from such programs may ultimately lead to the essential causes of job stress.

DEFINITION OF STRESS

Although the ultimate definition of job stress is yet to be determined, many facts about stressful conditions on the job are commonly mentioned by investigators in the field. The following is a list of some of the major factors said to cause psychological stress among white-collar workers as summarized by Cooper and Marshall.[5] (See Table 1.) At first glance items 11 to 18 in Table 1 seem to fall under the general category of poor interpersonal relations, items 19 to 21 are job specific, but items 1 to 10 seem to be filled with antitheses.

McLean has reviewed the literature on job stress[6] and cites reports that, while the stress of work overload is associated with increases in both cholesterol level and heart rate, the correlations between perceived occupational stressors and disease and the risk of disease is curvilinear or U-shaped. McLean resolves this relationship by explaining that those who are bored or understimulated and those who feel highly pressured represent the two ends of the continuum, each with a significantly elevated risk of disease. This so-called curvilinear relationship must be considered in any comprehensive definition of job stress and in any program designed to manage job stress.

In McLean's view, whether or not a worker will feel stressed depends upon two factors: the external environment and the particular vulnerability of the individual at that particular time. Of the two, McLean considers the vulnerability of the individual the more important factor. Only a stress management program utilizing the combined talents of industrial medicine, psychology, and management could hope to deal with both the job environment and the particular vulnerability of the individual.

TABLE 1.   Factors Which Cause Job Stress

1. Time pressures and deadlines
2. Boredom
3. Exorbitant work demands
4. Role ambiguity
5. Underpromotion
6. Overpromotion
7. Thwarted ambitions
8. Success
9. Information overload
10. Lack of participation in management of the organization
11. Responsibility for people
12. Territorial boundaries
13. Role conflict
14. Poor relationships with peers, subordinates, and boss
15. Threats from below
16. Bureaucratic pettiness
17. Pressures toward conformity
18. Lack of responsiveness
19. Lack of job security
20. Physical working conditions
21. Job design and technical problems

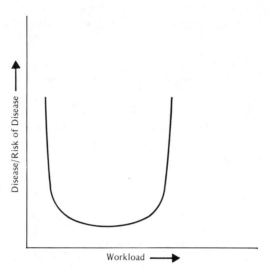

FIGURE 10-1.   Relationship of stress to workload.

Blue-Collar Stress

E. C. Poulton[7] discussed the factors which cause job stress in blue-collar workers. He lists insufficient light, too much light, and flickering light as job stress factors. Noise can interfere with work by masking auditory feedback cues coming from the equipment one is using and by distracting one's attention from one's work. But noise can enhance one's ability to work by causing behavioral arousal which can improve one's ability to concentrate. Music can decrease the stress of boring and routine jobs.

Vibration interferes with work by blurring vision and interfering with delicate movements, but vertical vibration at 5 Hz helps to keep people alert. Heat is an extremely dangerous stress. If the core temperature of the body reaches $40°C$ ($104°F$) heat stroke or heat collapse often occurs. But the initial effect of a hot working environment is behavioral arousal which can increase productivity. As we examine the effect of these job factors on the blue-collar worker we can see the wisdom of McLean's statement that stress results from the interaction of the person with the work environment, but the list of blue-collar stress factors again points out antitheses such as too much light and too little light. Some of this discrepancy can be attributed to subjective interpretation, but there is a special relationship between stress or arousal and performance.

Numerous studies over the years have shown that the relationship between stress and performance is also curvilinear but[8] in an inverted U. This relationship shows that our performance is best when moderate demands (stress) are placed upon us. Too little or too much stress will diminish performance.

It can be concluded from this relationship that any blue-collar stress factor which causes behavioral arousal (stress) has the potential to be either beneficial or harmful depending upon it's intensity and the worker's subjective interpretation. It is clear from the inverted U stress performance curve that the aim of any stress management program must not be to simply reduce stress, but to optimize stress.

White-Collar Stress

One unique problem facing white-collar workers is that they must be able to work with other people. More than half of the job stress factors listed in Table 1 involve or potentially involve interpersonal relationships. Blue-collar workers can be highly competent in a technical skill, be deficient in their interpersonal relationships, and still be productive for their organizations. White-collar workers seldom reach their full potential without skill in interpersonal relationships. A major effect of job stress in white-collar workers is a poor relationship with superiors, subordinates, and colleagues. Poor interpersonal relationships can lead to mistrust of one's working group, high role ambiguity, inadequate communications, and psychological stress due to low job satisfaction and feelings of job-related threat to one's well being.[9] The effects of poor interpersonal relationships limit the white-collar worker's opportunity for promotion.

Research in the field of job stress has repeatedly shown that one of the essential causes of job stress (especially in white-collar workers) is a lack of fit between the worker and the job environment.[10] The white-collar worker's first attempt at a good fit begins upon selection of a major course of study when he or she enters college. The corporation attempts to enhance the fit by the job interview and selection of the individual for a particular position with the company. In the past, standard management practice was to assume that the new employee could adapt his or her needs to the needs of the company.

According to R. Van Harrison[10] a job is stressful to the extent that it does not meet the needs of the individual and to the extent that the demands of the job exceed the ability of the individual to meet those demands. Both of these components of job stress are indicative of a poor person-job-environment fit (P-E fit). A poor P-E fit leads to job dissatisfaction, anxiety, complaints of insomnia and restlessness, high blood pressure, hypercholesterolemia, excessive smoking, and overeating.[10]

A good P-E fit enhances the worker's feelings of competence, efficacy, and self-worth. Continuously enhanced and increased feelings of self-worth contribute to the individual's total personality growth. It would seem cost effective for corporations to give more attention to P-E fit in order to decrease job dissatisfaction, anxiety, high blood pressure, hypercholesterolemia, and the risk of cardiovascular and mental disease in their work force. Sales has shown that enjoyment of a task is associated with lower levels of serum cholesterol in experimental subjects and that job satisfaction of work groups is correlated with lower rates of coronary artery disease.[11] This is one clear-cut example of how management can interact and aid the psychologist and the physician in the prevention of cardiovascular disease.

Likert, in his studies on productivity in business and industry, cites evidence that in professional workers there is a positive relationship between job satisfaction and performance.[12] Welford[13] discusses the "inverted-U" hypothesis of stress and performance. He explains this relationship by the hypothesis that job stress increases one's awareness of problems within one's environment which must be dealt with in order to be successful. As stress increases, the ability to distinguish between problems which must be solved to be successful and the minor problems which have no relation to one's success is diminished.

Weirman[14] studied the relationship between the incidence of disease/risk and stress experienced in the workplace. He found the same curvilinear U-shaped relationship between stress and disease/risk as was noted by McLean. A higher incidence of disease and risk of disease was found at both high and low stress ranges but was lowest with

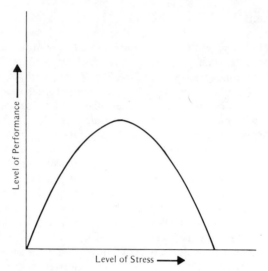

FIGURE 10-2. **Relationship between stress and performance.**

moderate stress. These relationships lead to the conclusion that some stress is beneficial not only to productivity, but also to one's health. It is important that a stress management program teach individuals to recognize the symptoms of job stress so that the employees may readjust their workloads in order to maintain maximum performance and health. Table 2 lists the warning signals that job stress is becoming excessive.[15]

In the late 1950s a particular behavior pattern was found to be common in patients with coronary artery disease.[16] This behavior pattern was described as enhanced hostility, ambitiousness, and competitiveness, and preoccupation with deadlines and with work. "Caught or placing themselves in a chronic struggle to reach an ever-expanding number of goals in the shortest period of time and/or against opposing environmental forces . . . ."[16] This behavior pattern was labeled *Type A* by Friedman and Rosenman and the absence of these symptoms as *Type B*.

The Type A person incessantly strives to accomplish too much or participate in too many events in the amount of time he or she allots for these purposes.[17] We have found that persons exhibiting Type A behavior characteristics experience more job stress than Type B's. A panel of biomedical and behavioral scientists commissioned by the National Heart, Lung, and Blood Institute has critically reviewed the association of

TABLE 2. **Warning Signals of Excessive Job Stress**

Overreacting to small irritations
Developing nervous habits
Gulping meals and smoking more
Feeling suspicious and distrustful of others without good reason
Getting no satisfaction from daily joys of life
Feeling trapped and doubtful of personal ability
Feeling chronically tired without good reason

Type A behavior and heart disease.[18] They concluded that Type A behavior is associated with an increased risk of heart disease in employed, middle-aged, U.S. citizens. "This risk is greater than that imposed by age, elevated blood pressure, and serum cholesterol and smoking..."

The Type A individual does not seem to be aware of the early symptoms of job stress and as a result questionnaires designed to detect job stress may be inaccurate in Type A individuals. This implies that job stress survey questionnaires will miss Type A individuals, and since the Type A individual is less aware of the symptoms of job stress, he or she will be less inclined to initiate action designed to diminish job stress.

Studies on occupational correlations with Type A behavior indicate that Type A individuals tend to have higher occupational status, faster career development, and work for companies with a more rapid growth rate. Thus, the Type A individual is not only less apt to attempt to cope with his or her stress but more prone to view attempts to modify Type A behavior as threatening to job status and current income. Indeed the work ethic of Western civilization encourages and rewards Type A behavior.

However, the short-term gains achieved for the company which rewards Type A behavior by the Type A individual may be overshadowed by the company's long-term loss. Coronary heart disease is one of the most prevalent forms of preretirement death in modern organizations.[19] Individuals responsible for the health of company employees should seriously consider job stress optimization as the cornerstone of any overall risk-reduction program. The relationships between stress and productivity indicate that stress optimization programs need not compromise worker productivity or company profits.

Reasonable goals of a stress optimization program are increased health of workers, increased worker productivity, increased job satisfaction, and decreased job turnover. These endpoints should be monitored carefully in any stress optimization program in order to convince Type A managers of the efficacy of the program for themselves and for others.

THE ESSENTIAL ELEMENTS OF A STRESS OPTIMIZATION PROGRAM

The most important element in planning any stress optimization program is the ability to demonstrate objectively measurable success. Increased health of workers can be demonstrated by medical examinations showing decreased measurable risk factors for coronary artery disease. Increased worker productivity can be measured by the management team. Finally, decreased job dissatisfaction can be implied from the results of job stress surveys by the psychologists and the surveys verified by a decreased labor turnover rate. The chief administrator's first concern in any organization is return on investment. Top management is interested in the health of the workers and in their job satisfaction, but they are even more interested in decreased labor turnover and increased productivity.

Once top management has agreed to support a stress optimization program, they should demonstrate their support by becoming actual participants in the program. Their personal participation will also help them assess the results of the data gathered at the end of the test phase of the program by the medical, management, and psychological surveys.

It is important that the chief administrator and the stress optimization program director agree on a reasonable time interval in which to test the program; otherwise it may be prematurely dismissed as ineffective. The time interval must include time to set up the program, time to gather base-line data, as well as a medical management, and psychological survey at the end of the test phase to assess the effectiveness of the program.

The entire medical department of the organization must agree to participate in the stress optimization program. There will be a natural resistance from the medical staff to any change in health care procedures. The assignment of a new medical assistant to the staff to help survey employees' health records for stress-related symptoms and diseases and to record base-line and test data will enable the medical staff to handle the increased work load generated by the stress optimization program. Assuming that the medical staff is dedicated to increased health of the workers, their acceptance or rejection of such a stress optimization program should be based upon the staff's ability to handle the increase in work load. If the support of the new program by the medical staff is not enthusiastic, the stress optimization program is doomed to failure.

The decision as to whether the medical, management, or psychological team should lead the stress optimization program should not be an arbitrary one. According to Warshaw[20] the medical department is in a unique position to lead the stress optimization program. "The routine medical examinations performed by the occupational physician provide excellent opportunities for the identification of unusual susceptibility to stress and the early detection of emotional difficulties" (p. 70). Reactions of the patients heart rate and blood pressure to the stress of the examination, the diagnosis, and the medical history of prior stress-related illnesses, as well as the measurements of serum cholesterol and uric acid are readily accessible to the industrial physician during a routine physical examination. An enormous amount of stress-related base-line data can be collected by the medical department without arousing the undue concern of employees. Once signs of stress or stress-related illnesses are detected in a worker; an orderly, voluntary system could be developed to utilize a job stress survey to survey the stress in the individual's work group. When stress or stress-related illnesses occur in an unusual frequency in certain departments or groups concomitant with a fall in productivity, the help of management is essential.

Basic Steps of Program

The following are the basic steps to setting up a stress optimization program once it has been approved by top management and the medical and management groups have agreed to work together in the program.

Notification of All Participants in the Program of the Absolute Confidentiality and Privacy of All Data: To quote Warshaw, "The confidentiality of all personal information acquired in the course of any program for dealing with work-related stress must be strictly and scrupulously maintained" (p. 37).[20] Anything less will destroy the program. Once company employees lose confidence in the ability of the medical staff to maintain confidentiality, they will conceal from the medical department any data they feel could embarrass them or affect their promotion status or job security. The code of ethical conduct for physicians providing occupational medical services adopted by the Board of Directors of the American Occupational Medical Association in 1976 states that confidential information should be released only when required by law or by overriding public health considerations. Medical counselors must consider employees first and employers second. Employers are entitled to information about the medical fitness of the individual in relation to work, but not to specific diagnoses or details of a specific nature (p. 40). [20]

The Mandatory Participation of All Employees in the Basic Stress Screening Battery: Some base-line data relating to stress should be recorded on all employees of the company. The tests that are required as a minimum are heart rate, blood pressure, height, weight, age, any family or past or present history of stress-related illnesses, and serum cholesterol and uric acid. These tests can usually be determined as part of a routine physical. (Additional tests which potentially indicate stress are ECG, serum cortisol, and serum catacholamines.) This mandatory screening and minimum data collection on all employees are required to determine the level of stress versus productivity of employees within sections or branches compared to other sections or branches within the company.

Participants Must Be Told That Their Involvement in the Stress Optimization Program Is Purely Voluntary: The base-line data on the stress/productivity that is gathered on initial screening should be made available to all employees. The various stress optimization programs should be explained to the employees and offered on a purely optional basis. Volunteers for the program will be more enthusiastic and desirous of change than nonvolunteers, and thus offer a better return on the time that the company invests in them to optimize their stress.

Time Commitment by Participants in Stress Optimization Program: Those who can benefit the most from a stress optimization program are typically very busy individuals. These individuals should be made to understand that part of the stress optimization program is learning how to use one's time more efficiently. If these busy individuals do not understand this, they will not volunteer for the program on the pretext that they are "too busy."

Once the base-line screening data indicate that an employee has a poor stress/productivity ratio, and the employee volunteers for the program, the employee should be given a series of written psychological tests. Tests for assertiveness, job satisfaction, and Type A behavior* can ensure that the stress optimization program will meet the individual needs of the program participants.

It is essential that the participants understand that their volunteer commitment to the program requires periodic rescreening. The intrepretation of the date derived from the rescreening should be made available to the participants as soon as possible to encourage their continued participation.

The medical staff must understand the need for immediate follow-up of rescreening data. The data should be analyzed for significant changes in the individual participants. If possible these changes should be analyzed in relation to the productivity of the individual. It is known that temporary job stressors such as tax deadlines are associated with elevations in serum cholesterol.[21] The serum cholesterol typically returns to its original level once the deadline has been met. Rescreening on a 1 to 2-month basis, resources permitting, will usually detect such trends. It is essential that the stress optimization team separate these temporary trends from the long-term effects of the stress optimization program. These temporary trends can best be differentiated from long-term effects of the program by analyzing the data by departments within the company. One would expect temporary organizational stressors within the department to correspond to an increase in the average levels of that group.

*Several Type A behavior tests are available. The most accepted is the Jenkins Activity Survey.

T-Group Discussions: Individuals who have particular difficulties responding to the classroom instruction given to the participants in the stress optimization program may benefit from the T-group technique. The members of the group must be carefully selected. Program participants having similar problems can meet with a knowledgeable, nonjudgmental group leader. The objectives of the T-group should be to discuss effective and noneffective coping techniques used to combat job stress. It is best to ask one individual employee who is particularly skilled at coping with job stress to sit in as an unofficial member of the group. It is important that this volunteer also be skilled in nonjudgmental group discussion.

Identification of Support Groups: If both the T-group discussion and the classroom lectures by the psychologist fail to help the employee cope with job stress, the employee's support group should be surveyed as a source of potential stress. Personality conflicts on the job or severe marital discord at home can thwart the best stress optimization program. Individuals who experience severe stress from their support groups may benefit from a referral to a private clinical psychologist.

CLASSROOM INSTRUCTION ON STRESS MANAGEMENT

The first author has given more than 150 lecture-workshops to military and civilian executives on the management of job stress. The main themes of the lectures are time management, effective delegation, and building self-esteem. These themes are ideally suited to the disciplines of management and psychology. The first author suggests that the classroom instruction on stress management should represent the shared efforts of the management and psychology members of the stress optimization team. The following points are excerpts from the lecture series which could be presented by the management team.

Time Management

The most important aspect of time management is to make a list of the things to be done during the day. The list should be prioritized by what will happen if the items are not accomplished. The length of the list should be realistic so that sufficient time is allotted to accomplish each item well. Concentrate on completing one item at a time before beginning another, study each item in depth, and avoid partial decisions. Without feeling guilty, take advantage of all work breaks which have been previously agreed upon. Get away from the work area at lunch time. Discuss other things besides business at lunch and while on coffee breaks. Find a hobby, during your off-duty hours, that demands your total concentration. While engaged in this hobby, resist any and all thoughts about work that may come to mind. Carefully plan off-duty hours to include some daily time with your spouse and children. Make sure that the daily time you allot to your family is long enough to listen to their problems, to help them find solutions, and to congratulate them on their accomplishments. If family time is neglected, small family problems will become bigger, family stress will increase, and ultimately job performance will suffer. Finally, vacation planning should not be rigid. A vacation schedule that demands that you be in a certain city on a certain day, see a previously agreed upon number of tourist attractions, and engage in a previously set number of hours of physical activity is not a vacation. It is not relaxing to follow a tight schedule.

Prerequisites to Effective Delegation

Workers under stress are often heard saying "only I can handle it" and "it's easier and faster to do it myself, than to teach someone else." Not only is their delegation ineffective, but they allow their subordinates to delegate to them. For those with the power to delegate, the question is "Why don't they delegate more of their work to others?"

There are prerequisites to effective delegation which improve our ability to delegate. We must have realistic goals clearly in mind before we can ask others to help us with them. We must realize that if we tend to be extremely critical of ourselves, we tend to treat our subordinates the same way. This causes them to be less cooperative when we attempt to delegate tasks to them. If we assume that our subordinates are going to do a poor job on a task we have given them, they will usually fulfill our expectations of them. Instead we should expect the best from others if they have sufficient time to do a good job. We should try to keep our sense of humor when things go wrong. The ability to laugh at one's mistakes lowers personal stress and prevents one from becoming angry. Angry people not only do not delegate effectively, but they also cause subordinates to conceal mistakes. We must learn to accept our limitations so that we know when to ask for help and learn the limitations of our subordinates so that we will know who to ask to help us. If we are quick to give negative feedback when a mistake is made, we must be equally quick with positive feedback when a subordinate has done a good job. Try to structure subordinates' jobs so that they will realize that their accomplishments contribute to the overall goals of the organization. Talk to the lowest ranking people in the organization periodically. Find out how they feel about how to improve the organization. If their concepts are totally different from your own, you have communication problems and, as a result, delegation problems. The higher anyone goes in an organization, the more aware he or she must be of communication with subordinates. Executives who exhibit Type A behavior are often poor listeners. Of the four communication skills—reading, writing, speaking, and listening—listening is most important to high-ranking executives because they cannot hire anyone to listen for them. Effective listening is essential in order to understand what particular difficulties our subordinates are having with the tasks we have delegated to them. (Effective listening also aids in making correct decisions.) Finally, we must make sure that our orders to our subordinates are clear and concise and that they understand what is expected of them.

The Relationship Between Work and Self-Esteem

For most workers, especially white collar, their job is a key factor in their self-image or self-esteem. The greater one's confidence or self-esteem, the better one is able to handle stress. In order to ensure that our job has a positive effect on our self-esteem, we must choose our jobs with great care with respect to our natural talents, abilities, and personal expectations of ourselves. Expecting too much too soon increases our job stress. Job goals should be specific, measurable, and attainable with a reasonable amount of effort. Acquire as much knowledge about your job as possible. Learn how to set goals for your subordinates that are mutually beneficial. When someone agrees to help you achieve a goal, make sure they get as much out of the accomplishment of the goal as you do. Try to enjoy helping others in your group succeed and give them positive feedback on their successes. Sincere positive feedback is the key to self-esteem. Mutually beneficial goals increase the likelihood of positive feedback and thus increased self-esteem.

The greater one's self-esteem, the more willing one is to take a risk. No great success in business is achieved without some degree of risk. Success builds self-esteem and thus one's tolerance for more risk. Groups which set mutually beneficial goals share both their successes and failures. Shared failure diminishes the detrimental effect of failure on one's self-esteem.

Shared success increases group loyalty. Group loyalty builds teamwork and increases the productivity of the group.[22] Maslow has introduced the concept of synergy and compared it to teamwork. Synergy (like teamwork) implies mutual interdependence, free and open communication, a congruence of the goals of the individual with the goals of the group, and mutual trust. Maslow states that individuals who possess synergy are more healthy psychologically.[23] Psychologically healthy individuals are less prone to the adverse effects of stress.

Physical Fitness Programs to Manage Stress

Almost every form of exercise performed regularly and rhythmically is useful in relieving the tension produced by stress.[24] Besides relieving the muscle spasms caused by job stress, exercise programs usually prevent the participants from thinking about their jobs, and increase the participant's feelings of well-being and self-esteem. Team activities may encourage group loyalties. Physical exercise helps one lose weight, lowers blood fat, and raises HDL cholesterol.

If the stress optimization team chooses to include exercise in its stress program, the emphasis can vary from a formal physical fitness program to simply encouraging supervisors to allow workers to have exercise breaks on a regular basis during working hours. Many reports now indicate that exercise breaks of almost any kind help alleviate job stress. However, a study presented at an annual meeting of the American Heart Association indicated that exercise programs must consume 2,000 calories per week in order to reduce the overall risk of heart attacks. Table 3 lists the amount of physical activity needed to burn 2,000 calories.

There are certain precautions which must be kept in mind before setting up a formal exercise program. The most important resource required, prior to establishing a fitness program, is knowledgeable personnel to suprevise physical conditioning. Prior to entering any strenuous exercise program, individuals over age 35 should have an electrocardiogram recorded under conditions of peak physical exercise. If the exercise ECG is normal, the individual can enter the program. But the exercise program must be graduated according to the physical condition of the individual. If the stress ECG is not done and the exercise program not graduated, the company may be held liable for a sudden cardiovascular event incurred during a company exercise program. It is well to keep in mind that excessively competitive (Type A) individuals may derive little stress reduction from formal exercise programs in comparison with Type B individuals.

In summary, exercise is clearly beneficial in any stress management program, but because of the excess competitiveness of coronary-prone (Type A) individuals, it cannot replace the other components of a stress optimization program. And, finally, one should never attempt to set up a formal program without personnel qualified to supervise physical conditioning.

The second author has designed a sample lesson plan on stress which could be given by the psychology members of the stress optimization team. It is especially structured

TABLE 3. Relationship of Physical Activity to Calorie Consumption

Activity	Time During Week Needed to Burn 2,000 Calories*
Good	
skating (moderate)	5 hrs. 48 min.
walking ($4\frac{1}{2}$ mph)	5 hrs.
tennis (moderate)	4 hrs. 45 min.
canoeing (4 mph)	4 hrs. 41 min.
Better	
swimming (crawl, 45 yards/min)	3 hrs. 47 min.
skating (vigorous)	3 hrs. 45 min.
downhill skiing	3 hrs. 25 min.
handball	3 hrs. 23 min.
tennis (vigorous)	3 hrs. 23 min.
squash	3 hrs. 10 min.
running (5.5 mph)	3 hrs. 4 min.
bicycling (13 mph)	3 hrs. 4 min.
Best	
cross-country skiing (5 mph)	2 hrs. 50 min.
karate	2 hrs. 34 min.
running (7 mph)	2 hrs. 22 min.

*These figures are for a 152-lb person. If you weigh more, you'll burn up more calories in the same time; if you weigh less, you'll burn fewer.

to deal with Type A behavior in general and with the anger and hostility of the Type A individual in particular. The disadvantages of Type A behavior in a management situation have been previously discussed.

General Description of Program

Provided here is an example of the topic sequence, the exercises, and the homework assignments which comprise a comprehensive stress management program.* The program is aimed at developing adaptive behavioral, physiological, and cognitive responses to stressful situations and includes six sessions of $1\frac{1}{2}$ to 2 hours in length. The initial sessions provide an overview of the program, introduce the concepts of stress, stressors, and adaptive responses, and provide descriptions and instruction in methods of relaxation. Subsequent sessions deal with the stressors individuals inflict upon themselves and stressors that can occur on the job and at home. Presentations relating to the job environment focus on improved management skills, "job-fit," and more effective interpersonal interactions. Instructions regarding stressors of the home environment emphasize the participants' relationship with his or her spouse and management of the household. Throughout all sessions, examples of anger responses and responses

*Present space limitations preclude an in-depth description. Interested readers may obtain additional information on how the topics are covered and how the exercises and homework are used from Tommie G. Cayton.

to anger are analyzed. The physiological changes associated with anger and the interpersonal consequences of anger expression are discussed and methods of adaptive communication of anger and responses to the expression of anger are presented. To maximize the application of stress management skills outside the training environment, the exercises provide participants with repeated opportunities to practice stress responses and to receive feedback from others on the appropriateness of their word selection, inflection, eye contact, nonverbal communication, and so on. The sequence of topics is a general one and different emphasis can be made and different exercises can be substituted, depending on the makeup of the participants and on the kinds of incidents or patterns of stress responses that are recorded in the homework assignments. Following the outline are more complete descriptions of a selection of the exercises used in the sessions.

Sample Curriculum—Session Descriptions

SESSION ONE
Objectives: To teach participants what stress is, how it influences their health, job, and home, and how to identify their own stressful events and situations and to encourage participation in discussion.
Topics Covered: (1) Definitions of stress, (2) differences between stressors and stress responses, (3) physiological response to stress (detail adapted for medical knowledge of group), (4) relation between stress and performance, (5) relation between stress and unhealthy behavior (e.g., smoking, overeating, etc.), (6) changing your own behavior, (8) recording of stressful events, (9) cognitions, behaviors, and physiological reactions.
Exercise Used: (1) Introduce your partner; (2) stress recording.
Homework: Recording of stressful events and situations.

SESSION TWO
Objectives: To review topics covered in Session 1 and to teach participants why they are not aware when they become stressed until after a stressful incident and to instruct participants on, and give practice in, different methods of relaxation.
Topics Covered: (1) Experiences of the past week relating to topics of Session 1, (2) perceptions of the state of your body, (3) the fight or flight response, (4) daily stress reactions, (5) the relaxation response, (6) hobbies, (7) progressive muscle relaxation, (8) autogenics, (9) imagery, (10) hypnosis.
Exercises Used: Relaxation methods most appropriate for respective groups (two of those presented).
Homework: (1) Recording of stressful events and situations, (2) recording of relaxation exercises.

SESSION THREE
Objectives: To review the topics covered in Session 2 and instruct participants in ways in which they stress themselves.
Topics Covered: (1) Overscheduling and overcommitment, (2) nonassertive behavior, (3) trying to please everyone, (4) unrealistic expectations, (5) irrational beliefs, (6) errors in reasoning and interpretation that lead to irrational beliefs, (7) the right to feel angry versus communicating anger effectively, (8) adaptive uses of anger.
Exercises: (1) "Old sayings," value clarification.

Homework: (1) Recording of stressful events and situations, (2) recording of relaxation practices, (3) recording of self-induced stressors.

SESSIOR FOUR

Objectives: To teach participants to identify and remediate (and/or seek additional training) areas of skill deficits or habit patterns that occur in the job environment.

Topics: (1) Inadequate planning, (2) priority setting, (3) establishing goals, (4) limiting the number of goals, (5) delegating authority, (6) giving positive feedback, (7) giving negative feedback, (8) nonassertiveness, (9) aggressiveness, (10) providing and receiving support, (11) uncritical-nonjudgmental listening.

Exercises: (1) Active listening, (2) positive feedback, (3) negative feedback, (4) skill deficit identification.*

Homework: (1) Recording of stressful situations, (2) recording of relaxation exercises, (3) goal setting, (4) priority setting.

SESSION FIVE

Objectives: To teach participants to identify and remediate areas of skill deficits or habit patterns that occur in the home environment.

Topics Covered: (1) Need communication, (2) child management, (3) monetary management, (4) providing and receiving support, (5) value clarification, (6) problem resolution.

Exercise: (1) Need communication, (2) value clarification, (3) problem resolution.†

Homework: (1) Recording of stressful situations, (2) recording of relaxation exercises, (3) communication exercises, (4) appreciation exercises.

*See following descriptions:

1. *Active listening*: receivers practice checking out the accuracy of interpretations of sender's goals (reasons for making statements).

2. *Positive feedback*: participants practice saying positive statements to each other while observers rate the appropriateness of eye contact, voice quality and intonation, word choice, specificity, sincerity, and distance. Participants then practice responding to the positive feedback in a similar manner.

3. *Negative feedback*: participants state something they do not like about themselves. Partners then restate the same information to the original stater as if it were the partner's original idea. An observer then rates the appropriateness of the feedback in terms of beginning with a positive statement, eye contact, specificity, word choice, voice quality and intonations, probability of resulting in an aggressive response. Participants then practice responding to the negative feedback in a similar manner.

4. *Skill deficit identification*: participants analyze scenerios for indications of skill deficits and then describe to their subgroup how they are different from these individuals in the scenerios and how they are similar. From this they develop a list of two areas that they might benefit most from additional training.

†*Need communication:* Participants identify different kinds of responses they need from their spouses in different situations, such as to listen without saying anything, to demonstrate love, to offer solutions, to tell participant they recognize how hard he or she has been working, and so on. Participants then pair off and practice communications to the partner what their need is at the moment. For example: "A spouse has just arrived home after an exasperating day at work in which several problem areas have been identified that need action. The spouse is keyed up, doesn't really want to hear how the day could have been run more effectively, nor what things should be done tomorrow, nor about all the family problems that need solving, unless they are true emergencies. What is really needed, at least at the moment of arriving home, is to have someone listen in a caring manner, understand how difficult the spouse's job is, and communicate to the spouse that he or she is working very hard and is a worthwhile individual." After being given this scenario, partners practice how they may indicate these needs to their spouses and how they might respond if a spouse acted in this manner toward them.

SESSION SIX

Objectives: To review content presented in prior sessions, to provide an opportunity for additional questions, and to obtain evaluations of stress management program.

Topics: (1) Definitions of stress, (2) stress and performance, (3) effects of cognitions on arousal level, (4) self-induced stress, (5) skill-deficit induced stress, (6) ways of relaxing, (7) health benefits of adaptive stress management, (8) individualized stress copying strategies developed from stress recordings.

Exercise: Evaluation questionnaire.

REFERENCES

1. Cooper, C. L. and Marshall, J., *Understanding Executive Stress*. New York: Petrocelli Books, 1977, p. 57.
2. Rosch, P. J., "Stress and Illness," *Journal of American Medical Association* 242 (1979), pp. 427–428.
3. Yates, J. E., *Managing Stress*. New York: AMACOM, 1979, p. 1.
4. Levi, Lennart M.D., *Preventing Work Stress*, Reading, Mass., Addison-Wesley Publishing Co., 1981, p. 75.
5. Cooper, C. L. and Marshall, J., Occupational Sources of Stress: A Review of the Literature Relating to Coronary Heart Disease and Mental Ill Health. *Journal of Occupational Psychology* 49 (1976), pp. 11–28.
6. McLean, A. A., *Work Stress*. Reading, Mass.: Addison-Wesley Publishing Co., 1979, p. 5.
7. Poulton, E. C., "Blue Collar Stressors." In *Stress at Work*, C. L. Cooper and R. Payne, eds. New York: John Wiley & Sons, 1978, pp. 51–66.
8. Morano, R. A., "How to Manage Change to Reduce Stress." *Management Review* 66 (1977), pp. 22–26.
9. Cooper, C. L. and Marshall, J., "Sources of Managerial and White Collar Stress." In *Stress at Work*, C. L. Cooper and R. Payne, eds. New York: John Wiley & Sons, 1978, p. 89.
10. Van Harrison, R., "Person-Environment Fit and Job Stress." In *Stress at Work*, C. L. Cooper and R. Payne, eds. New York: John Wiley & Sons, 1978, p. 175.
11. Sales, S. M. and House, J., "Job Dissatisfaction as a Possible Risk Factor in Coronary Heart Disease." *Journal of Chronic Diseases* 23 (1971), pp. 861–873.
12. Likert, R., *New Patterns of Management*. New York: McGraw-Hill, 1961, p. 16.
13. Welford, A. T., "Stress and Performance." *Ergonomics* 16 (1973), pp. 567–580.
14. Weirman, C. G., "A Study of Occupational Stressors and the Incidence of Disease Risk." *Journal of Occupational Medicine* 19 (1977), pp. 119–122.
15. "Five Antidotes for Job Tension." *Supervisory Management* 14(1969), pp. 32–32.
16. Chesney, M. A. and Rosenman, R. H., "Type A Behavior in the Work Setting. In Current Concerns in Occupational Stress. C. L. Cooper and R. Payne, eds. New York: John Wiley & Sons, 1980, p. 188.
17. Friedman, M. and Rosenman, R. H., *Type A Behavior and Your Heart*. Greenwich, Conn.: Fawcett Publications, p. 87.
18. Review Panel on Coronary-prone Behavior and Coronary Heart Disease "Coronary-prone Behavior and Coronary Heart Disease: A Critical Review." *Circulation* 63 (1981), pp. 1199–1215.
19. French, J. R. P. and caplan, R. D., "Psychosocial Factors in Coronary Heart Disease." *Industrial Medicine* 39 (1970), pp. 31–45.
20. Warshaw, L. J. *Managing Stress*. Menlo Park, Calif.: Addison-Wesley Publishing Co., Series on Occupational Stress, 1979, pp. 68-75.

21. Friedman, M., Rosenman, R. H., and Carrol, V., "Changes in Serum Cholesterol and Blood Clotting Time in Men Subjected to Cyclic Variation of Occupational Stress" *Circulation* 17, 1958, pp. 852–861.
22. Ibid., 12, pp. 30–31.
23. Maslow, A. H., *Eupsychian Management*. Homewood, Ill.: Dorsey Press, 1965, pp. 98–99.
24. Ibid., 20, p. 164.

11 / Environmental Health Risks and Their Reduction

Turkan K. Gardenier, Ph.D. *

The environment is enormously complex and constantly changing. Toxic factors exist ubiquitously in the environment and threaten all of us. We require society to satisfy ever increasing demands to improve life, and the unavoidable accompaniments to this are unforeseen environmental hazards associated with such material gain. As the economy produces goods and services that contribute to our standard of living, it simultaneously produces polluted rivers and streams, poisonous pesticides, toxic substances, hazardous wastes, radiation, unsafe drinking water, and noise pollution, all of which detract from our quality of life. Increased population, urban growth, and industrial and technological development present a myriad of challenges to health. The most important identified hazard of these toxic substances is cancer. It has been determined that environmental factors, directly or indirectly, cause the great majority of all cancers. Many do not realize that this danger exists because toxic substances in our air, food and water often require many years to produce a negative impact on health. By the time a disease due to pollution manifests itself, the original insult may be long forgotten or perhaps was not noticed at its inception.

Preventing hazards in the modern technological society has been receiving major attention from federal, state, and public-based environmental organizations. Since 1970 when the U.S. Environmental Protection Agency was formed with the mandate to coordinate and implement program in pollution control, several regulations have been initiated or amended. Among them are the following:

1. The Toxic Substances Control Act and Resource Conservation and Recovery Act of 1976 to control toxic chemicals suspected of health risk;
2. The Endangered Species Act of 1973 to prevent extinction of endangered plant and animal species;
3. The Safe Drinking Water Act promulgated in 1974 and the Water Pollution Control Act promulgated in 1972 in order to clean water resources;
4. Amendments to the Clean Air Act which set air quality standards at the national level and interfaced with the Occupational Safety and Health Act to establish workplace-oriented safety and air pollution standards.

Managing hazards for health in our technological society demands an evaluation of the nature and source of the risk, methodology used to conclude or suspect that there is a risk, and measures used to reduce it.

*The opinions and factual accuracy of material contained in this manuscript are the sole responsibility of the author; they do not necessarily reflect official views or policy of the U.S. Environmental Protection Agency.

IDENTIFICATION CRITERIA AND DEFINITIONS

A systems approach to environmental risks as they impact on human health is taken in a study[1] which aims at identifying total body burden from:

(I)   Discharge sources of toxic chemicals which impact on human health;
(II) Sources for monitoring pollutant levels and the way they act as statistical indicators to levels of pollution;
(III) Modular data units impacting on exposure level such as human activity patterns which need to be considered in modeling efforts;
(IV) Sources of data for a profiling analysis, such as simultaneous samples for the same pollutant obtained from air, water, and food;
(V)   Data sources within the human metabolism to identify concentrations of the pollutant impact as total body burden.

Figure 1 is a graphic representation of this global approach to data gathering and modeling of human exposure. However, efforts to link health effects with environmental pollution have involved a number of different approaches. Futhermore, terminology has been defined and used often by toxicologists and risk assessment personnel which associate health hazard with environmental concentrations of a pollutant. Some of these are the following:

1. LD_{50}, LD_{10}, LD_{90}: *Lethal dose* or dose which will kill respectively, 50, 10, and 90 per cent of a specific type of organism. This term is used in experimentally designed studies which explore the toxicity of a specific chemical. It is used as input for extrapolations from the animal studies to human risk estimation. Dose is defined by amount administered to the animal by oral, intravenous, or inhalation methods.
2. LC_{50}, LC_{10}, LC_{90},: *Lethal concentration* of a substance which will be fatal to 50, 10, and 90 per cent of a particular species. These terms are often used in aquatic studies in setting water quality criteria for selected pollutants. Data collection involves collecting samples of water over time and counting the number of organisms of a specific type which inhabit the water resources. Designed laboratory studies are also conducted tracing the number of organisms which die over time after exposure to a specific concentration of a pollutant.
3. TLV_{50}, TLV_{10}, TLV_{90}: *Threshold limit value* defined similar to previous proportion of organisms affected but defined in terms of units of volume. This index is often encountered with studies dealing with toxicity of a particular substance in the air using units related to the volume of the substance inhaled.
4. Concentration $/m^3$, /l, /dl, or /ppm: Specific concentration of a pollutant expressed as *per meter cubed*, which is a volume index usually used with concentrations in air, *per liter or deciliter* used with concentrations in body fluids, and *parts per million* often used as an index related to volume, such as the tolerable level of a substance mixed with the medium which will be exposed to humans.

Environmental surveillance of health effects and associated pollution levels has also been studied through an epidemiological approach. Population registries, environmental monitoring systems, and disease registries have proved useful in identifying exposure cohorts, such as survivors of the atomic bombings in Japan. Genetic predisposition heightens susceptibility to environmental hazards[2] as in genes which in-

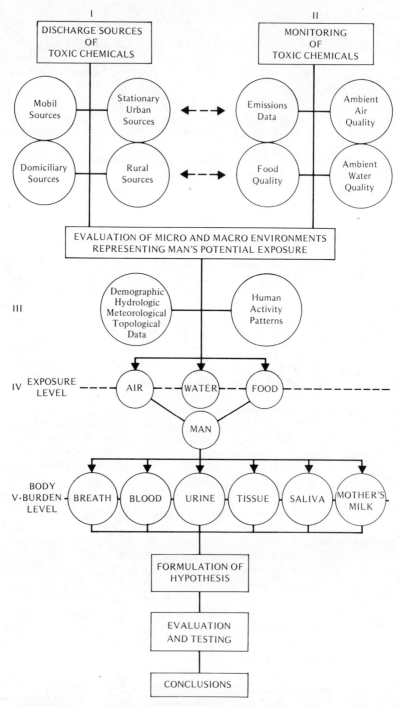

FIGURE 11-1. Relationships between micro- and macro-environmental pollution sources, exposure routes and body-burden. (Source: Erickson, M. D. et al. *Preliminary Study on Toxic Chemicals on Environmental and Human Samples.* Part I. U.S. Environmental Protection Agency Contract Report 68-01-3849, Washington, D.C., 1980, p. 9.)

crease an individual's susceptibility to cancer heightening the observed effect of environmental factors. Table 1 presents a summary of observable health effects, and interactive environmental and genetic predispositions which place the individual at a heightened risk level.

There are various sources of occupational data which have been used to make two-tier estimates of exposure and associated health effects[3] as input to the Occupational Safety and Health Act (OSHA). Data from occupational surveillance has had methodological advantages in that:

1. Exposure level to pollutants is higher among occupational groups than among the general public; thus, disease elicitation is more frequent and earlier than in nationwide samples;
2. The worker sample usually has additional records from employment files identifying employment duration and more specific levels of the contaminant.

On the other hand, in all epidemiological analyses the following difficulties with any inference relating health and environmental exposure links need to be acknowledged:

1. Unidentifiable and long latency necessary between exposure and onset of health effect. Most cancer latency is between 10 and 30 years.
2. Difficulty in separating total exposure into long-term low-dose exposure, usually referred to as chronic exposure, versus short-term exposure to high doses, usually referred to as acute exposure. The latter is encountered mostly in accidents.
3. Existence of multipollutant exposure in many settings, particularly in worker environments, and probably existence of synergistic effects.
4. Nonspecificity of a particular disease; for example, exposure to asbestos or cigarette smoking may cause lung cancer. In both cases the clinical and pathological symptoms are identical. Furthermore, a particular individual may be a cigarette-smoker *and* exposed to asbestos.

PRIORITY CHEMICALS SELECTED FOR POSSIBLE HEALTH HAZARD

As a result of priority setting and selection under several environmental regulations as well as integrating literature from a number of studies and multimedia sources, a number of chemicals have been identified as possible health hazards. They are presented in Table 2 in matrix form identifying where they are most often found in the environmental media.[1] The information is taken from the profiling study to analyze interactive and synergistic effects of pollutants found in multimedia, traceable in human body fluids, and in other sites such as hair and nails and for which biological assays have been formulated.

Evaluation of health risks emanating from the environment has recently followed two orientations, the first a research orientation and the second a regulatory decision approach. Among studies with a research orientation are the epidemiological and follow-up designs discussed earlier, controlled studies with animals, and clinical experiments with humans. In addition, the impetus to reach nationwide regulations has recently spurred an interest in using larger and more diversified data sets in attempting to associate health and environmental indexes. Lave and Seskin[4] used socioeconomic data from census statistics at the standard metropolitan statistical areas (SMSA) level

TABLE 1. Some Inherited Disorders Placing Individuals at Altered Risk in Particular Environments

Enzyme System or Genetic Trait Involved	Environmental Agent(s)	Sign or Symptom of Individual Effect	Mode of Inheritance
Glucose-6-phosphate dehydrogenase (some mutations)	Primaquine, sulfonamides, fava bean, naphthylene	Red cell hemolysis	X-linked recessive
6-Phosphogluconic dehydrogenase	Fava bean, naphthylene	Red cell hemolysis	Autosomal recessive
Glutathione reductase	Fava bean, naphthylene	Red cell hemolysis	Dominant
Abnormal response to CS_2 exposure	Carbon disulfide	Polyneuritis	Unknown
Mixed function oxidase that de-ethylates acetophenetidin	Acetophenetidin	Hemolysis and methemoglobinemia	Autosomal recessive
Microsomal "oxidases"	Dicumarol (antipyrine, phenylbutaxone)	Hemorrhage	Unknown
Tyrosinemia	Tyrosine	Hepatocellular carcinoma	Autosomal recessive
Hemochromatosis	Iron	Hepatocellular carcinoma cirrhosis	Autosomal dominant
Cutaneous albinism	Untraviolet radiation	Skin cancer	Autosomal recessive
Xerodema pigmentosa	Ultraviolet radiation	Skin cancer	Autosomal recessive
Turner syndrome	Stilbesterol	Endometrial carcinoma	Chromosomal
Hemoglobin H disease	Sulfonamides, nitrates	Red cell hemolysis	Autosomal dominant
Hemaglobin zurich	Sulfonamides, primaquine	Red cell hemolysis	Autosomal dominant
Diaphorase (methemoglobin reductase)	Sulfonamides, nitrites, acetanilide, amines	Methemoglobinemia	Autosomal recessive
Plasma atypical pseudocholinesterase	Succinylcholine	Apnea	Autosomal recessive
Glucoronide transferase (Gilbert's disease; Crigler Najiar syndrome)	Salicylates, tetrahydrocortisone, menthol	Jaundice and/or drug toxicity	Autosomal recessive
Isoniazid acetylase (slow acetylators)	Isoniazid phenelzine, hydralazine, dapsone, sulfadimidine	Polyneuritis and side effects of specific drugs	Autosomal recessive
Porphyria (variegata and hepatic types)	Barbiturates	Polyneuritis, neurosis, psychosis	Autosomal dominant
Resistance to warfarin anticoagulation	Oral anticoagulants	Increased resistance to anticoagulation	Autosomal recessive
Catalase (acatalasia)	Hydrogen peroxide	Mouth ulcers	Autosomal recessive

Source: National Academy of Sciences, *Report of the Committee for a Planning Study for an Ongoing Study of Costs of Environment-Related Health Effects,* Washington, D.C., 1981, Appendix F prepared by Paul Marks and Robert Murray.

TABLE 2. Toxic Chemicals Selected For Monitoring In Environmental Media

Air		Drinking Water	Beverages	Food (tent.)	Household Dust
Vapors	*Particulate*				
Benzene	Arsenic	Benzene	Chloroform	Arsenic	Arsenic
Chloroform	Cadmium	Chloroform	1,2-Dichloroethane	Cadmium	Cadmium
1,2-Dichloroethane	Lead	1,2-Dichloroethane	1,1,1-Trichloroethane	Lead	Lead
1,1,1-Trichloroethane	—	1,1,2-Trichloroethane	1,1,2-Trichloroethane	—	—
Carbon tetrachloride	Benzo(a)pyrene	Carbon tetrachloride	Vinylidene chloride	α-BHC	Benzo(a)pyrene
Vinylidene chloride	Pyrene	Vinylidene chloride	Trichloroethylene	Lindane	Fluoranthene
Trichloroethylene	Chrysene	Trichloroethylene	Tetrachloroethylene	Heptachlor	Benzo(k)fluoranthene
Tetrachloroethylene	Benzo(a)anthrene	Tetrachloroethylene	Bromodichloromethane	Heptachlor epoxide	Pyrene
Bromodichloromethane	Fluoranthene	Bromodichloromethane	Chlorobenzena	Chlordane	Chrysena
Chlorobenzene	Benzo(k)fluoranthene	Chlorobenzene	Vinyl chloride	t-Nonachlor	Benzo(a)anthrene
1,1,2-Trichloroethane		Vinyl chloride		Oxychlordane	—
—		1,1,1-Trichloroethane		HCB	α-BHC
Vinyl chloride		—		DDT/DDD/DDE	Lindane
—		Arsenic		PCBS	Heptachlor
α-BHG		Cadmium			Chlordane
Lindane		Lead			HCB
Heptachlor		—			DDT/DDD/DDE
Chlordane		Benzo(a)pyrene			PCBS
HCB		Fluoranthene			
DDT/DDD/DDE		Benzo(k)fluoranthene			
PCBS		Pyrene			
		Chrysena			
		Benzo(a)anthrene			

Source: 1980 Preliminary Study on Toxic Chemicals on Environmental and Human Samples. Part 1. U.S. Environmental Protection Agency Contract Report 68-01-3849, Washington, D.C., p. 158.

as well as the concentration of sulfate and suspended particulates in ambient air, and they used the method of regression analysis to relate the results to overall death rates or to selected causes of death in the area. In addition, the effect of several indicators of climate, such as minimum and maximum daily temperature, precipitation, and wind-speed, were used along with characteristics related to usage of gas versus electricity for home heating and type of heating equipment. Table 3 shows a summary of some of the data used in terms of the averages observed in the data (means) and an index of statistical variation (standard deviation).

Lake et al.[5] used the method of statistical factor analysis to identify significant characteristic sets from environmental and demographic indicators. Groups of "similar" cities were thus formed based upon how they clustered in terms of their air, water, and demographic indexes. The mathematical modeling approaches by Lave et al. and Lake et al. have both been subjected to criticism because of the existence of the high degree of dependence among the variables associated with death rates, a statistical term denoted as multicollinearity.

The second, regulatory decision approach, to selecting hazardous pollutants combines exposure assessment, biological studies, and a mandate for identifying major regulations by the U.S. Environmental Protection Agency (1979). Major regulations are those that address major health or ecological problems and have economic and urban impact. A decision package is prepared to analyze (*a*) environmental, (*b*) economic, (*c*) urban, (*d*) resource, and (*e*) paperwork effects for each such rule. Several agencywide and interagency committees have been formed to assist in health-effect–related input and decisions. Among them are the Interagency Testing Committee (ITC) and the Inter-Regulatory Liaison Group (IRLG). The decision framework followed in the Toxic Substances Control Act (TSCA) provides a case for the analysis in the definition of health risk and input documents for reaching the regulatory decisions.

Let us review some of the criteria which determine the classification of chemicals as hazardous to human health.

Carcinogenicity: According to recent theories, substances which are carcinogenic damage or alter cells and their growth and replacement cycle. More than 100 cancer types have been identified. Statistics tell us that one out of every four Americans is likely to develop cancer; at present almost 20 per cent of all deaths are cancer-related.

Difficulties with testing for carcinogens arise since it is difficult to test for cancer at every possible target site and, as mentioned earlier, some chemicals may be cancer promoters since they cause damage to some body cells that would then be sensitized to known carcinogens. The presence of more than one toxic substance may enhance the probability of cancer, as discussed in a recent *Toxics Primer.*[6] Some agents are not carcinogenic per se but are converted to carcinogens after ingestion; for example, sodium nitrite, a food preservative becomes nitrosamine, a potent carcinogen.

Mutagenicity: A mutagen causes change in the genes of the sperm and egg and leads to birth defects or more subtle but dangerous mutations. Identifying mutagens and evaluating their potential in the human population are of as much concern as calculating the probability of increase in genetic disorders which can be traced to the exposure. Estimating the increment in probability further demands a knowledge of the underlying genetic variation prior to exposure. This is often referred to as background rate of incidence.

Teratogenicity: This term refers to toxic pollutants which cause birth defects by affecting the fetus during its formation. Perhaps the most publicized case is that of thalidomide which was prescribed as a sedative during pregnancy but caused severe malformations in babies. Exposure to heavy metals and pesticides have recently been linked to teratogenic effects.

Neurological and Behavioral Effects: Toxic substances can affect nerve cells and often cause irreversible damage, such as brain damage in children exposed to lead. Certain food additives have been found to cause hyperactivity in children. We may well remember the kepone incident in 1975 in Hopewell, Virginia, which caused loss of memory, headaches, and tremors among exposed workers.

TSCA, promultaged in 1976, authorizes the U.S. Environmental Protection Agency to require industry to test selected chemicals following guidelines of testing protocols and standards. How to select these priority chemicals has become a concern. As stated by the Council of Environmental Quality[7] the American Chemical Society listed over 4 million chemical compounds compiled since 1965. At present more than 70,000 chemicals are being produced by over 115,000 companies, accounting for a business that exceeds an annual $113 billion. Prior to TSCA, the National Cancer Institute was actively involved in testing chemicals as to carcinogenic potential on the basis of long-term animal experiments. As of 1978, 19 out of the 29 chemicals selected for testing were found to cause cancer. Priorities for chemicals under TSCA consider an assessment of potential exposure through the use of production data as well as hazard, as estimated from animal studies. The task has become vast—a staff of over 600 was authorized to work on this act after its promulgation. Under presidential direction, the Toxic Substances Strategy Committee was formed with members from 17 agencies to supplant gaps in toxicity data, eliminate duplication in data collection, and coordinate activities in research and implementation of the regulation.

The next question becomes: What are some statistical estimating procedures in arriving at the conclusion of health risk from the environment?

STATISTICAL AND COMPUTER TECHNIQUES FOR ANALYSIS OF ENVIRONMENTAL INDICATORS

With the advent of inter- and intraagency collaborative efforts, a new trend has emerged for data banking of toxicity and environmental health hazards. Some have been in the form of monitoring actual levels of ambient concentrations of pollutants in the air and water. Examples are the STORET data base of water quality and SOROAD data base of air quality of the U.S. Environmental Protection Agency, NASQUAN data base of the U.S. Geological Survey. Others are in the form of literature abstracts and compilation of basic results relating to toxicity, such as TOXLINE (Toxicology Information On-Line) of the National Library of Medicine which contains interactive subfiles of Chemical-Biological Activities (CBAC), Abstracts of Health Effects of Environmental Pollutants (HEEP), Pesticides Abstracts (PESTAB), Environmental Mutagen Information Center file (EMIC), and Environmental Teratology Information Center file (ETIC). The on-line data base contains more than 450,000 records dating back to 1971; older data may also be retrieved through computer batch processing commands.

The Toxicology Data Bank (TDB) also developed by the national Library of Medicine with support contracts to Oak Ridge National Laboratory has computerized data relating to health hazards of pollutants subsequent to review by a panel of scientists. The records contain information on whether the chemical was found to be or is suspected of being a carcinogen by the National Cancer Institute.

TABLE 3. Variables Selected for Analysis of Environmental, Demographic, and Health Effects

Variable	Description	1960 (117 SMSAs) Mean	Standard Deviation	1961 (117 SMSAs) Mean	Standard Deviation
Air Pollution	Min S: Smallest biweekly sulfate reading (μg per cubic meter × 10)	47.239	31.276	47.598	30.796
	Mean S: Arithmetic mean of biweekly sulfate readings (μg per cubic meter × 10)	99.649	52.885	102.342	57.773
	Max S: Largest biweekly sulfate reading (μg per cubic meter × 10)	228.393	124.411	237.427	131.655
	Min P: Smallest biweekly suspended particulate reading (μg per cubic meter	45.479	18.571	44.658	18.592
	Mean P: Arithmetic mean of biweekly suspended particulate readings (μg per cubic meter)	118.145	40.942	113.786	39.573
	Max P: Largest biweekly suspended particulate reading (μg per cubic meter)	268.359	132.073	265.145	131.386
Socioeconomic	P/M^2: SMSA population density (per square mile × 0.1)	69.965	135.443	70.738	135.178
	≥65: Percentage of SMSA population at least 65 years old (× 10)	83.872	21.072	84.376	20.733
	NW: Percentage of nonwhites in SMSA population (× 10)	124.812	104.099	125.726	103.290
	Poor: Percentage of SMSA families with incomes below the poverty level (× 10)	181.120	65.236	172.581	62.208
	Log Pop: The logarithm of SMSA population (× 100)	565.717	40.663	566.401	40.721
Mortality	Unadjusted total mortality rate (per 100,000)	912.316	153.282	895.043	154.014
	Age-sex-race adjusted total mortality rate (per 100,000)	1015.974	78.045	988.470	74.870

Unadjusted infant mortality rate (per 10,000 live births)	254.034	36.462	250.325	33.683
Race-adjusted infant mortality rate (per 10,000 live births)	251.436	30.953	247.162	25.350
White infant mortality rate (per 10,000 live births)	224.205	27.637		
Nonwhite infant mortality rate (per 10,000 live births)	382.564	121.279		

Home-heating characteristic

Water-heating fuels (percentage of occupied housing units × 10)		
Gas: utility gas	534.529	280.055
Electricity	220.082	218.334
Coal: coal or coke	28.138	86.339
Bottled gas: bottled tank, or low-pressure gas	42.697	24.324
Oil: fuel oil, kerosine, etc.	90.136	158.771
Other: other water-heating fuel	4.780	7.645
None: without water-heating fuel	79.642	60.941
Home-heating fuels (percentage of occupied housing units × 10)		
Gas: utility gas	491.987	329.679
Oil: fuel oil, kerosine, etc.	315.074	291.318
Coal: coal or coke	110.683	149.846
Electricity	23.666	73.616
Bottled gas: bottled, tank, or low-pressure gas	31.488	32.623
Other: other home-heating fuel	21.340	27.943
None: without home-heating fuel	5.772	23.541
Heating equipment (percentage of total housing units × 10)		
Steam or hot water	192.807	218.110
Warm-air furnace	355.873	222.767
Floor, wall, or pipeless furnace	125.964	125.317
Electric: built-in electric units	17.449	54.767
Flue: other means with flue	178.160	119.940
Without flue: other means without flue	118.811	181.913
None: without heating equipment	10.938	27.088
Without air conditioning (percentage of total housing units × 10)	843.521	115.488

Source: Lave, Lester B. and Seskin, Eugene P., *Air Pollution and Human Health*. Baltimore: Resources for the Future, Johns Hopkins University Press, 1977, pp. 324, 330.

The Chemical Information System (CIS) which is in process of development jointly by the National Institutes of Health and the U.S. Environmental Protection Agency integrates data bases and computer programs accessible to a variety of users for retrieval of chemical and toxicological data and scientific/regulatory support through literature search. It contains the following four basic components:

1. Catalog and referral list of chemicals including the Chemical Abstracts Service Number;
2. Structure search for chemicals and mass spectral search;
3. Numerical data bases such as LD_{50} and LC_{50} values for chemicals;
4. Analysis software such as MLAB (Mathematical Modeling System) developed by the National Institutes of Health and used for statistical analysis.

The CIS system is being used nationwide and abroad through satellite networking and is available to many organizations, public and private, in over ten countries.[8] Figure 2 is a diagram showing the interrelationship between the various files accessed through the module of the Chemical Abstracts Service (CAS) Registry Number which may also be linked to the Structure and Nomenclature Search System (SANSS) to access information such as molecular formula, structure, and weight.[9]

A summary of information sources for the number of compounds for which environmental risk data exists is given in Table 4. Since they were developed by different data base designers, their search strategy and access methodology differ. The CIS system just discussed aims at providing a uniform format for access and utilization by providing a centralized host software which interacts with the user.

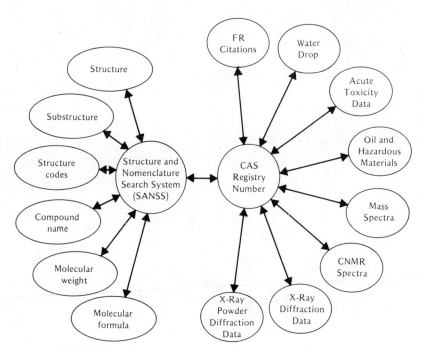

FIGURE 11-2.   Chemical Information System Network.

TABLE 4.   Database Resources for Suspect Pollutants

Organization	File Type and Contents	Approximate Number of Compounds
1. *Environmental Protection Agency* (EPA)	Active Ingredients in Pesticides	1,500
	AEROS/SAROAD (Air Quality)	65
	Chemical Producers	400
	Pesticides Standards	400
	STORET (Water Quality)	250
	TSCA (Toxic Sustances Control Act) Candidate List	33,000
2. *Food and Drug Administration* (FDA)	Pesticide Reference Standards	600
3. *Merck*	Merck Index	8,900
4. *National Institute of Mental Health* (NIMH)	Psychotropic Drugs	1,700
5. *National Institute for Occupational Safety and Health (NIOSH)*	Registry of Toxic Effects of Chemical Substances	20,000
6. *National Science Foundation*	RANN Pollutant File	230
7. *Stanford Research Institute/ Public Health Service*	List 149 of Carcinogens	4,500

The use of graphics and mapping capabilities has also interacted with the interagency data sharing trends. The Domestic Information Display System (DIDS) which was initially developed at NASA's Goddard Space Flight Center has received environment, demographic, and economic data from over 20 agencies in a collaborative effort to compile, integrate, and retrieve data modules to interested users on a county, state, or SMSA level.[10] They include

1. Bureau of the Census with population statistics, birth and death rates;
2. Department of Energy with data relating to fuel consumption;
3. Environmental Protection Agency with air and water quality data and mortality rates from various diseases;
4. U.S. Geological Survey with coal production data by method.

The DIDS system produces a color-coded United States map with selected variables displayed in units selected by the user. Geographical coverage may be varied through a progressive zoom option; data ranges and colors may be varied. Single variables may be mapped; or two variables may be cross-tabulated for subsequent mapping. A histogram of the data may be requested for display on the cathode ray tube which serves as the medium for input to the menu-driven system.

Data banking, retrieval, mapping and graphics, and dissemination of risk data have aided in the awareness of etiology and control of risk factors. Information scientists have also been concerned with the methodology for statistical evaluation of health and environmental effects. Some statistical measures of association will be presented here with selected formulas for computation and program codes written in the FORTRAN computer language. The program is shown in the Appendix.

Arcsine Transformation for Comparing Two Percentages: This procedure is used in testing the statistical significance between percentages in two sets of data that do not belong to the same population. The Arcsine transformation makes it possible to apply the assumptions underlying the Normal distribution, commonly used with statistical data. The computer program in Appendix A uses two percentages as input— for example, the percentage of individuals afflicted with a certain disease in populations exposed to a hazardous pollutant versus those who have not—and prints the Z value, the significance of which may be tested by referring to tables of the Normal distribution. The computation formula is

$$Z = \frac{\text{arc } \sqrt{p_1} - \text{arc } \sqrt{p_2}}{\sqrt{\dfrac{0.25}{N_1} + \dfrac{0.25}{N_2}}}$$

where p_1 and p_2 refer to the two percentages and N_2 and N_2 refer to the sample size.

t-Test for Independent Samples: This test is often used to test the statistical significance between average values of two independently distributed samples. In addition to the two means or averages, the programs uses as input the variances or square of the standard deviations and the number of samples in each group. It calculates a t value, refers to a "degrees of freedom" table, and prints out the probability of error in testing the statistical significance between the two means.

The computation formula, if the two sample sizes are not very small, is

$$t = \frac{\bar{X}_1 - \bar{X}_2}{\sqrt{\dfrac{\sigma_1^2}{N_1} + \dfrac{\sigma_2^2}{N_2}}}$$

where $\bar{X}_1$ and $\bar{X}_2$ refer to the averages in the two samples, σ_1^2 and σ_2^2 to the two variances, and N_1 and N_2 to the two sample sizes.

7-11-13 Rule: This is a nonparametric test initially quoted by Mosteller and Tukey[11] and which does not use any assumptions as to the underlying statistical distribution in the two samples being compared. The user combines both data sets, marking to which data set each observation belongs. Then the observations are ranked and a count is made of how many cases fall outside the range of overlap between the two data sets. If the sum totals at least 7, there is a "significant difference" between the two groups with 5 per cent probability of error; if the sum equals at least 11, the probability of error is 1 per cent, if it is at least 13, the associated error is 0.1 per cent.

There are statistical software packages such as the Bio-Medical Computer Programs (BMDP), Statistical Analysis System (SAS) and Statistical Package for the Social Sciences (SPSS). Analysis routines fall into the following categories:

A. Descriptive statistics, including mean, standard deviation, minimum, maximum, frequency distribution, and cumulative frequency distribution;
B. Two sample comparisons as discussed previously, using t-tests, percentage comparisons, incorporating degrees of freedom and F statistics;
C. Univariate and bivariate plots and histograms with flexibility for logarithmic transformation of data;
D. Cross-tabulation of a data matrix (two-way and multi-way) with statistics for measures of association;
E. Regression analysis, including simple linear regression, multiple regression, stepwise regression, all possible subsets regression, and nonlinear regression;

F. Analysis of variance, including one-way and two-way analysis of variance and co-variance with repeated measures;
G. Nonparametric statistics, including Wilcoxon statistics, Kendall's coefficient of concordance, Mann-Whitney rank sums test, and Spearman-Brown rank correlation coefficient.[12-14]

In environmental health surveillance, important inputs are provided to the development of regulatory standards through the use of simulation models. Time series analysis has been essential in models analyzing monitoring data. Some examples are

A. Evaluating how various pollutants show simultaneous increases or decreases or periodic peaks and lags;
B. Associating fluctuations in death rates, disease incidence, hospital visits, and occurrence of symptoms to pollutant concentrations in air, water, soil, and other sources of contamination;
C. Extrapolating to determine exposure and health effects in the future in order to assess the impact of intervention or regulation;
D. Evaluating differences between new pollution control devices as compared with standard equipment and adjacent monitoring devices.

A RISK/BENEFIT APPROACH

Identification of environment-related health effects is insufficient to prevent and control risk. Environmental regulation aims at reducing risks to human health. Yet, statistical uncertainties in defining cause and effect, the economic impacts of pollution control on industry, and individual differences in perceived risk[15] makes it difficult to have a consensus of opinion of how much or what type of control is needed. The value of statistical information gathering should be assessed in view of the incremental gain to public welfare of a policy action impact. We often find *benefit* defined as a reduction in the number of people exposed to specific levels of a hazardous chemical. This definition gives no credit to the individual. The person himself or herself should be aware of existing risks and actively participate in designing environmental systems and products which

1. Conserve the resources of the natural environment;
2. Meet the production and employment needs of the economy; and
3. Have competitive production and distribution costs.

New trends in dissemination of information to the public have emerged and have cyrstallized in the existence of hotlines, accessible through the telephone, and clearinghouses. The Cancer Information Clearinghouse, Clearinghouse for Occupational Safety and Health, Office of Smoking and Health, and Toxicology Information Response Center are among the 20 such clearinghouses which serve as sources of general information to the public and media for interface of common data resources.[16]

The rapid rate of information growth also makes it imperative for health professionals to be familiar with the most recent findings related to toxicity and health hazard likely to emanate from environmental pollutants. A new directive for periodic physician recertification in many states demands the accumulation of continuing medical education (CME) credits. These points may be obtained through formal courses, attendance at professional meetings, or with computerized on-line instruction with patient–

physician simulations, many of which incorporate recent findings relating to diagnosis and treatment.

Although they deal with data base confidentiality issues, reliability of statistical results and sensitivity in exposure and body burden estimation would be enhanced through more adequate systems for health effects surveillance. Some systems involve establishment of registries, consistent reporting and coding of industry and occupation data on death certificates, and liaison efforts between the National Institute for Occupational Safety and Health (NIOSH) and data from the Internal Revenue Service.

ROLE OF INDIVIDUALS AND HEALTH CARE PROFESSIONALS IN MINIMIZING HEALTH RISKS

Knowledge about health risks and accessibility of health care play a major role in helping individuals prevent risk. A Surgeon General's Report entitled *Healthy People* stresses the importance of greater effort by individuals in reducing the probability that they will contract health problems.[17] This includes choice of personal lifestyles, such as avoiding unhealthful products, drunken driving and smoking.

Community surveillance can also yield valuable ideas for local educational programs identifying those issues peculiar to a specific community. The programs would then pinpoint those remedial risk prevention for a specific area rather than risk prevention in general. For example, localities where citrus groves exist are more commonly exposed to pesticide spraying. Thus, they would particularly benefit from information related to chemical effects of pesticides.

In the spring 1980 meeting of the Operations Research Research Society of America held in Washington, D.C. a debate was held about how much individuals themselves should decide about risk prevention versus risk prevention at the national or state level. Some participants felt that as much as individuals voluntarily expose themselves to high risk activities, such as skiing, they should decide upon how much risk they allow in their own lives after adequate knowledge of the risk consequences. This raises the importance of the concept of perceived risk and the concept of risk/benefit at the individual level.[18] Yet, it also emphasizes how significant it is to familarize individuals with existing hazards in as quantifiable a way as possible. This, in turn, demands research, facts and figures, and widely disseminated information through not only formal training programs but also centers such as the American Cancer Society, American Diabetes Association and American Heart Association.

WHERE ARE WE IN ENVIRONMENTAL HEALTH RISK REDUCTION

The impetus for environmental protection is to reduce health risks emanating from hazardous pollutants, whether they emanate from smoke stacks, industrial dumping or any other source. According to a recent report entitled "State of the Environment" the following trends are observed since 1972.[19]

1. Air quality has improved in general; particularly in carbon monoxide and sulfur dioxide levels. Metropolitan area statistics in 25 areas show a 15 per cent decline in unhealthful days and 32 per cent decline in very unhealthful days between 1974 and 1977.

2. Statistics for water quality show improvement in dissolved oxygen and phosphorus levels as well as ambient water quality; secondary treatment was achieved in about half of major municipal discharge sources.
3. More than 300 hazardous waste disposal sites have been investigated; the Environmental Protection Agency issued standards for disposal which states will use to prevent health hazards such as Love Canal.
4. As of 1979 chemical substances are also being reviewed by the Environmental Protection Agency prior to their manufacture in order to identify any human health risks. This constitutes a volume of about 400 new chemicals which are released annually into the market. This activity is mandated under the Toxic Substances Control Act and aims at preventing potential risks prior to exposure.

In parallel to these encouraging observations, are the following results which project implications of environmental trends.[20]

1. Rapid increase in coal use will triple sulfur dioxide emissions in southern central U.S. Electric utilities and industrial boilers will generate increased emissions from fossil fuel combustion and offset transportation source reductions.
2. A "greenhouse effect" generated by forecasted increase in carbon dioxide in the atmosphere will probably impact hydrology and agriculture. This is due to deforestation and increased fossil fuel combustion.
3. Hazardous wastes are expected to double in the quarter of a century 1975-2000, causing further land degradation, air and surface water pollution. Prolonged exposure to toxic substances and the finding of residue in human tissue and mother's milk causes concern about continued exposure.

Combined with the above are shortcomings related to inadequate data and methodology used to profile health hazards emanating from exposure to pollutants. Most statistics reporting the impact of regulation are geared to depict decreases in pollution levels without showing their impact upon reducing health hazard. The latency concept in onset of disease further complicates the issue of associating health and environmental data. It is thus very important to utilize as many resources as possible in encouraging collaborative efforts in environmental health risk reduction.

REFERENCES

1. Erickson, M.D., et al., *Preliminary Study on Toxic Chemicals in Environmental and Human Samples. Part II: Protocols for Environmental and Human Sampling and Analysis.* EPA Contract No. 68-01-3849, RTI/1521/00, Washington, D.C.: U.S. Environmental Protection Agency, 1980.
2. National Academy of Sciences, *Report of the Committee for a Planning Study for an Ongoing Study of Costs of Environment-Related Health Effects,* Institute of Medicine Washington, D.C.: 1981. Appendix F prepared by Paul Marks and Robert Murray.
3. Discher, D. P., Raymond, M. A., and Witwer, C. R., "Evaluation of Existing Data Sources of Occupational Injury and Illness Statistics." SRI Project 4434, Stanford, Calif.: Stanford Research Institute, 1976.
4. Lave, Lester B. and Seskin, Eugene P., *Air Pollution and Human Health.* Resources for the Future, Baltimore: Johns Hopkins University Press, 1977.
5. Lake, E., et al., *Classification of American Cities for Case Study Analysis.* EPA-

600/5-77-008 a, b. Washington, D.C.: Office of Research and Development, U.S. Environmental Protection Agency, 1977.

6. Sasnett, Sam K., *A Toxics Primer.* Pub. No. 545, Washington, D.C.: League of Women Voters of the United States, 1979.

7. Council on Environmental Quality, 1978, *Environmental Quality: The Ninth Annual Report of the Council on Environmental Quality.* Washington, D.C.: Executive Office of the President.

8. Heller, S. L., Milne, G. W., and Feldman, R. J., "A Computer-Based Chemical Information System," *Science* 195 (January 21, 1977), pp. 253-259.

9. *NIH/EPA Chemical Information System, User's Guide,* Washington, D.C., Inter-active Sciences Corporation, 1979, p. 1.

10. Domestic Information Display System, *Domestic Information for Decision Making: A New Alternative.* Washington, D.C.: Office of Federal Statistical Policy and Standards, U.S. Department of Commerce, 1979.

11. Mosteller, Frederick and Tukey, John W., *Data Analysis and Regression: A Second Course in Statistics.* Reading, Mass.: Addison-Wesley, 1977.

12. Nie, Norman H. et al., *SPSS: Statistical Package for the Social Sciences.* New York McGraw-Hill, 1975.

13. SAS Institute, Inc., *SAS User's Guide: 1979 Edition.* Raleigh, N.C.: SAS Institute, Inc., 1979.

14. University of California, *BMDP: Biomedical Computer Programs, P Series.* Los Angeles, Calif.: University of California Press, 1977.

15. Slovic, Paul, Fischhoff, Baruch, and Lichtenstein, Sarah, "Rating the Risks." *Environment* 21: 3 (1979), pp. 14-20.

16. Duncan, Laurie and Heatwole, Roy, "A Clearinghouse for Environmental Health Statistics and Information." NCHS Report to the Subcommittee on Environmental Health of the National Committee on Vital and Health Statistics, Washington, D.C., 1980, unpublished.

17. U.S. Department of Health, Education and Welfare, *Healthy People: The Surgeon General's Report on Health Promotion and Disease Prevention,* Washington, D.C.: U.S. Government Printing Office, 1979, p. 7.

18. Slovic, Paul, Fischhoff, Baruch, Lichtenstein, Sarah, "Facts and Fears: Under-standing Perceived Risk," In Richard Schwing and Walter Albers, Jr. (ed), *Societal Risk Assessment: How Safe is Safe Enough?* New York, Plenum Publications, 1980, pp. 181-216.

19. U.S. Environmental Protection Agency, *State of the Environment.* EPA Journal Reprint, Vol. 6, No. 1, Washington, D.C.: Office of Public Awareness, 1980, pp. 32-33.

25. U.S. Environmental Protection Agency, *Environmental Outlook 1980. Summary Report,* EPA 600/8-80-003, Washington, D.C.: Office of Research and Development, December, 1979.

Appendix A

Program Listing

```
.TYPE ARCZ
C      TEST PRGRM FOR THE ARCSIN TRANSFORM
100   FORMAT ( ' TITLE:'$)
       ACCEPT 12,JUNK
10    TYPE 11
11    FORMAT ( ' TYPE P1,P2 :'$)
       ACCEPT 1,P1,P2
```

```
1     FORMAT (2F)
      T1=ASIN(SORT(P1))
      T2=ASIN (SORT(P2))
      TOP=T1-T2
      TYPE 15
15    FORMAT( ' TYPE N1,N2: '$)
      ACCEPT 1,XN1,XN2
      SN1=0.25/XN1
      XN2=0.25/XN2
      BOT=SORT(XN1+XN2)
      Z=TOP/BOT
      TYPE 2,Z
2     FORMAT('   Z=',1F)
      TYPE 3
3     FORMAT ( ' ANY MORE?'$)
      ACCEPT 12,ANS
12    FORMAT (A1)
      IF (ANS.EQ.'Y') GO TO 10
      CALL EXIT
      STOP
      END
```

12 / Nutrition and Risk Reduction

Christopher Hitt, M.S.

OVERVIEW

In the United States health care generally means medical care. Health insurance is in reality disease insurance. Millions of dollars are invested to develop synthetic body parts—hearts, kidneys, arteries—while scant attention is given to keeping the originals in good running order. Billions of dollars are spent annually on sophisticated medical technology directed toward curative and ameliorative care while almost nothing is spent on disease prevention and health promotion. Yet increasingly we are finding that life-style is probably more important to maintaining health than all the medical care that modern medicine can provide. And diet looms large as one of the life-style factors that affects health. In general, the overconsumption of foods high in fats, particularly saturated fat, refined and processed sugars, cholesterol, salt, or alcohol has been associated in varying degrees with the major degenerative illnesses of society.

After introducing a rationale for adopting a population-oriented risk reduction strategy, this chapter focuses on why the strategy is appropriate for attempting to reduce morbidity and mortality from the diet-related killer diseases. It discusses why health professionals should be prepared to respond to the growing public interest in nutrition. It presents the scientific consensus indicating that many Americans are eating themselves to premature illnesses and deaths. It outlines life-long nutrition principles and practices by which Americans can improve their chances of remaining healthy. Its dietary recommendations are not a panacea for all of our ills but could prevent or delay untold personal pain and tragedy. Its message is the value of reducing dietary risks among healthy individuals in order to further the overall objective of staying healthy as late in life as possible.

THE CASE FOR CHANGING THE AMERICAN DIET

The Rationale for Adopting a Population-Oriented Risk Reduction Strategy

Risk reduction is not a new idea. Health practitioners have always sought to lessen or eliminate an individual's risk of illness. When infectious diseases were the scourge of society, health professionals would intervene on a community-wide basis if the majority of the population was determined to be at risk from a particular illness, and significant benefits would result from intervening on a societal scale. Broad-brush, public health interventions, were well accepted and utilized when the causal relationship was determined for a specific disease (diphtheria, smallpox, polio, and others), or when a consensus existed as to the probable cause of a specific illness and its risk factors (cholera, yellow fever, bubonic plague, and so on). Such interventions were not well accepted, and thus rarely were utilized in those instances where neither the causal relationship nor the risk factors had yet been well elucidated. In these cases, it was argued that until more evidence was available, no action should be taken because the risks of intervening were either unknown or were greater than maintaining the status quo. However, the crisis nature and usually epidemic scale of communicable diseases placed great pressure on the take-no-action position.

The need for some kind of intermediate response undoubtedly led to the utilization of a third kind of intervention in which the health care provider, after concluding than an individual was at risk, would recommend a course of action for the individual to reduce the risk factors associated with the already apparent or predicted malady. Such a prescription might carry other risks, but they were of less consequence than the risk from the given illness. This medically oriented, practitioner–patient approach was particularly useful when the low prevalence or incidence of the illness did not create pressure for implementing a communitywide intervention. In such instances this approach could be used even if a clear causal relationship had not yet been determined.

These three modes of intervention, plus ongoing scientific research, achieved great success in reducing and in some cases totally eradicating the acute, communicable diseases as well as the nutrient-deficiency diseases such as scurvy, pellagra, rickets, and beriberi. However, we then found ourselves with the much more difficult task of combating the chronic degenerative diseases, which had become the more prevalent menaces to health. Because these diseases were exceedingly complex in their etiology, had a long developmental time period, and had no known causes, health care providers were forced to look to risk-factor modification as the principal means of attacking them. Even though some degenerative illnesses, such as heart disease, were epidemic in proportion, the lack of a causal relationship or even very well defined risk factors led to the adoption of the medical approach as the principal means to attempt to lessen their incidence. Screening people to assess what, if any, risk factors they might have become the normal practice.

Screening and then counseling only high-risk individuals proved to be an acceptable procedure for many years. But as we continued to fail to find the causes of these diseases, it became apparent that this level of intervention was insufficient. We began to realize that a more aggressive, primary prevention strategy was necessary to help control the degenerative diseases. At the same time, our understanding of risk factors had become more sophisticated, thereby stimulating renewed interest in greater use of risk-reduction methods for the general population.

Unfortunately for the American public, much energy was and continues to be wasted and valuable time lost over needless debate as to whether a public health or a medical intervention strategy should now be used against a particular degenerative disease. Fortunately, meshing the two approaches provides an optimal solution that builds on their complementary strengths and mutes their respective weaknesses. In particular, medicine's orientation towards the individual can result in a tendency to understate the benefits and overstate the risks to *populations*. Public health's population focus can result in a tendency to overstate the benefits and understate the risks for individuals. Therefore, incorporating medical thinking into deliberations on societal interventions directed toward lessening the incidence of chronic degenerative illness ensures that we do not overstate the benefits to the population. Adding in a public health perspective protects us from overstating the risks to the individual. By combining both approaches, it is possible to reach a comfortable middle ground on which to provide sound advice even though a probable cause-and-effect relationship is not yet firmly established. Anyone who follows such advice would incur no known risks. Anyone who is at risk and follows such advice would increase his or her probability of improved protection from a given illness or illnesses.

Adopting this population-oriented strategy acknowledges the value of risk factors in predicting later degenerative illness. It shifts our initial intervention strategy for a degenerative disease, where appropriate, from the individual to the population by addressing life-style changes in all healthy individuals rather than waiting until a particular person has made use of the medical care system and has been identified as exhibiting either specific risk factors or manifest illness. The population-oriented approach to helping to control a degenerative illness provides a primary prevention strategy comparable to our well-established programs for combating infectious and nutrient-deficiency diseases. The next few sections, beginning with diet and the diseases of longevity, will explain why implementing a population-oriented, dietary risk reduction strategy to reduce or delay the incidence of the major diet-related degenerative diseases is in the best interest of the American public and the health profession.

Diet and the Diseases of Longevity

Biomedical research and medical necessity have solved the easy problems. Infectious and nutrient-deficiency diseases are no longer a concern for most Americans. Now we are confronted with the diseases of longevity whose complex etiologies continue to confound our scientists' best attempts to determine definitive cause-and-effect relationships for these plagues on our society. Millions of dollars, thousands of scientist man-years, and decades of research have, however, provided much greater insights into the risk factors associated with most of these diseases. In fact, modification of the known primary risk factors—high blood cholesterol, high blood pressure, and smoking—has contributed to the dramatic decline over the last 10 years in mortality from the number-one killer of Americans—heart disease.[1] But even with this good news, we have made almost no headway against reducing the overall mortality from our major causes of death. With respect to those illnesses for which diet is a factor, mortality statistics indicate that six out of ten Americans die from such illnesses.[2] These are heart disease, some cancers, stroke and hypertension, diabetes, and cirrhosis of the liver.

These are diseases that develop slowly over many years and then cripple or kill, frequently without any warning. These are diseases for which no lasting cure has been found. These are diseases that swallow most of the dollars expended on costly medical care. But these diseases are not an inevitable fact of aging. These diseases are not necessarily the fate of nations that have eradicated deaths from infectious illnesses. These are not diseases that we must simply expect as a concomitant of increased longevity and affluence. Dr. Theodore Cooper, the assistant secretary of health under the Ford administration, in testimony in 1976 to the Senate Select Committee on Nutrition and Human Needs, said:

> Many of today's health problems are caused by a variety of factors not susceptible to medical solutions or to direct intervention by the health provider.
> While scientists do not yet agree on the specific causal relationships, evidence is mounting and there appears to be general agreement that the kinds and amounts of food and beverages we consume and the style of living common in our generally af-

fluent, sedentary society may be the major factors associated with the causes of cancer, cardiovascular disease, and other chronic illnesses.[2]

Statements like Dr. Cooper's have become increasingly more common. Once again we are beginning to appreciate that the true advances in the overall health of the nation have come from preventing illness rather than from either curing or more often only ameliorating our physical maladies.

At the same time Americans have never been healthier. Our nation's increased longevity is given as an indication of how healthy Americans are, often implying that we should be thankful and satisfied with our good fortune. However, our lengthened life span is primarily a result of the dramatic decline in the infant mortality rate in the twentieth century. It is important to recognize that the life expectancy of an adult in the United States has remained essentially the same throughout this century. For example, in 1900 a man aged 40 could expect to live on average 31.2 years longer, whereas in 1970 a man aged 40 could expect to live 31.7 years longer.[3] Most important of all is that a long life is much less enjoyable if one is stricken with heart disease at 55, diabetes at 40, or nondeath-dealing but constantly aggravating afflictions such as arthritis or osteoporosis before age 50.

A long life span should not be the acknowledged standard. Rather an overall, measureable improvement in the quality of our basic health indexes particularly among older Americans, should be the measure of excellence for this country. If our past record is any indication of the potential for achieving such a quality standard in a health care system that is dominated by medical care and curative methods that attempt to restore an individual's health, then it is apparent that national priorities for enhancing the health of all Americans must be realigned to include greater emphasis on preventing disease by promoting health.

In striving to alter health care priorities, whether it concerns national health insurance, or the adoption of the most healthful dietary pattern that this country's farmers and food processors can produce, the final decision must depend on the evidence at hand. Unfortunately, because we still have an incomplete understanding of the possible causes of our major killing diseases, determining the best course of action to reduce the risk of these diseases can be a difficult and controversial endeavor. This is compounded even further when diet is a risk factor because we still have much more to learn about nutrition as it relates to maintaining health. Nevertheless, the failure to solve the degenerative diseases in our society, in conjunction with the prevalence and extremely long developmental time frame for these illnesses, has lent greater urgency to modifying those risk factors, including diet, that are strongly associated with our principal causes of death. In 1979 Dr. Donald Fredrickson, the director of the National Institutes of Health, said with respect to the diet and health issue:

> We've more or less become adjusted to the fact that we probably will never be able to get the ideal proof that we want. . . . The weight of the evidence seems to be strong enough so that we can now direct people toward a kind of set of guidelines.[4]

The Evolution of Dietary Guidance

For the first half of this century, nutrition scientists spent most of their time discovering what nutrients were essential for maintaining an individual's health. To apply their findings meant basically that each individual should eat a varied diet that r vided sufficient energy, protein, vitamins, and minerals. This concern was incorporated into national priorities in the 1940s with the establishment of the Recommended Dietary Allowances (RDA) by the Food and Nutrition Board of the National Academy of Sciences:

> Recommended Dietary Allowances (RDA) are the levels of intake of essential nutrients considered, in the judgment of the Committee on Dietary Allowances of the Food and Nutrition Board on the basis of available scientific knowledge, to be adequate to meet the known nutritional needs of practically all healthy persons.
>
> RDA are recommendations for the average daily amounts of nutrients that population groups should consume over a period of time. RDA should not be confused with requirements for a specific individual. Differences in the nutrient requirements of individuals are ordinarily unknown. Therefore, RDA (except for energy) are estimated to exceed the requirements of most individuals and thereby to insure that the needs of nearly all in the population are met.[5]

Quite clearly the RDA was established as a public health approach for preventing the recurrence of the known nutrient deficiency diseases such as pellagra, rickets, and scurvy.

Scientists throughtout this century also were discovering that many of our chronic degenerative diseases were associated with our dietary pattern, and the association had nothing to do with the traditional nutrient-deficiency diseases we had already conquered. Furthermore, because the origins of these diseases were far from understood, how to attack them was a much more complicated problem. Rather than apply a public health approach to these diseases, initially the medical approach of recommending that only high-risk individuals should alter their diet was used. As a cause-and-effect relationship continued to elude us, and as we ascertained that diet was a risk factor for some of the chronic degenerative illnesses, the public health approach was put forward once again as being potentially a more appropriate intervention strategy.

Which intervention strategy to follow became a matter of national inportance when the Senate Select Committee on Nutrition and Human Needs published in 1977 the report, *Dietary Goals for the United States*. In the foreword, Senator George McGovern said:

> The purpose of this report is to point out that the eating patterns of this century represent as critical a public health concern as any now before us.
>
> We must acknowledge and recognize that the public is confused about what to eat to maximize health. If we as a Government want to reduce health costs and maximize the quality of life for all Americans, we have an obligation to provide practical guides to the individual consumer as well as set national dietary goals for the country as a whole.
>
> These recommendations, based on current scientific evidence, provide guidance for making personal decisions about one's diet. They are not a legislative iniative. Rather, they simply provide nutrition knowledge with which Americans can begin to take responsibility for maintaining their health and reducing their risk of illness.[6]

This report extended the concept of the RDA to include carbohydrates, fats, sodium, and cholesterol. By providing dietary guidance for both micro- and macronutrients, the committee believed the American people would be in an even better position to develop sound food use practices. The report outlined for the first time at the federal level a population-oriented intervention strategy to combat some of society's major killers.

Its publication created great controversy and allegations that such a course of action was premature. The public debate initiated by the Dietary Goads report was further enflammed by the subsequent release of two similar and yet also conflicting sets of dietary advice. The first was the report released in February 1980 by the Departments of Agriculture (USDA) and Health and Human Services (HHS) entitled, *Nutrition and Your Health, Dietary Guidelines for Americans.*[7] The second was the May 1980 report, *Toward Healthful Diets* published by the Food and Nutrition Board of the National Academy of Sciences.[8]

The two reports advised Americans to eat a variety of foods; to maintain an ideal body weight; to avoid too much sodium; and to moderate alcohol intake. But with respect to the appropriate amounts of fat, cholesterol, and carbohydrates in the diet, they parted ways. Specifically, USDA and HHS suggested that the general public should avoid too much fat, cholesterol, and sugar and increase the amount of complex carbohydrates. The Food and Nutrition Board said that only people at risk for heart disease should worry about cholesterol; only obese individuals and those at risk of heart disease should be concerned about fat; and only diabetics should be concerned about fat and the mix of sugars and complex carbohydrates. Fluoride would protect us from dental caries that could result from sugar consumption.

Since both bodies examined the same scientific evidence, the key question to be asked is why are there differences in their recommendations? Undoubtedly there are many factors that affected the two sets of recommendations, not the least of which the personal biases of the various individuals involved. One major factor that helps to explain the discrepancies is the different assumptions on which the authors based their respective reports. Whereas the two government departments employed a population-oriented strategy, the Food and Nutrition Board's findings were apparently derived from a medically oriented perspective. Whereas the government looked at the total population and what could be done to improve the health of the aggregate person, the board approached the matter clinically as a physician treating a single patient.

More specifically, the Food and Nutrition Board found the evidence regarding the benefits of altering an individual's diet to be less than convincing. USDA and HHS, after examing the scientific evidence, assumed change was beneficial to the population if no risks to the individual might result from making a modest dietary shift. Most simply stated, the Food and Nutrition Board appeared to have concluded that if it isn't indisputably broken, then don't try to fix it. The government said, since the ponderance of the evidence indicates it's going to break unless some action is taken, then let's offer guidance that could prevent or delay its breaking. Thus, because of the lack of a casual relationship for the diet-regulated degenerative diseases, we are faced with a dispute over at what point and to what extent dietary intervention is appropriate. Further evaluation of the possible reasoning behind the conclusions of the two reports will provide additional insights to this dispute.

With respect to the USDA/HHS Dietary Guidelines, I would suggest that the question asked of each guideline was what are the risks to the individual from making such a recommendation to the general public? Obviously, counseling everyone to eat a variety of foods, maintain ideal body weight, and moderate the intake of alcohol poses no known health risks. Avoiding excess sodium intake is more questionable, but since Americans eat daily an average of 20 times the required intake of sodium, reduced sodium consumption would appear to be a risk-free recommendation.

The same reasoning could apply to fat intake since we require only 1 to 2 per cent of our calories to consist of essential fatty acids, but we consume currently about 40 per cent of our total calories as fat. With respect to cholesterol, because the body normally manufacturers all the cholesterol it requires to function, it is not necessary to eat cholesterol to remain healthy.

If one decides to reduce fat and cholesterol intake, then one must examine the sources of these dietary constituents to determine if reduced consumption would have any negative nutritional effects. Foods from animal sources are the major contributors of cholesterol and fat, particularly saturated fat, in our diet. But they also are our primary sources of protein. Since Americans eat on average about twice the daily requirement for protein, a reduction in animal protein that might result from a reduction in fat and cholesterol would carry no risk.

How about the vitamins and minerals that would be lost if animal protein foods were modestly reduced? Some, if not all, as well as some protein, would be replaced bu the increased consumption of complex carbohydrates as recommended in the USDA/HHS Dietary Guidelines. Finally, since refined and processed sugars provide nothing but calories, a modest reduction in their intake would present no risks either.

In analyzing *Toward Healthful Diets*, one finds that its conclusions reflect the predominant clinical orientation that pervades the report. Specifically, although, the amount of biomedical research is negligble on which to base such recommendations, a clinician knows from experience that ideal weight and modest alcohol intake are healthy for a patient. obtaining sufficient vitamins, minerals, and protein is essential to good health and can be achieved if a patient eats a variety of foods. A patient who is on a weight-reduction regimen needs to alter his or her food intake, particularly with respect to highly caloric but nutrient-scarce components such as fats, sugars, and alcohol. Cholesterol consumption is not a consideration in treating obesity, whereas increased exercise will help burn off excess calories in the diet. Finally, while the evidence is quite meager, the clinical findings do support the efficacy without risk of reduced salt intake in lowering blood pressure.

Therefore, while weight control, modest alcohol intake, and reduced sodium consumption are all population-oriented recommendations, these recommendations, like the Food and Nutrition Board's RDA, were principally based on clinical practice, and basic research demonstrating that benefits *will result* without any attendant risks. Even though the preponderance of the scientific evidence indicates that benefits without any risks also *may result* from a reduced consumption of fats, cholesterol, and refined sugars, the board found the clinical evidence insufficient for making these additonal population-oriented diet recommendations. Instead, they fell back to the medical intervention strategy of prescribing dietary modification where appropriate for each individual who comes into contact with the medical care system. That the board generally prefers the medical intervention strategy is exemplified in the following first sentence from the chapter "Decision-making in Public Health":

> Good public health practice depends upon the application of sound principles of *preventive medicine to* population groups.[8]

If a public health intervention strategy were the objective of this report, then I suggest this sentence would have read as follows:

> Good public health practice depends upon the application of sound principles of *health maintenance and promotion by* population groups.

In the first sentence, the practitioner–patient approach is apparent, whereas in the second, educating people to care for themselves is the message.

Overall, then, it is not surprising that the Food and Nutrition Board reached the conclusions spelled out in *Toward Healthful Diets*. However, given the increasing public demand for nutrition advice, it is imperative that we reconcile conflicting viewpoints on what is the most appropriate dietary advice for the general public. Until we do, people will continue to be confused by the inconsistent nutrition signals coming from its most trusted sources of health advice. The population-oriented strategy provides the opportunity to achieve just such a reconciliation.

Increased Public Interest in Nutrition

The 1970s has seen an upsurge of public interest in nutrition. A 1980 survey conducted by Yankelovich, Skelly, and White found that 72 per cent of those surveyed were more concerned about nutrition than they had been 5 years ago.[9] Another 1980 survey undertaken for *Self Magazine* found that 50 per cent of U.S. women had a greater interest in nutrition compared to 3 years earlier.[10]

The public has become aware that during this centrury there has in effect been an ongoing experiment with the American diet. As food availability and variety has increased, our diet has gone through a marked evolution. In the early 1900s fruits, vegetables, and grain products were the mainstay of the diet. Fats and refined and processed sugars provided only 40 per cent of our total caloric intake.

Today 60 per cent of total calories are obtained from fats and refined and processed sugars. Processed foods and food products now contribute over half of the dietary intake. Ironically, in a world where the word malnutrition has always brought forth images of hungry, often starving people, Americans are faced with a new form of malnutrition that may partially result from our success in making food so abundant.

The following two tables from *The Changing American Diet*, document the kind of shift that has occurred.[11]

The surveys also have found that the vast majority of Americans are not well-informed about nutrition. Furthermore, partly because of their lack of knowledge, the public has come to question and even have some fears about the food supply. That such fears exist is indicated by the fact that one out of two Americans today think chemical food additives are a major cause of cancer.

One reason the American people have fears about their food supply is because nutrition science cannot provide them with the kind of precise answers that they want and have come to expect from science. But they still want advice, which explains why the *National Enquirer* now carries more stories on food, nutrition, and health than on sex. Both the Yankelovich and *Self Magazine* surveys found that magazines and newspapers were the main source of nutrition information. Health professionals, particularly physicians, were ranked second in the Yankelovich report and fourth in the *Self Magazine* study.

The public is looking more to the media and books precisely because they believe that health professionals are not giving them useful advice. Simply reassuring someone about his or her diet is not nearly sufficient when the media are constantly providing a smorgasbord of so-called dietary wisdom. In general the public no longer wants to be told what to do. Instead they want meaningful recommendations on which to base their own dietary decisions.

The reluctance of health professionals to adopt a population-oriented risk reduction approach encourages the proliferation of misleading and, unfortunately, at times, harmful diet advice, which partially explains why we continue to have a multibillion-dollar a year "diet of the week," "miracle cure" business. Most important, those at greatest risk from all types of malnutrition, the poor people of this country, receive their di-

TABLE 1. Changes in Food Consumption

Food		Change in ·Consumption per Person (Percent)
Apples, fresh	1910 to 1976	-70
Beef	1910 to 1976	+72
	1950 to 1976	+90
Butter	1910 to 1976	-76
Cabbage, fresh	1920 to 1976	-65
Candy	1968 to 1976	-18
Chicken	1910 to 1976	+179
Coffee	1910 to 1976	+22
	1946 to 1976	-44
Corn syrup	1960 to 1976	+224
Fish, fresh and frozen	1960 to 1976	+42
Food colors (certified dyes)	1940 to 1977	+995
Fruit, fresh	1910 to 1976	-33
Grapefruit, fresh	1910 to 1976	+800
Margarine	1910 to 1976	+681
Potatoes, fresh	1910 to 1976	-74
Potatoes, frozen	1960 to 1976	+465
Soft drinks	1960 to 1976	+157
Sugar and other caloric sweetners	1909 to 1976	+33
Tuna, canned	1926 to 1976	+1,300
Turkey	1910 to 1976	+820
Vegetables, frozen	1960 to 1976	+44
Wheat flour (including flour used in bread, spaghetti, etc.)	1910 to 1976	-48

TABLE 2. Changes in Nutrient Consumption

Nutrients		Change in Consumption per Person (Percent)
Calories	1910 to 1976	-3
Fat	1910 to 1976	+28
Carbohydrates	1910 to 1976	-21
Protein	1910 to 1976	+1
Dietary fat from separated fats and oils (butter, margarine, oil, etc.)	1921 to 1976	+56
Grams of carbohydrates from sugars	1909–13 to 1976	+31
Grams of carbohydrates from starches	1909–13 to 1976	-45

etary advice from the media because they cannot afford to go to a health professional. As long as we insist on screening people for dietary risk factors, rather than applying a population-oriented intervention, millions of poor Americans will not receive adequate nutrition information.

Respect for the health professional can only be increased by an honest straightforward presentation of the facts, the controversies, and the risk-reduction possibilities that might result from a modified diet. The American people are not gullible enough to think that immortality can be achieved through diet modification. They are savvy enough to understand that diet alteration can only change the probabilities of later illness but can not guarantee improved protection. Thus, no one is going to suggest, because risk modification is possible, that we should cut back on research and simply declare victory against our major killing diseases.

On the other hand, there is a real potential for a loss of credibility to the profession by continuing with the current diet and health advice. For example, seeking to modify risk factors after they are apparent for diseases that take 20 to 30 years to develop is not particularly useful. Even more absurd, though, is to recommend a modest 5 to 10 per cent reduction in dietary fat consumption, plus reduced cholesterol and sodium consumption once a person has heart disease. If all the clinical and animal research to date has taught us anything, it should be that such a minor diet modification, which can create unrealistic expectations, is a cruel hoax on anyone who already has heart disease.

The Yankelovich, *Self Magazine* and other surveys indicate clearly that Americans will be seeking more dietary advice in the 1980s, and health professionals will be asked for their counsel. However, the stark reality is that most health professionals receive inadequate nutrition training. Even the registered dietitian is generally unprepared to address the primary focus of this chapter—reducing risk among healthy individuals in order to prevent or at least delay serious and often chronic afflictions.

Thus we are caught in a dilemma. On the one hand, because health professionals so affect public opinion, our devaluation of nutrition is harmful to the health of the American people. On the other hand, as people renew their commitment to more healthful practices, health professionals' disregard of nutrition may cause a loss of the respect now accorded our profession by the public.

A resolution of this dilemma is possible by adopting a population-oriented strategy to help reduce those risk factors in the diet that appear to contribute to our degenerative diseases. Accepting such a population-oriented strategy not only will help all Americans, it should also provide the impetus to develop and implement relevant and practical nutrition programs as part of the core, and clinical curricula of the various schools that train health professionals. The need for such training has been the topic of countless conferences for at least 20 years and has been documented in hearings before the Senate.[12] However, to date little has been accomplished principally because most health professionals have not yet been convinced of the importance of nutrition to their practice.

While many factors have contributed to our marginal interest in nutrition, two in particular are at the crux of the matter. The first is the relative lack of knowledge about the complex diet and health relationships as compared with the levels of knowledge in the other medical specialties. The second is that the direction and character of our medically dominated health care system pushes health professionals toward viewing the world from a clinical/treatment orientation. But nutrition is primarily a means by which the individual can take some responsibility for preventing illness by establishing health-promoting dietary practices in his or her everyday life. As a result of these two factors, nutrition has continued to play a very small part in the practice of medicine. Nevertheless, when it is a matter of health, the public prefers to takes its cues from health professionals, and health professionals prefer to offer advice based upon at least a scientific consensus.

The Scientific Basis of Consensus

Obviously in the short space provided in this chapter, it is not possible to lay out the kind of documentation that one would find in reports such as the Ninth Edition (1980) of the Food and Nutrition Board's *Recommended Dietary Allowances*, or the Select Committee's *Dietary Goals for the United States*. It is useful to know, though, that since the late 1960s, 17 scientific bodies from around the world have made dietary recommendations similar to those in the Dietary Goals Report.[13] Even more useful with respect to the question of scientific consensus is the 1978 study by the American Society for Clinical Nutrition (ASCN). The ASCN, which is one of our most pretigious bodies of clinical nutrition scientists, spent a year and a half analyzing the scientific data regarding six components of the nation's diet to determine if a consensus message about diet and health could be developed. The six components studied included fat, cholesterol, carbohydrates, calories, alcohol, and sodium. In the introduction to its report, *The Evidence Relating Six Dietary Factors to the Nation's Health*, Dr. E. H. Ahrens explained the reasoning behind the report's existence:

> Public policy relating to alterations in established patterns in the nation's food intake is made by government officials guided by their perception of the relevant body of scientific information. Unfortunately, this process of communication between scientists and government officials often takes the form of an advocacy proceeding in which interested scientists, either in oral or written testimony, put forth those elements of the total body of data that support the change in public policy that they favor.
>
> In order to produce a series of documents that would present the basic facts a about several issues that relate to the role of nutrition in the nation's health, the American Society for Clinical Nutrition (ASCN) . . . . undertook this mission so as to ensure that such documents would avoid the advocacy role and would constitute a consensus that would be of help to public officials in formulating national nutrition policy.
>
> It was evident from the start that there are important limitations to this process. It is clear that the scientists with sufficient involvement in these issues to produce such documents have developed their own biases about the data and have strong feelings about the type and degree of intervention in this area that would be of most value to the population. It is hoped that, by having on the committee individuals with a full range of convictions, a consensus document could be produced that would not be dominated by a single point of view.[14]

The ASCN report provides six consensus statements plus numerical ratings of the degree of consensus on ten diet and health associations. Those ratings are as follows in Table 3.

The nine scientists chosen by the council of the ASCN to prepare the report weighed the evidence on each issue in relation to the following five categories:

> For this evaluation the evidence on each issue was weighed in still another manner than by kinds and quality, namely:
>
> 1. Associations among various population groups.

TABLE 3.   ASCN Ratings of the Degree of Consensus on Ten
Diet and Health Associations

Issue	Mean Score	Standard Deviation
1. Cholesterol	62	20
2. Saturated fat	58	15
3. Cholesterol and fat	73	15
4. Carbohydrate and atherosclerosis	11	8
5. Carbohydrate and diabetes	13	17
6. Carbohydrate and dental caries	87	6
7. Alcohol and liver disease	88	8
8. Alcohol and atherosclerosis	13	15
9. Salt	74	9
10. Excess calories	68	18

2. Associations among individuals within a given population. In each of these two categories, the net weight of the evidence was considered in terms of consistency, autopsy data, strength and independence of the association, temporal association, and effect of new exposure.
3. Intervention studies. In this category, all available evidence was assessed in terms of preventive and improvement effects of removal, i.e., an evaluation of the results obtained in primary and in secondary prevention studies.
4. Animal models.
5. Biological explanation.[14]

The maximum score that could be assigned to a category was 20 points. A score of 100 would indicate total agreement that the dietary factor is associated with a particular disease. A score of 0 would indicate total agreement that the dietary factor is *not* associated with a particular disease. The panel of nine scientists in its introduction emphasized that the rating system was arbitrary, and that different weights could be assigned to each of the five categories depending upon the relative importance or value one wished to place on each category. Nevertheless, the introduction concluded by indicating that it was the panel's hope that this approach might serve as a model for other interactions between scientists, the government, and the public.

The ASCN methodology clearly demonstrates that the medical bias toward placing greater value on clinical evidence can be balanced against the tendency of public health practitioners to overvalue epidemiological findings. Furthermore, because of its design and choice of diverse viewpoints, the ASCN study is the best indication that substantial scientific consensus does exist regarding the degree of dietary association between certain dietary factors and health status.

Scientific Consensus Does Not Ensure That the Same Intervention Strategy Will Be Employed

Notwithstanding the existence of a scientific consensus, the lack of a causal relationship for a given illness can result in different groups proposing different intervention strategies. For example, the ASCN report reached the same degree of consensus for fat and cholesterol (73 per cent) and sodium (74 per cent), and a slightly lower degree of consensus on excess calories (68 per cent). Nevertheless, the Food and Nutrition Board, which has members who also belong to the ASCN, including the chariman of the board, Dr. Alfred Harper, and the principal author of *Toward Healthful Diets*, Dr. Robert Olson, made population-oriented recommendations for sodium and obesity but not for fat and cholesterol.

Even when there is a scientific consensus, lack of a causal relationship can also provide the smoke screen of "scientific controversy" behind which scientists and health professionals can hide. All too frequently this smoke screen is employed effectively by food interests in their efforts to maintain the status quo. The meat, egg, and sugar industries have used "scientific controversy" as a means of attacking the Dietary Goals report. The USDA/HHS Dietary Guidelines, which initially were criticized in some quarters for saying nothing new and for being nonspecific, also have come under attack from agricultural groups. *Toward Healthful Diets* has been a valuable weapon to create the appearance that the USDA/HHS Dietary Guidelines do not represent a scientific consensus.

It makes sense that a small or even large farmer who specializes in a few products should worry that any decline in consumption of these products could put him or her out of business. Nevertheless, like those health professionals who do not yet see that simply waiting for risk factors to manifest themselves before taking action is shortsighted, farmers could benefit from a longer term perspective. Dr. Theodore Cooper provided that vital insight in the following statement made at a 1978 hearing before the Senate Nutrition Subcommittee:

> Somehow there is a widespread feeling, probably fostered by the good and sometimes zealous intentions of various advocates, that change of dietary habits must be rapid, or at least as rapid as possible. This conjures up images of dietary changes drastically imposed or taking place over a few months of intensified campaigns. To me it is clear that changes in dietary patterns are likely to develop in rather slow trends, over periods of several years, in a dynamic interplay of educational pressures, food demand shifts, production incentives and regulatory policies. The long time required for this process is likely to give ample opportunity for policy corrections in mid-course, persuasive behavioral changes, and changes in food production practices that should not cause economic disruption.[15]

The responsibility of the government was aptly presented in the preface of the Second Edition of *Dietary Goals for the United States:*

> Nutrition and health considerations must be in the forefront of the development of this Nation's agriculture and food policy. In accepting such a policy position, instead of ignoring or clouding the scientific facts in order to prevent any shift in the economic status quo, we must be willing to make economic and market adjustments to meet the scientific evidence that will, or probably will provide improved health benefits to the Nation.[6]

It is time that we, as health professionals, begin to exercise our critical cultural role as health advisors. We need to understand that simply opting to hide behind "scientific controversy," either by doing nothing until there is unequivocal evidence or simply treating and counseling those who can afford medical care, is an inadequate response to coping with those chronic degenerative diseases that are linked to our diet. We need to recognize that when there is a scientific consensus, our willingness to hide behind "scientific controversy" allows powerful food producers and processors to use that smoke screen to protect their economic interests to the detriment of the nation as a whole. In order to act responsibly, we need to implement a population-oriented risk reduction agenda to help prevent or delay the diet-related degenerative illnesses.

A DIET TO KEEP US HEALTHY AS LATE
IN LIFE AS POSSIBLE

A diet to keep healthy people healthy must be based on the principles of variety, moderation, and balance if it is to be successful in reducing dietary risks while also maximizing the pleasure of eating. Even before the science of nutrition was born, having a variety of foods in the diet was most likely important because it provided greater enjoyment, and it helped increase the probability that sufficient food would be available. As nutrition scientists began to learn about the vital links between nutrients and human health, variety was reaffirmed as a critical principle.

When we became successful in producing an abundance of food, and our caloric requirements were reduced as a result of our becoming a more sedentary society, obesity became a significant problem. As a result, moderation in food intake in order to balance energy intake and expenditure was added to the first principle of variety. Today nutrition science appears to be ready to recognize fully the third dietary principle—balance. Most simply stated, *excesses as well as deficiencies* of nutrient intake must be considered as potentially damaging to human health.

Balanced diets have long been standard jargon, but a full appreciation of the term from a scientific perspective has yet to take hold. A lengthy discussion of the balance principle is not possible in this chapter, but a couple of points should be made. First, adoption of the balance principle not only can be a boon for nutrition research, but it also can provide nutrition science with the critical, all-encompassing concept it has lacked up until now. Second, its value lies in the ability to acknowledge that there is probably no one perfect diet but that we can better understand how diet affects our health if we recognize that the more out of balance one major element is, the greater the shifts that must occur in other elements to compensate. For example, because some types of fiber affect fat and cholesterol absorption, raising fiber intake might compensate for a higher fat and cholesterol diet. Similarly, a higher protein intake requires greater calcium consumption. Thus the principle of balance underscores the importance of viewing a diet in its totality and recognizing that each modification will affect the impact of other elements in a diet.

The establishment of the Dietary Goals was the first government attempt to examine the total diet and set forth recommendations that would provide greater direction than simply the words variety, moderation, and balance. The USDA/HHS Dietary Guidelines was the second such attempt. However, unlike the Dietary Goals, they had no specific numbers such as 30 per cent of calories from fat to 10 per cent calories from refined sugars but only suggested that too much fat, cholesterol, sugar, and salt are not conducive to optimum health. The same general approach to making diet recommendations was used in October 1979, when Dr. Arthur Upton, then director of the National Cancer Institute (NCI), set forth the following Diet and Cancer Principles:

1. Maintain optimal body weight
2. Eat a lower fat diet
3. Eat a higher fiber diet
4. Eat a balanced diet in order to ensure adequate intake of vitamins and minerals, without needing additional supplementation
5. Moderate consumption of alcohol[16]

The recommendations provided here represent a combination of the Dietary Goals report, the NCI Diet and Cancer Principles, and the USDA/HHS Dietary Guidelines.

They are not therapeutic. They are not a panacea or the key to immortality. They cannot guarantee that an individual who follows them will never experience a disease that is associated with either a nutrient excess or deficiency. They simply increase the probability of improved protection from such diseases. Children under age 2, pregnant women, and the elderly are subgroups in the population who should be given additional nutritional guidance.

Individuals who already are afflicted by an illness require special nutritional care. For example, the Longevity Center in Santa Monica, California has employed what to most Americans would be an austere diet regimen as part of its treatment for heart disease, diabetes, and other chronic illnesses. The caloric composition of the diet is 80 per cent complex carbohydrates, 10 per cent fat, and 10 per cent protein. Apparently the center's highly motivated patients find the diet to be reasonable. In addition some Americans who don't have a chronic illness are adopting the center's diet, which has been popularized in the very successful book, *The Pritikin Program for Diet and Exercise*.[17] While eating the Pritikin diet may prove to be very healthy, consuming such a diet probably is not necessary if one's lifelong dietary pattern is similar to the following risk-reduction diet:

RISK-REDUCTION DIET

1. Maintain ideal weight.
2. Increase the consumption of complex carbohydrates and "naturally occurring"* sugars to about 50 per cent of total calories.
3. Reduce the consumption of refined and processed sugars, including alcohol, to about 10 per cent of total calories.**
4. Reduce overall fat consumption to about 30 per cent of total calories, and reduce saturated fat intake to account for no more than 10 per cent of total calories.
5. Reduce cholesterol intake to a level of 300 mg or less a day.
6. Limit the intake of sodium by consuming no more than 5 gm of salt a day.

Meeting these guidelines or goals requires the following shifts in food consumption patterns:

1. Increase consumption of fruits, vegetables, and whole grains.
2. Decrease consumption of refined and other processed sugars and foods high in such sugars.
3. Decrease consumption of foods high in total fat, particularly saturated fat, by reducing the portions consumed of these foods high in total fat and substituting lower fat alternatives such as lean meats, poultry or fish, or low-fat and nonfat dairy products.
4. Decrease consumption of foods high in cholesterol by reducing the portions consumed of those foods high in cholesterol such as egg yolks and organ meats.
5. Decrease consumption of sodium and foods high in sodium content, and reduce the use of salt to season foods in the home, both in the kitchen and at the table.

*"Naturally occurring" sugars that are indigenous to a food as opposed to refined (cane and beet) and processed (corn sugar, syrups, molasses, and honey) sugars that may be added to a food product.
**Alcoholic beverages affect the diet in much the same way as refined and other processed sugars. Both add calories but contribute little or no vitamins or minerals.

Although these shifts in consumption patterns are quite moderate, a healthy person should not expect to make them all at once or overnight. Because a healthy person is not in immediate risk of illness, he or she has the luxury of making these kinds of diet alterations more gradually. By so doing, one is more likely to continue to follow the new diet. Of course such advice can become an excuse to do nothing, but that is each person's free choice. Our only responsibility as health professionals is to convey clearly the reasons for a healthy person to lessen his or her dietary risks, and to provide assistance, if asked, in making the suggested dietary changes. For example, it will be necessary to provide information about the specific kinds of food that should be increased or decreased. In addition, some people, because of allergies or simply because they want to lessen their risk of illness even further, will want information about food additives, particularly those that are nonessential or possibly carcinogenic. It will also be necessary to encourage people to read food labels carefully in order to identify food additives and hidden sources of fats, sugars, and sodium.

The following list of materials would be useful resources for all health professionals:

Dietary Goals for the United States, 2nd ed.
Senate Select Committee on Nutrition and Human Needs
December 1977
Stock No. 052-070-04376-8.

Food, A Publication on Food and Nutrition
U.S. Department of Agriculture, Home and Garden Bulletin no. 228, Science and Education Administration, 1979
Stock No. 001-000-03881-8

Healthy People: The Surgeon General's Report on Health Promotion and Disease Prevention
Public Health Service, Department of Health and Human Services, 1979
Stock No. 017-001-00416-2.

To obtain copies of these three publications, write to:
Superintendent of Documents
U.S. Government Printing Office
Washington, D.C. 20402.

Nutrition and Your Health, Dietary Guidelines for Americans
USDA/HHS
(Copies can be obtained from either department).

Jane Brody's Nutrition Book
Jane E. Brody
W.W. Norton
New York, N.Y. 1981

Recommended Dietary Allowances
Food and Nutrition Board, 1980
(Copies are available from the office of Publications, National Academy of Sciences, 2101 Constitution Ave., N.W., Washington, D.C. 20418.)

Nutrition Scores: a chart and booklet that provides nutrient density information on almost all basic foods. (Copies are available from the Basic and Traditional Food Association, 1707 "N" Street, N.W., Washington, D.C. 20036.)

A useful book for information about sodium in foods is the *Brand Name Nutrition Counter* by Jean Carper, New York: Bantam Books, 1975.

The Changing American Diet
Letitia Brewster and Michael Jacobson, Ph. D.
Center for Science in the Public Interest, 1978

Jack Sprat's Legacy: The Science and Politics of Fat and Cholesterol
Patricia Hausman, M.S.
Center for Science in the Public Interest
Richard Marek (publisher), 1981

To obtain copies of these publications, write to:
Center for Science in the Public Interest*
1755 "S" Street, N.W.
Washington, D.C. 20009.

In conclusion, by actively implementing a dietary risk reduction strategy for the diet-related degenerative diseases, we can counter many of the existing fears about the food supply and one's diet. In turn, we encourage the public to adopt sensible living habits that could protect them from unnecessary risks which may contribute to an untimely illness or death.

*Editor's Note: The Center for Science in the Public Interest is one of the most active groups in the country in focusing public attention on important issues in consumer health and safety.

REFERENCES

1. Committee on Agriculture, Nutrition, and Forestry, U.S. Senate, *Hearing on Heart Disease: Public Health Enemy No. 1*. Washington, D.C.: U.S. Government Printing Office, May 22, 1979.
2. Select Committee on Nutrition and Human Needs, U.S. Senate, *Hearing on Diet Related to Killer Diseases*, Vol. I. Washington, D.C.: U.S. Government Printing Office, July 27–28, 1976.
3. Blackburn, H., *Progress in the Epidemiology and Prevention of Coronary Heart Disease*, P. N. Yu and J. F. Goodwin, eds. New York: Lea & Febiger, 1974, chap 3.
4. Broad, W. J., "NIH Deals Gingerly with Diet-Disease Link." *Science* 204 (June 1979), pp. 1175–1178.
5. Food and Nutrition Board, National Research Council, *Recommended Dietary Allowances*, 9th ed. Washington, D.C.: National Academy of Sciences, 1980.
6. Select Committee on Nutrition and Human Needs, U.S. Senate, *Dietary Goals for the United States*, 2nd ed. Washington, D.C.: U.S. Government Printing Office, December 1977.
7. U.S. Department of Agriculture and U.S. Department of Health and Human Services, *Nutrition and Your Health, Dietary Guidelines for Americans*. Washington, D.C.: U.S. Government Printing Office, 1980.
8. Food and Nutrition Board, National Research Council, *Toward Healthful Diets*. Washington, D.C.: National Academy of Sciences, 1980.
9. Yankelovich, Skelly, and White, *Nutrition vs. Inflation: The Battle of the Eighties*. New York: Woman's Day, 1980.

10. Mark Clements Research, Inc., *Trends in Nutrition*, New York: Self Magazine, 1980.
11. Brewster, L. and Jacobson, M., *The Changing American Diet*. Washington, D.C.: Center for Science in the Public Interest, 1978.
12. Committee on Agriculture, Nutrition, and Forestry, *Hearings on Nutrition Education in Medical Schools*. Washington, D.C.: U.S. Government Printing Office, Part I, September 20, 1978; Part II, January 30, 1979.
13. Turner, R. W. D., "Perspectives in Coronary Prevention." *Postgraduate Medical Journal* 54 (1978), pp. 141–148.
14. Ahrens, E. A., "Introduction to the Report of the Task Force on the Evidence Relating Six Dietary Factors to the Nation's Health." *American Journal of Clinical Nutrition, and Supplement* 32:12 (December 1979).
15. Committee on Agriculture, Nutrition, and Forestry, *Hearing on Nutrition and Cancer Research*. Washington, D.C.: U.S. Government Printing Office, June 12–13, 1978.
16. Committee of Agriculture, Nutrition, and Forestry, *Hearing on the Diet and Cancer Relationship*. Washington, D.C.: U.S. Government Printing Office, October 2, 1979.
17. Pritikin, N., *The Pritikin Program for Diet and Exercise*. New York: Grosset & Dunlap, 1979.

PART III
Present Programs for Risk Reduction
and Health Promotion

Innovative programs specifically aimed at health promotion and risk reduction are the focus of several chapters included in Part Three. In addition, this part contains chapters describing one state's experiences with development and implementation of an advisory committee on prevention and wellness and a chapter that provides comprehensive background information on the Centers for Disease Control and its Bureau of Health Education. This chapter is descriptive of focal points of the federal government's efforts in health promotion activities.

In Chapter 13, Christine Williams, M.D., describes the rationale and operation of a unique model of a risk reduction and health education program presently being conducted in public schools in the New York area. There are four major components to the "Know Your Body" program:

1. A health profile for selected risk factors (or a minihealth screening):
2. A personal health passport containing results of the health screening;
3. A behaviorally oriented health education curriculum; and
4. Specific high-risk intervention activities.

The methods by which these components are implemented and integrated into a total program are described in an absorbing manner. Hopefully, this model program could be adopted by health educators and health care professionals in many school programs. Certainly, judging by the early results of the program as described here, such efforts to implement programs modeled after this one should bear positive results for the younger generation.

Williams points out that many school districts currently offer health education curricula which tend to be didactic, limited in scope, and often perceived by youngsters as unrelated to their own personal health. Williams's innovative program applies risk reduction and health promotion principles utilizing student participation in learning their personal risk factors and options for adopting preventive behaviors and methods of achieving measurably improved wellness levels. The students are more strongly influenced by becoming involved in assessing their own health risks and are more likely to modify their health behavior in positive directions. It is to be hoped that more such health education program curricula will be designed and implemented throughout the country in the coming decade.

A unique wellness promotion program, ongoing since 1972, is described by Bill Hettler, M.D., in Chapter 14. Dr. Hettler is the director of the University Health Service and Lifestyle Improvement Program at the University of Wisconsin—Stevens Point, Wisconsin. The editors are impressed with the comprehensive nature of the philosophy guiding this program. This philosophy may be summarized by the program's definition of wellness as a "positive approach to living—an approach that emphasizes the whole person." In this view, wellness is conceptualized as six dimensional: intellectual, emotional, physical (fitness, nutrition), social (family, community, environmental), occupational (vocational), and spiritual (value orientations). The editors recommend that health care professionals associated with universities study this program in terms of developing and implementing such a program at their own college or university.

Techniques for organizing health promotion activities and programs in a rural community are described and illustrated by authors–contributors Rentmeester and Hall in Chapter 15. In absorbing detail, this chapter introduces the reader to a community-based health promotion program that is presently being implemented in Stevens Point, Wisconsin. This chapter describes the major organizational and programmatical components present in a successful community-based project. The authors provide definitions of health promotion in their community and delineate the steps required to initiate a project of this nature. The major elements of leadership support, current health environment, development of specific task forces, high involvment in the process, the local support groups, and evaluation of the project are examined. The project descibed was intended to focus primarily on family units within the community. This focus was achieved through concentration of program efforts on the major influences upon the family, that is, employer groups, schools, churches and civic organizations.

An example of a comprehensive lobbying effort by public health officials, educators, other community leaders, and groups resulted in the establishment of a health planning and promotion task force in Wisconsin. This task force reviewed public health practices and formulated recommendations emphasizing how the public could become better informed about health and its maintenance through improved methods of health education.

This report resulted in the creation of the Wisconsin Advisory Commission on Prevention and Wellness. In Chapter 16, William Blockstein, Ph.D., describes the problems of political realities and financial barriers encountered. As funding of this project came from a tax base, it was subject to (and the target of) the vagaries of political and priority changes. This chapter factually illustrates the accomplishments of cooperative efforts of community leaders and health professionals and also the problems of limited immediate political rewards in the short-term view.

The overriding message of this chapter is that the health educator or health professional attempting to establish a community or state wide health promotion program must continually cultivate support of the program from all community groups who, in the final analysis, are capable of influencing continued financial support of such programs. With common recognition of the value of prevention and health promotion programs, such programs are less likely to be set aside in the continuing jockeying for funding. Consumer health education is potentially the most cost-effective means of disease prevention and health promotion.

In Chapter17, Charles Althafer has contributed a historical background and perspective on the Centers for Disease Control and its role in health promotion through its Bureau of Health Education. He details programs that are currently underway and those in the planning stages. Many of these programs will be undertaken in collaboration with one or more of other public health service agencies at the federal level.

13 / Risk Reduction in the Schools: The "Know Your Body" Program

Christine L. Williams, M.D., M.P.H.

There seems little doubt that precursors of heart disease, cancer, and stroke can be identified in childhood, and that by age 10 years 30 to 60 per cent of the population will exhibit at least one risk factor for one or more of these diseases.[1,2,3] Since a major proportion of the pediatric population is involved, both in terms of the proportion currently at risk and those who may be expected to die of these diseases as adults if the current mortality trends continue in this country, programs of screening and intervention to be most effective should involve the maximum number of children possible.

Public schools provide an extremely efficient vehicle for risk-factor screening, intervention, and health education. They not only involve large numbers of children in one geographic location, provide access to parents and educators, but are also best equipped to provide the health education which forms a foundation on which to motivate behavior change toward healthier life-styles. In addition, intervention strategies based in the schools can take advantage of important peer pressure phenomena which are essential to the success of programs aimed at modifying health behavior.

The majority of chronic disease risk factors are directly related to habits acquired early in life, such as overeating and eating the wrong foods, inactivity, and cigarette smoking. Efforts to prevent chronic disease must also begin early in life and attempts should be made to encourage the adoption of healthy life-styles. In the past, educational attempts to influence behavior by merely providing information (for example, past antismoking campaigns in schools utilizing "show and tell" programs run by adults) have been largely unsuccessful. Despite an awarness of the health hazard of cigarette smoking, the behavior continues at high levels.

The goal of any health education program must be to motivate adoption of health behaviors aimed at reducing premature morbidity and mortality from known preventable causes, including major chronic disease (heart disease, cancer, and stroke) and accidents. Such motivation requires an innovative health education approach capable of achieving a maximal degree of personal involvement.

The following section describes the Know Your Body program, a model school health education "system" which combines health screening, a health passport concept, a behaviorally oriented health curriculum, and special interventions for high-risk students. The primary objective of "KYB" is to promote health maintenance by motivating adoption of healthy life-styles, particularly in the areas of nutrition, avoidance of cigarette smoking and substance abuse, and accident prevention.

THE KNOW YOUR BODY PROGRAM

By design, the "Know Your Body" Program consists of four major components which are repeated each successive year. These major components are as follows:

189

1. Health profile for selected risk factors, conducted in the schools (minihealth screen).
2. Return of screening results directly to the child in the form of a personal health passport.
3. Provision of a behaviorally oriented health education curriculum for subsequent classroom use with appropriate teacher training.
4. Specific high-risk intervention activities aimed at anti-smoking and weight-cholesterol control.

These four basic program components evolved over the course of 5 years of pilot studies in public schools in the New York area. It was found that certain essential steps are necessary to motivate children to reduce their own risk for future disease. They must be medically screened to become aware of their own risk status. Students are told that they will have the opportunity of conducting a "scientific experiment" on themselves—to discover what their own blood pressure, cholesterol, height, weight, skinfold, and pulse rate recovery scores are. They must be provided with a personal health passport to impress upon them their own personal health profile in terms of risk factors. This is more meaningful than being informed by a parent or physician that their blood pressure or cholesterol is on the "high side." Educators have referred to this exercise as the reality factor. Following the health profile and health passport experiences, children must be provided with additional educational activities describing the significance of elevated risk factors as well as steps needed to reduce them. And, finally, it's obvious that they must be channeled into active intervention programs within a peer setting so that healthy behavior becomes the norm rather than the exception.

Positive Health Profile

Before a health education program such as Know Your Body is begun it is important to develop a broad base of community support including that of the school board, the superintendent, the teachers, physician, parents, and finally the children themselves. The children themselves are first introduced to the Know Your Body program after completing the Health Knowledge Questionnaire designed to provide baseline information levels on selected topics which would be stressed in the curriculum material. Following this, a discussion of the program takes place focused on self-care concepts, including, for example, how individual life-styles and personal habits are related to risk for disease later in life. The theme "Nobody Takes Better Care of You Than You" is stressed. A live demonstration of the complete screening is shown to the students using teacher volunteers. This is followed by questions and answers about specific tests. A parent meeting is held to discuss the health profile and curriculum strategies with parents. The nutrition goals and smoking prevention units are highlighted with emphasis on how parents can encourage positive health habits at home. Students take part in the actual medical screening or positive health profile only with written parental consent. Teachers are encouraged to be screened along with their classes. This not only provides a good role model of health interest for the children but frequently stimulates further individual study on the part of the teacher, particulary if personal risk factors are elevated as is frequently the case.

The health profile is conducted in school in any convienient room such as the library, cafeteria, or gymnasium. The first station consists of height, weight, and triceps skinfold thickness (measured twice and averaged); the second station consists of three resting blood pressures (recording an average of the second two readings); the third station consists of a health habits survey, where the child reports on smoking, alcohol, exercise, nutrition, and dental health habits. This is a confidential questionnaire identified by number only and placed in a slotted ballot box after completion. At the fourth station a blood sample is drawn for total cholesterol and also in some cases HDL cholesterol, glucose, and hematocrit. At the final station an exercise test is conducted to determine a pulse recovery score. A modified Harvard step test is generally used since it requires a minimum of equipment to test several children at one time and also can be repeated periodically in gym classes to follow progress in fitness.

The screening is conducted at a leisurely pace, approximately 30 minutes per child, by a team of registered nurses and licensed medical technicians with clerical support. All team members follow a detailed protocol and must complete an annual training workshop. Students are encouraged to ask questions and actively participate in the health profile as a learning activity which is a critical component of the KYB curriculum. It is stressed that the health profile is not a medical screening. Rather it utilizes medical technology in an educational way in order to make the curriculum more personal and meaningful. A summary of the Know Your Body screening tests and interpretation is provided in Table 1. In addition, the results of the health profile tests are given separately in each chapter. Overall, 36 per cent of the junior high school students and 33 per cent of the first-through third-grade students had one or more elevated clinical value of "risk factor." The most common elevation was cholesterol followed by overweight and cigarette smoking (Figure 1).

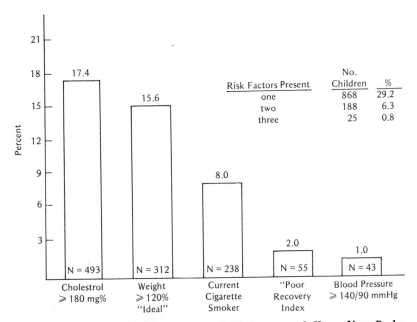

FIGURE 13-1. **Risk factor status of children screened: Know Your Body Project, 1976 (n = 2962, ages 11 to 14 years).**

TABLE 1. Know Your Body—U.S.A.—Methodology for Screening Procedures, 1978-1979

Measurement	Equipment	Technique	Value Considered Abnormal or "Undesirable" for Children Ages 11-14 Years	References
Blood pressure	Mercury sphyg-momanometer (Baumanometer Model No. 300) Child, adult, and obese cuff sizes.	With child seated, BP is measured on right arm three consecutive times with 30 seconds between measurements (taking care that bladder is completely deflated between measurements and child pumps hand between measurements to reduce venous stasis. A cuff is chosen which covers at least two thirds of the length of the upper arm and completely encircles the limb with the center of the bladder over the brachial artery. The sphygmomanometer rests on a table at heart level. First and fourth Korotkoff sounds are recorded. BP is recorded to the nearest mmHG. An average of the second and third of three readings is reported for the child.	≥140/90 mmHG "definitely" too high Upper 5th percentile considered as possible potential risk	"Report of the Task Force on Blood Pressure Control in Children." *Pediatrics* 5 9:5 Supplement (May 1977).
Cholesterol	Autoteknikon II Beaton Dickenson	With child seated and non-fasting 4 ml of venous blood is obtained from	180–199 mg/dl "probably" too high total ≥200 mg/dl "definitely" too high total	Abell, L. L., Levy, B. B., Brody, B. P., and Kendall, F. E., "A Simplified Method for the Esti-

Variable	Instrument	Procedure	Criteria	Reference
	Vacutainers 4-ml purple top	the antecubital vein into a purple top vacutainer tube. The citrated blood is mixed and placed on ice. Plasma cholesterol is measured on the Autoteknikon II with the Liebermann-Bruchard reagent. Standardization of CDC, Lipid Standardization Laboratory is routine.		mation of Total Cholesterol in Serum and a Demonstration of Its Specificity." *Journal of Biological Chemistry*, 195 (1952), pp. 357–366.
Weight	Standard medical balance beam scale	Scale is placed on firm level surface and calibrated at zero and 50 lb daily. Students remove shoes and heavy outer clothes only. They stand in the center of the scale facing the vertical bar. Weight is recorded to the nearest half pound.	≥120% of ideal weight (by age and sex)	*Height and Weight of Children 6 to 11 and Youths 12-17 Years.* U.S. Vital and Health Statistics. U.S. Department of Health, Education and Welfare Series 10, Nos. 104 and 124, 1970 and 1973.
Height	Standard medical balance beam scale	Scale positioned as above; student dressed as above. Student stands in center of scale facing away from vertical bar, posture erect, and head held steady with horizontal gaze directly ahead. The height bar is placed on the child's head without undue pressure, and height is measured to the nearest quarter inch.	≥120% of ideal height (by age and sex)	
Skinfold	Lange skinfold caliper	With right arm flexed to 90° angle (hand on abdomen) the	According to sex and age of child, referring to standards chart	Seltzer, C. C. and Mayer, John A., "A Simple Criterion of

TABLE 1. (Continued)

Measurement	Equipment	Technique	Value Considered Abnormal or "Undesirable" for Children Ages 11–14 Years				References
			BOYS		GIRLS		
			Age	Too High*	Age	Too High*	
			yrs	mm	yrs	mm	
		acromium to olecranon distance is measured with nylon tape measure and midpoint marked. With the arm released and hanging extended loosely at side the skin and subcutaneous tissue is grasped about 1 cm above the mark and the caliper applied to the marked midpoint while maintaining the pinch. Skinfold is reported to the nearest half millimeter. An average of two measurements is recorded.	5	12	5	14	Obesity." *Postgraduate Medicine*, 38 (1965), pp. A101–107.
			6	12	6	15	
			7	13	7	16	
			8	14	8	17	
			9	15	9	18	
			10	16	10	20	
			11	17	11	21	
			12	18	12	22	
			13	18	13	23	
			14	17	14	23	
			15	16	15	24	
			16	15	16	25	
			17	14	17	26	
HDL cholesterol		On the same plasma sample, HDL cholesterol is measured in the supernatant after precipitation of VLDL and LDL according to the method of Burstein et al. (heparin/manganese-chloride precipitation method)					Burstein, M., Scholnick, H. R., and Morfin R., "Rapid Method for the Isolation of Lipoproteins from Human Serum by Precipitation with Polyanions," *Journal of Lipid Research*, 11 (1970), p. 583.
Recovery Index	Plywood box platform—12 inches high	The Recovery Index test consists of stepping up and down	≥199 score = Poor				*Youth Physical Fitness*. President's Council on Physical Fit-

by 4 feet long by 18 inches wide, covered with 1-inch (tight low pile) carpeting. Stopwatches. Tape recording of "up-two-three-four" at proper speed for 4 minutes.

on a platform 12 inches high, 30 times a minute for 4 minutes. The subject faces the platform, and, starting with either foot at the signal "up" places his or her foot on the platform, then steps up so that both feet are on the platform, then immediately steps down again in the same rhythm. The subject then continues stepping up and down in a marching count, "up-two-three-four." The signal "up" comes every 2 seconds. After 4 minutes of this exercise, the subject sits down and remains quiet. One minute later, the pulse rates are taken.

1. One minute after the exercise for 30 seconds.
2. Two minutes after the exercise for 30 seconds.
3. Three minutes after the exercise for 30 seconds.

To determine the Recovery Index, add the 3 pulse counts and refer to the table.

See scoring system below:

When the 3 30-second pulse counts total:	Then the response to this is:
199 or more	needs activity
171 to 198	can improve
150 to 170	average
133 to 149	good shape
132 or less	super fit

ness and Sports. No. 4000-00297. Washington, D.C.: U.S. Government Printing Office, September, 1973.

*≥85%.

Health Passport

The second step after screening, and a key step in motivating behavior change in children, is to give the students their own results in school. This is based on the belief that individuals must first know what needs to be changed, and then learn how to do it. Unfortunately, health education in the past has tended to omit both this personal element and the essential steps in motivating behavioral change.

In didactic lessons, schools have advocated eat right, don't smoke, and don't drink unless you want to "ruin your health." But to the students this usually means some-one else and not them. A strong "illusion of immortality" is common to all healthy persons and is felt particularly keenly by adolescents who tend to believe that chronic disease is something you get when you are over 30 and "old." Many believe they can smoke for a while and quit before it's too late, or eat what they please without ill effects on their health. In contrast, the exercise of giving students their screening results provides a reality factor. It clearly says this passport contains your own personal results and what you do about it is up to you. In practical terms the screening results are re-turned to the students in the form of a computer printout distributed during science class or homeroom period. The results are recorded into a health passport designed so that it may be updated annually to follow progress in each area. Individual results can be kept confidential by each student, and health habit information is not reported at all. Students in the early elementary school grades receive only a few of their test results based on their ability to comprehend certain concepts at each age. First-grade students may receive only height and weight results. In second grade exercise test results and skinfold might be added. In third grade blood pressure would be included, and by fourth grade and on all results are returned to the child.[4]

The students have the option of reporting their cigarette smoking habits on their passports if they so desire. Teachers discuss general results with the children with the aid of certain explanatory materials which suggest optimal values for lowest risk at the particular age of the child. This is part of a whole unit of learning activities in the cur-riculum which prepares the child for and explains the meaning of the health profile tests. The positive aspects are stressed at all times emphasizing that these values can be improved by adopting healthier everyday habits, particularly better nutrition, avoidance of cigarettes, and daily exercise. Parents also receive all health profile results in the mail generally a day or two before students receive the passport in school. If indicated on the consent form, the child's physician also receives all screening results.

The possibility of creating undue anxiety among children through returning their screening results to them and "labeling" them as abnormal has been raised. The task of preventing such anxiety lies with meticulous attention to detail, maintenance of superior quality of personnel in all areas of program managment, and nurturing the positive relationships between teachers, parents, children, and health professionals. Preliminary data from administration of an anxiety inventory (State-Trait Anxiety Inventory)[5] in a subsample of 41 seventh-grade (age 12 year) students indicated that state anxiety scores, designed to measure reaction to a particular immediate event, did not change significantly before and after the students received their health training re-sults in school. The mean score decreased in the directon of lowered anxiety (34.4 to 33.5) although not to a statistically significant degree. All results are described in positive terms to minimize possible stigmatization from abnormal values. The value of learning about the body's warning signals (risk factors) while there is still plenty of time to improve is emphasized. It is felt that giving children their own results is important in motivating appropriate behavioral change toward healthier life-styles, especially if one or more risk factors is elevated.

Children referred for medical attention are those who are overweight (20 per cent or greater than ideal weight for height), have elevated cholesterol levels ($\geqslant$200 mg/dl), poor ratings for the recovery index of the Harvard Step Test (as recommended by the President's Council on Physical Fitness), and elevated blood pressure (top 5 per cent for age and sex).[6] Physicians who are sent copies of screening results are asked to keep a record of children examined or retested by them for any screening result. Occasional difficulty may arise in that many physicians still base their interpretation of cholesterol levels on average population values, as published in standard textbooks, rather than on risk levels determined in prospective epidemiologic studies such as the Framingham study. Such a practice causes confusion and anxiety unless area physicians understand the basis for risk level determination in the KYB program. Hence a level of total cholesterol of 260 mg per cent may be "normal" by a standard medical laboratory's criteria; however, by results based on the Framingham study it would be a level at increased risk of disease (threefold that of a comparably aged man with cholesterol under 220). The determination of "positive" then on screening must take into consideration these epidemiologic findings if the goal of the research activities is to reduce risk factor levels. Preliminary discussions with school physicians and area pediatricians before the health profile generally clarifies this point of view.

It is obvious that one treads a fine line between creating concern in the individual enough to motivate behavior change to reduce risk and at the same time to avoid creating anxiety. It is probably true, however, that children are much more objective about medical results than their elders. Unfortunately, society has classically felt that medical news, particularly bad news, should be shielded from the patient. In the case of chronic disease risk factors such shielding is counterproductive. Children must want to eat a more prudent diet, exercise more, control their weight, and abstain from smoking in order to reduce their own risks for future disease. Being aware of one's risks and being responsible for one's own body is the first step in creating this desire.[7]

Teacher Training

Teachers are introduced to the KYB curriculum during a 1 to 2-day workshop covering development, implementation, and evaluation of the learning activities and basic units of the curriculum. The workshop topics vary depending on grade level and previous experience with the KYB or similar type of curriculum. Background information is covered in the areas of epidemiology of chronic disease risk factors, basic nutrition goals and prudent diet concepts, teaching techniques based on behaviorally oriented learning activities, smoking prevention strategies, health decision models, short-term rewards for desired behavior changes, and other topics.

Teachers from several districts (generally 30 to 50 persons) actively participate in sample learning activities, role play situations involving return of health profile results, contribute ideas for new units, suggest modifications needed for their own districts or for special situations related to ethnic, socioeconomic, or physical conditions of students.

Teacher evaluations of the training workshops have tended to be very positive with highest ratings recorded for those in the program for several years. This suggests that though initially skeptical and somewhat resistant to the addition of a major new curriculum area (in which they feel personally inadequate to teach) experience provides a gradual increase in knowledge, confidence, and willingness to actively pursue health education.

Know Your Body Curriculum

The KYB curriculum currently consists of teacher's guides and student workbooks for grades 1 through 8. It has been designed around a health decision-making model, progressing developmentally from the more simple to the more complex. Health concepts are taught in relation to life-style behavior patterns. The units stressed during the year after screening are also related to the relative prevalence of risk factors and the type of health decisions the children are making at that particular age. For example, children in early grades would spend a great deal of time on nutrition and dental health. As children get into the middle elementary age grades they would then be introduced to more complex ideas involving substance abuse, blood pressure, cancer control, heart disease prevention, and other topics. Teachers are encouraged to use the materials and to capitalize on the personal screening experience and the results of the screening.[8]

Besides the classroom learning activities in the KYB curriculum units, teachers also utilize variations of antismoking campaigns, field trips, health fairs, junior olympics, prudent bake sales, parent breakfasts, cafeteria surveys, newsletters, and poster contests. School districts must form parent advisory boards, student advisory boards, and implement special programs for high-risk students such as those who are overweight, have high cholesterol levels, or poor physical fitness.

The KYB curriculum material is divided into two levels—an *elementary* school level appropriate for students ages 6 to 10 years and a *junior high school* level appropriate for students ages 10 to 14 years. Within each level the material is divided into ten units. The different teaching levels provide a sequential development of concepts, objectives, and activities aimed toward attaining the overall objectives of the curriculum listed previously. This progression from simple to more complex learning takes into consideration the cognitive development level of the students, patterns of growth and development, intrinsic needs and activities of the students themselves, specific contemporary health needs, local and national health problems, and the ability of the student to take on self-responsibility for making health decisions.

The elementary school level focuses on learning the basic skills necessary to practice health measures. In addition, specific core knowledge stressing certain cognitive factors is taught from a personalized self-behavior perspective utilizing the minihealth screening as its focal point. Students have experience making health choices based on likes, dislikes, and attitudes concerning their bodies.

In junior high school, students examine the influence of *peers* on their health decisions. In addition the middle school–junior high school units assist the students in looking at the decisions they are currently making concerning their health behaviors. Specific interventions that deal with nutrition and substance abuse are key units that are focal points at this level. Additional units serve as a support system and continue to reinforce the learning that has taken place on the previous level.

More specifically, the overall objectives of the curriculum at all levels are to

1. Increase health knowledge about selected personalized health factors;
2. Develop and reinforce positive feelings about one's body;

3. Promote increased responsibility for maintaining one's own health;
4. Increase students' ability to monitor and change their own health practices to reduce their health risks;
5. Promote specific healthy life-style behaviors that students will actively practice.

The general response from school districts has been that the type of health education program represented by the Know Your Body program is a feasible, acceptable, safe, and effective approach to modifying health habits in childhood in a positive direction.

Evaluation

Evaluation of the overall effectiveness of the Know Your Body program has involved measurement of cognitive, behavioral, and clinical changes over time. Six school districts took part in this 3-year evaluation study to determine if the KYB system could be effective in actually producing measurable changes in these areas. The three experimental junior high schools (two suburban and one inner city) were compared with three similar schools serving as age and socioeconomically matched controls. Treatment in the experimental and control schools is summarized in Table 2. Basically, all schools were treated identically up to the point of returning students' screening results in school. After that, only experimental schools taught the curriculum, conducted the antismoking and overweight interventions, and took part in the special projects described later. The project continued for 3 years, with annual health profile screening and administration of health knowledge and health habit surveys. These measurements provided the base line for evaluation of program effectiveness.

Cognitive Changes

Health knowledge increased significantly for both experimental and control groups on the junior high school level.[9] However, the students participating in the screening and the curriculum did significantly better than those involved only in the screening. This was the case for the overall questionnaire scores as well as for the individual subscores of smoking, nutrition, and blood pressure knowledge. The mean pretest and posttest

TABLE 2. KYB Evaluation Study Design—Junior High School, 1975–1978

Program Content	Experimental Schools	Control Schools
Initial parent meeting	√	√
Initial teacher meetings	√	√
Prescreening demonstration to students	√	√
Annual health profile screening	√	√
Return results to parents, students, and physicians	√	√
Teacher training workshops	√	
Classroom curriculum units	√	
Antismoking intensive program	√	
Weight control groups	√	
Special projects (contests, etc.)	√	
Parent educational meetings	√	

increase in knowledge for the experimental group was about 30 per cent higher (6.37 compared with 4.51 for the screening-only group [t (3109) = 6.88, $p < 0.01$] than for the control group. Similarly, there were significantly greater pretest–posttest changes for the experimental group on the nutrition (t [3109] = 5.17, $p < 0.01$), smoking (t [3109] = 3.72, $p < 0.01$), and blood pressure (t [3109] = 7.08, $p < 0.01$) subscores. These results suggest that a risk factor screening, particularly when combined with a formal curriculum, may facilitate the acquisition of health knowledge by personalizing what is frequently conceived of as abstract health information.

Behavioral Changes

The general health education curriculum intervention was not able to effect changes in risk factor levels in children as measured by clinical indexes on repeat screening. The one exception was in the area of cholesterol levels which did change significantly greater in the experimental group compared with the control group. That is, there were 30 per cent fewer children with cholesterol levels above 180 mg/dl after 3 years in the experimental group compared with no change in the control group.

The most significant behavioral changes were seen in the intensive small group intervention activities—that is, the obesity treatment group and the cigarette smoking prevention group. For example, in the weight-loss program an intensive 16-week program was conducted for 119 overweight students in junior high school. Ten to 12 students in a group met weekly with one trained faculty member under the supervision of a staff nutritionist. No specific diets were prescribed. Instead, reduction of nutrition-related risk factors will be sought through behavior change by means of specific learning activities such as risk-factor quiz, nutrition IQ, food selection sheets, food-exercise logs, diet-feeling checklist, calorie-cholesterol booklets, diet plans, weigh-ins, group goals, group progress records, food comparison cards, portion control, hunger ratings, exercise strategies, pedometers, task solution cards, fast food items, and creative projects. Posttest measurements after the 16 weeks indicated that over half (51 per cent) of this experimental group had lost weight compared with only 16 per cent of the control group. There was also a significant shift from obese to nonobese in the experimental group whereas the slight decline in the control group was not significant (Figure 2). In addition, 70 per cent of the experimental group had lower triceps skinfold measurements on posttest compared with 43 per cent of controls, also a significant difference. Recently a 1-year follow-up study of these students has shown that after

	Pretest	Posttest (16 weeks)	Follow-Up (1 year)
Study (n)	38% (24)	17% (6)	13% (4)
Control (n)	37% (27)	35% (24)	29% (18)

FIGURE 13-2.   Percent of students who were ≤ 130% of ideal weight "nonobese" in intensive weight loss program.

one year with no booster sessions, the advantage gained by the experimental students was slowly lost but remained borderline significance.[10]

In the intensive smoking prevention program it was found that 12 one-hour sessions held weekly for 10 weeks was effective in preventing the onset of cigarette smoking behavior in eighth, ninth, and tenth-grade students.[11] Approximately 250 students took part in this intensive smoking intervention program. Each weekly session in this program builds upon the others during the course of the 10 weeks. Sessions include both group discussion and formal initial sessions dealing with immediate and long-term physiological effects of smoking. This unit is designed to provide students with basic background information about the hazards of smoking so students will understand how smoking affects their bodies. The reasons for and against smoking as well as common situations in which people smoke will also be covered. Subsequent sessions deal with decision making, values clarification, and understanding the various influences to smoke and how to resist them. In addition, the social acceptability of smoking and society's changing attitudes toward smoking will be covered. Further along topics focus on promoting a positive self-image through acquisition of basic life skills. Some of the topics included will be the relationship between self-image and behavior, self-improvement strategies, coping with anxiety, assertiveness, and resisting peer pressure. Time is also devoted to social skills training to help students feel more competent in social situations and thereby reduce their social anxiety. The major focus of this is on communication skills and dating skills. The final sessions include modified sessions from each of the previous areas covered in order to reinforce the decision not to smoke. The apparent effectiveness of the antismoking activities was inversely related to grade level. It was highest among eighth graders (100 per cent), midlevel for ninth graders (77 per cent), and lowest for tenth graders (53 per cent). This finding suggests that better results should occur when such programs are initiated earlier in elementary school. Again, a 1-year follow-up was done which showed that the advantage gained by the experimental group was slowly lost to the point of a nonsignificant difference between the experimental control group (Figure 3). This would be expected at this age level without any booster sessions, since the children are still being exposed to a great deal of social and

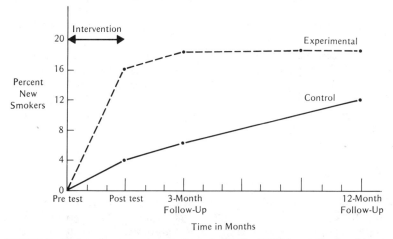

FIGURE 13-3. Percent new smokers following KYB intensive smoking prevention program—252 students in grades 8, 9, and 10.

TABLE 3. Self-Reported Cigarette Smoking Status and Plasma Cotinine Levels in 137 Students, 14 to 17 years, in New York, 1978.

Self-Reported Cigarette Smoking		Plasma Cotinine Level (ng/ml)		Number of Students
		Detectable	Nondetectable (nd)	
"Daily" Cigarette Smoking	Mean Continine:	158 ng/ml	N.D.	
	Range:	5–616 ng/ml	N.D.	
	No. Students:	19 (95%)	1 (5%)	20 (100%)
	No. Cigarettes/ Week	50 per week	50 per week	
"Occasional" Cigarette Smoking	Mean Cotinine:	80 ng/ml	N.D.	
	Range:	29–131 ng/ml	N.D.	
	No. Students:	4 (21%)	15 (79%)	19 (100%)
	No. Cigarettes/ Week:	16 per week	1 per week	
"Never" Smoke Cigarettes	Mean Cotinine:	4 ng/ml	N.D.	
	Range:	3–5 ng/ml	N.D.	
	No. Students:	2 (2%)	96 (98%)	98 (100%)
	No. Cigarettes/ Week:	0	0	
Total Number of Students				137

psychological pressure to begin smoking cigarettes. It seems clear that both for cigarette smoking and obesity intervention a long-term maintenance phase needs to be incorporated into the program.

A subsample of 137 students was randomly selected for validation of the self-reported smoking data.[12] Samples of blood drawn for cholesterol determinations were also analyzed for cotinine. Cotinine values were matched with self-reported smoking frequency reported on the health habits survey completed within 20 minutes of venipuncture. Ninety-five per cent of the students who reported "daily" cigarette smoking had detectable cotinine levels (mean 158 ng/ml). This was compared with only 2 of the 98 students reporting they never smoked who had any cotinine in their blood. Since plasma cotinine has a relatively short half life (30 hours) it was unable to validate the responses of "occasional" smokers since many of these smoked only 1 or 2 cigarettes per week. As Table 3 indicates, however, cotinine values were detectable for students reporting occasional smoking (mean 16 cigarettes per week), and nondetectable for students reporting only 1 cigarette per week. This data suggests that adolescents can report accurately on their own smoking status if sufficient assurance of confidentiality is stressed.

Curriculum Evaluation

Behavioral and clinical changes for students who were exposed to the KYB classroom curriculum for 2 years (but did not take part in the intensive small group interventions), were limited in scope. Overall there were no significant changes in the proportion of students who were at risk for weight, blood pressure, or cigarette smoking. A significant decrease in the proportion of students at risk for elevated cholesterol was seen for the experimental schools after 2 years, compared with no change for the control group. In addition more students in the experimental schools who were initially at risk for poor exercise tolerance improved their scores in relation to the comparison group. No difference in change in overall proportion of students at risk for any risk factor was seen for experimental versus control groups.

In reviewing the experience of the classroom teachers who had actually taught the KYB curriculum during the 2-year period, it was obvious that the area given most time and emphasis was nutrition. This may have accounted for the change in cholesterol "risk" status.

Other Changes in School

SCHOOL LUNCH PROGRAM

An effort to change the school lunch program was the target of several parent-teacher organizations in the six initial school districts involved in the KYB evaluation study. Project nutritionists outlined a strategy for change and provided technical assistance to parent and teacher leaders without actually directing the effort. An initial nutritional survey and analysis of current menus was developed into a proposal for specific changes that school made to: (1) reduce the sale of nonnutritious snack and dessert items which competed with more nutritious foods, (2) reduce the total and saturated fat content of foods served, (3) serve more high-fiber foods like whole-grain cereals, (4) provide healthier dessert items such as raisin-nut mixes, frozen low-fat yogurt, fresh fruits, and salad plates.

Significant changes were made in two of the three experimental school districts. These changes occurred slowly and often in small steps. A major resistance was often the economic benefits to a school derived from the sale of snack/dessert/candy items (e.g., proceeds may support the football team). Parents and teachers, however, were quick to realize the futility of teaching good nutrition in the classroom and then not providing healthier food choices in the school's own cafeteria.

The kind of typical school lunch changes made were as follows:

District A: Changed all school milk in the district from regular to low fat (26 per cent). Provided more salad plates, yogurt, and whole wheat bread in addition to usual menu. These new additions proved to be very popular and cafeteria sales increased.

District B: Changed food items sold in machines from nonnutritious to nutritious (e.g., replaced soda pop with juice, candy with raisins, nuts, and fresh fruit).

District C: This was an inner-city school whose school lunch program was part of the huge New York contract. This, combined with the difficulty of developing parent action groups, accounted for the lack of official change in the school lunch program here. Teachers and administrators reported that more students seemed to be eating breakfast and fewer candy items were observed at school. Students themselves reported a shift away from high-fat and highly salted foods, although this was not validated.

Special Projects

Activities were planned to contribute to the enthusiastic momentum of the program which began after the initial screening. Poster contests were very popular; scientific fairs or essay contests were held. A "Health Happening" in Central Park provided an opportunity for students from several districts to display gymnastic or dramatic skills and display winning posters. "Prudent" picnic lunches were served on frisbees. Bake sales in school shifted from the usual cake and cookies to healthier fare like zucchini bread, carrot cake, bran muffins, raisin-nut snack bags, sesame squares, and other foods. A local department store hosted an awards evening for parents and students, displaying video tapes made by students on an antismoking theme. A newsletter for students reported on KYB activities in other districts and gave student reporters a chance to write their own health columns.

International Collaboration

As a contribution to the "Year of the Child" 15 countries around the world conducted pilot studies replicating the KYB model on the junior high school level. These countries included Finland, Norway, Holland, Germany, France, Italy, Yugoslavia, Greece, Japan, Taiwan, Thailand, Kuwait, Kenya, Nigeria, and the United States. Risk-factor comparison for these 10- to 15-year-old children provided interesting data with respect to pediatric risk-factor levels, adult levels, and current mortality rates from coronary heart disease, cancer, and stroke. These data are currently being analyzed, and some preliminary comparisons are given in the individual sections of this book.

CONCLUSION

One of the basic strengths of the Know Your Body project is its innovative approach and its ability to captivate the attention and the support of the community and the schools and the students. It's well known to all of us that health education is one of the least popular topics in any school. In contrast, the Know Your Body program has been consistently able to develop keen interest and cooperation among students and teachers and to elevate health education to the level of other major curriculum areas in elementary and junior high school. In a number of schools the program has been able to initiate significant changes in the school cafeteria as well, indicating that the type of approach is effective in slowly changing behavior and general health atmosphere of the school

It has been significant that this project, which was begun in six school districts in the New York City area, is still operational in four of these districts, and using funds from the districts themselves rather than continuation of research funding. All of the districts who have been involved with the program have indicated a growing support and desire for expansion. This is relatively surprising in view of the significant amount of time and energy that must be devoted to a program and curriculum of this type in any school.

One of the key factors in getting teacher support has been the inclusion of teachers in the screening health profile itself and also in conducting teacher workshops which involve a certain amount of competition among several districts and fruitful exchange of ideas. A major strength of this type of approach is the personalizing of the curriculum with the health profile itself which in general has not been used before.

There are, however, a number of drawbacks to the Know Your Body type of health education approach. The major factor is cost. A program which includes a health profile in school naturally will be more expensive than a comparable program which offers only curriculum materials. Even though the average New York school district (for example) spends between \$3,000 and \$5,000 per pupil per year, they are unwilling to commit even \$25 per pupil on an effective health education system. It has been suggested that different versions of the Know Your Body approach could be used. Some simple versions would consist of only the curriculum, that is, teacher's guide and student workbook. In comparison, the total program would include not only the curriculum materials but also the health screening, health passport, and intensive intervention activities (weight control, blood pressure control, cholesterol reduction, and special smoking prevention groups) as well.

It's obvious that school districts differ a great deal in the type of health education curriculum that they currently teach. In general it tends to be didactic in nature, limited in scope, and ineffective in producing behavioral change. Only a few progressive school districts are willing or financially able to cast off the old and take on a large new health education program as comprehensive and innovative as the Know Your Body project. On the other hand, it's not clear whether separating the Know Your Body type of approach into individual components would be as effective as the whole program together.

The Know Your Body project was originally developed on the junior-high-school level and has since been adapted for elementary school. It's been interesting that in the earlier elementary grades there seems to be more positive initial teacher receptivity and also a much greater degree of parental involvement. The interventions and the activities that are planned for the younger grades also involve parents and teachers to a greater degree than with the older children. Continuing development, refinement, and evaluation of the elementary level KYB program is in progress.

In many ways, implementation of the Know Your Body project in any particular school district initiates a slow process of social change and an increasing level of knowledge and health activity within the entire community, involving students as well as parents, physicians, teachers, and principals.

ACKNOWLEDGMENTS

The author wishes to acknowledge the invaluable support of all those whose teamwork has made the "Know Your Body" program, from which this study emanates, a successful project. Sincere appreciation is expressed to the students, parents, teachers, and administrators in the cooperating school districts, without whose support this study could not have been possible.

This work was supported in part by the National Cancer Institute Grant No. CA-17867 and in part by Grant No. CA-17613.

REFERENCES

1. Williams, C. L., Arnold, C. B., and Wynder, E. L., "Primary Prevention of Chronic Disease Beginning in Childhood: The Know Your Body Program–Design of Study." *Preventive Medicine* 6:2 (June 1977), pp. 344–357.
2. Williams, C. L., Carter, B. J., Wynder, E. L., and Blumenfeld, T. A., "Selected Chronic Disease Risk Factors in Two Elementary School Populations: A Pilot Study." *American Journal of Diseases of Children* 133 (1979), pp. 704–708.
3. Willmore, J. H. and McNamara, J. J., "Prevalence of Coronary Heart Disease Risk Factors in Boys 8 to 12 Years of Age." *Journal of Pediatrics* 84 (1974), pp. 527–533.

4. Williams, C. L., Carter, B. J., and Eng, A., "The Know Your Body Program: A Developmental Approach to Health Education and Disease Prevention." *Preventive Medicine* 9 (1980), pp. 371–383.
5. Spielberger C. D., Gorauch R. L., Lushene, R. E., *The State-Trait Anxiety Inventory (STAI)*. Palo Alto, Calif.: Consulting Psychologists Press, 1970.
6. Williams, C. L., Arnold, C. B., and Wynder, E. L., "Chronic Disease Risk Factors Among Children: The Know Your Body Study." *Journal of Chronic Diseases* 32 (1979), pp. 505–513.
7. Williams, C. L. and Wynder, E. L., "Motivating Adolescents to Reduce Risk for Chronic Disease." *Postgraduate Medical Journal* 54 (1978), pp. 212–214.
8. Eng A., Carter B. J., Williams C. L.: "Personalizing Primary Cancer Prevention Education for Students." *Health Values* 3: 304–309, 1979.
9. Eng, A., Botvin, G. J., Carter, B. J., and Williams, C. L., "Increasing Students' Knowledge of Cancer and Cardiovascular Disease Prevention Through a Risk Factor Education Program." *Journal of School Health* 49 (1979), pp. 505–597.
10. Botvin, G. J., Cantlon, A., Carter, B. J., and Williams, C. L., "Reducing Adolescent Obesity Through a School Health Program." *Journal of Pediatrics* 95 (1979), pp. 1060–1064.
11. Botvin, G. J., Eng, A., and Williams, C. L., "Preventing the Onset of Cigarette Smoking Through Life Skills Training." *Preventive Medicine* 9 (1980), pp. 135–143.
12. Williams, C. L., Eng, A., Botvin, G. J., Hill, P., and Wynder, E. L., "Validation of Students' Self-Reported Cigarette Smoking Status with Plasma Cotinine Levels." *American Journal of Public Health* 69: 12 (1979), pp. 1272–1274.

14 / Wellness Promotion and Risk Reduction on a University Campus*

Bill Hettler, M.D.

Eight years ago there was launched at the University of Wisconsin–Stevens Point (UW–SP) a new program devoted to life-style improvement. That undertaking, most of which was initiated by the staff of the Student Life Division of University Services, continues with increased emphasis today.

The guiding philosophy of the student life program is the pursuit of high-level wellness, which Halbert Dunn first defined in 1959 as "integrated method of functioning which is oriented toward maximizing the potential of which the individual is capable, within the environment where he is functioning."[1]

Wellness can also be defined as an active process through which the individual becomes aware of and makes choices toward a more successful existence. These choices are greatly influenced by one's self-concept and the parameters of one's culture and environment. Each individual develops a unique life-style that changes daily in the reflection of his or her intellectual, emotional, physical, social, occupational, and spiritual dimensions. Wellness is a positive approach to living—an approach that emphasizes the whole person. As shown in Figure 1, wellness can be divided into six basic dimensions:

1. *Intellectual*—Measures the degree to which one engages his or her mind in creative, stimulating mental activities. An intellectually well person uses the resources available to expand his or her knowledge in improved skills, along with expanding potential for sharing with others.
2. *Emotional*—Measures the degree to which one has an awareness and acceptance of one's feelings. This includes the degree to which one feels positive and enthusiastic about oneself and life. It measures the capacity to appropriately control one's feelings and related behavior, including the realistic assessment of one's limitations.
3. *Physical*—Measures the degree to which one maintains cardiovascular flexibility and strength. Measures the behaviors that help one to prevent or detect early illness. Measures the degree to which one chooses foods that are consistent with the dietary goals of the United States as reported by the Senate Select Committee on Nutrition (Sup. of Doc. No. 052-07003913-2).
4. *Social*—Measures the degree to which one contrbutes to the common welfare of one's community. This emphasizes the interdependence with others and with nature.
5. *Occupational*—Measures the satisfaction gained from one's work and the degree to which one is enriched by that work.
6. *Spiritual*—Measures one's ongoing involvement in seeking meaning and purpose in human existence. It includes a deep appreciation for the depth and expanse of life and natural forces that exist in the universe.

*Reprinted from *Family and Community Health* 3 : 1, May 1980, by permission of Aspen Systems Corporation, Germantown, MD, © 1980.

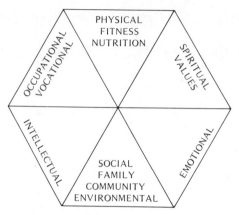

FIGURE 14-1.   **Six dimensions of wellness.**

Figure 2 provides a graphic representation of the high-level wellness to premature death continuum. This continuum was modified from early works by Sorochan,[2] Diesendorf and Furnass,[3] and Travies.[4] Diesendorf and Furnass have suggested that each dimension of wellness be viewed separately in a vertical configuration with optimal functioning as a base line.

A three-dimensional presentation of high-level wellness would be a tetrahedron with each of the six edges representing one of the six dimensions. This is more consistent with the whole-person concept. Buckminster Fuller has discussed the universal stability of the tetrahedron.[5] The stability and integrity of the tetrahedron depends on the presence of each of the six edges. A tetrahedron is more easily recognized as that particular structure if the edges are close to equal length. This same principle can support the proposition that the stability of the human depends on the integrity of each dimension of wellness.

The function of a university is to provide an atmosphere and physical environment in which the students have an opportunity to improve their knowledge, skills, and attitudes. Most colleges and universities provide the atmosphere and physical environment for intellectual development. Few colleges and universities, however, provide equal resources for improving the other five dimensions. There even exists on some campuses disdain for physical fitness. Yet comprehensive wellness promotion on the university campus has the potential to increase students' retention in academic programs (thus increasing faculty retention). These programs also improve student chances for success once they have been graduated. There are now over 1,000 companies in the United

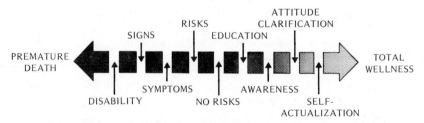

FIGURE 14-2.   **Continuum of high-level wellness to premature death.**

TABLE 1.   Leading Causes of Death: Ages 20-24 (1976)

Causes of Death	Rate*	Percent†	Chance in 100,000 of the Individual Dying from This Cause
Motor vehicle accidents	40.7	31.0	202.9
All other accidents	21.6	16.5	108.0
Homicide	16.6	12.6	82.5
Suicide	16.4	12.5	81.8
Malignant neoplasms	7.3	5.6	36.7
Diseases of heart	3.3	2.5	16.4
Other external causes	3.1	2.4	15.7
Influenza and pneumonia	1.7	1.3	8.5
Cerebrovascular diseases	1.5	1.1	7.2
Congenital anomalies	1.4	1.0	6.5
All other causes	17.7	13.5	88.3
All causes	131.3	100.0	654.5

*Rates per 100,000 population.
†Percent of total deaths.
Source: Center for Disease Control, Public Health Service. *Leading Causes of Death and Probabilities of Dying, United States, 1975 and 1976.* Atlanta: Center for Disease Control, 1979.

States that have full-time fitness directors. These companies believe that health promotion is cost effective. Many companies now realize that it is even more cost effective to hire a healthy employee in the first place. Therefore students exhibiting healthy lifestyles would have a competitive edge given equal academic credentials.

There is good evidence that many of the causes of death at age 40 are the result of behaviors that were established during the adolescent and young adult years. Tables 1 to 3 clearly indicate that the most significant contribution to premature mortality

TABLE 2.   Leading Causes of Death: Ages 40-44 (1976)

Causes of Death	Rate*	Percent†	Chance in 100,000 of the Individual Dying from This Cause
Diseases of heart	72.8	23.2	360.9
Malignant neoplasma	68.9	22.0	342.3
Cirrhosis of liver	22.1	7.1	110.5
All other accidents	19.8	6.3	98.0
Motor vehicle accidents	18.3	5.8	90.2
Suicide	16.7	5.3	82.5
Cerebrovascular diseases	15.0	4.8	74.7
Homicide	13.6	4.3	66.9
Influenza and pneumonia	6.4	2.0	31.1
Diabetes	4.6	1.5	23.3
All other causes	55.2	17.7	275.3
All causes	313.4	100.0	1,555.7

*Rates per 100,000 population.
†Percent of total deaths.
Source: Center for Disease Control, Public Health Service. *Leading Causes of Dealth and Probabilities of Dying, United States, 1975 and 1976.* Atlanta: Center for Disease Control, 1979.

TABLE 3. **Estimated Proportion of Factors Contributing to Premature Mortality to the Four Elements of the Health Field (1975)**

Cause of Death	Health System	Life-Style	Environment	Human Biology
Heart disease	12	54	9	28
Cancer	10	37	24	29
Cerebrovascular disease	7	50	22	21
All other accidents	14	51	31	4
Influenza and pneumonia	18	23	20	39
Motor vehicle accidents	12	69	18	0.6
Diabetes	6	26	0	68
Cirrhosis of the liver	3	70	9	18
Arteriosclerosis	18	49	8	26
Suicide	3	60	35	2
Average	10.8	48.5	15.8	26.3

Source: Center for Disease Control, Public Health Service. *Ten Leading Causes of Death in the United States, 1975.* Atlanta: Center for Disease Control, 1979.

in America is the result of individual choices. Collectively, these choices can be described as the life-style. Universities can assist students in establishing life-styles that will serve them well into their later years and will not lead to premature death or disability.

Of course, one sure sign of effectiveness on the job is for the individual to remain alive. Other signs of success after graduation would include minimizing sick time and illness-care expense. People with positive self-concepts, high energy levels, and positive human relationship skills have a competitive edge in the modern Western world.

The academic programs of most colleges and universities could be enhanced by wellness promotion efforts. Life-style issues such as physical fitness, social skills, nutrition, spiritual development, and emotional development may be touched on in the academic classroom, but there can also be practical programs that give the students in-depth assessment and empirical learning opportunities for their personal development. The Student Life Division of UW–SP has actively been promoting wellness for the past 5 years.

The Student Life Division consists of: (1) University Health Services, (2) University Counseling Services, (3) Residence Hall Program, and (4) University Centers. The directors of Student Life meet for 2 hours every week to inform each other of activities of the individual units; minimize competition for the student's time; arrange for sharing personnel and resources whenever possible; provide ongoing planning and evaluation activities; and discuss problem-solving difficulties that arise.

The leadership of Student Life met in January 1979 and established the following six goals:

1. Assist the UW–SP community in the creation of a healthy and safe environment and one that provides stimulation, order, privacy, and freedom;
2. Provide opportunities that enhance the personal growth and development of students intellectually, socially, emotionally, physically, spiritually, and vocationally;
3. Provide services that support the academic mission of our community as well as services that enhance a student's comfort in the community;
4. Provide through research, assessment of the efficacy of our current program and the direction for our future program;

5. Maintain an effective and efficient delivery through resource responsibility—both fiscal and personnel; and
6. Maintain an ongoing professional development thrust, reaching into the university community as well as outside of the community to collaborate with colleagues.

These six goals have been simplified for health services by the author to include three broad missions:

1. Student services → traditional illness care.
2. Student development → wellness promotion.
3. Outreach → creating a supportive environment on a local, state, and national basis.

LIFE-STYLE ASSESSMENT QUESTIONNAIRE

The Life-style Assessment Questionnaire (LAQ) is an important component of the total health promotion program. It was first developed by the author in 1976 and has undergone continuous revision for the past 3 years. Suggestions from professionals and LAQ users throughout the United States have been evaluated and selectively incorporated by a committee of the Student Life Division. The LAQ is recommended to the students as their entrance health assessment instrument. (See Appendix B.)

In the fall of 1974 UW–SP modified its entrance requirement concerning health assessment. At that time students were given the option of completing a Data Automated Student History (DASH) questionnaire provided by Medical Datamation of Bellevue, Ohio, or a traditional history and physical examination. One of the main reasons for the modification of the requirement was increasing evidence that it was not cost effective to require a history and physical examination for young, healthy adults. Blankenbaker has demonstrated that it is more cost effective to do a health hazard appraisal than history and physical examinations when the goal is to identify significant health problems.[6] Table 4, a summary of the data presented by Blankenbaker in 1977, indicates the cost per unique problem from a variety of screening efforts.

TABLE 4.   Cost to Identify Unique Problems from a Variety of Screening Efforts

Screen	Number of Tests Performed	Total Problems Found	Number of Problems/ Screened	Cost per Problem	Unique Problems Found	Cost per Unique Problem
History, physical	357	889	2.49	$14.06	678	$18.43
VDRL	251	2	0.01	251.00	2	251.00
Chest x-ray	155	31	0.20	75.00	25	93.00
PPD	76	18	0.24	16.89	16	19.00
ECG	109	42	0.39	44.12	29	63.90
Chem-12	235	195	0.83	14.46	183	15.41
Pap smear (with pelvic)	318	76	0.24	66.95	70	72.68
Urinalysis	313	155	0.50	6.06	147	6.39
CBC	327	122	0.37	16.08	117	16.76
HHA	474	2801	5.91	1.36	2616	1.36

Source: Blankenbaker, R., "Total Care the Cost-Effective Way." *Thirteenth Annual Meeting of the Society of Prospective Medicine Proceedings.* Bethesda, Md.: Health and Education Resources, 1977.

The DASH system was in use at UW–SP from 1974 through 1977. By the spring of 1976 the price had increased from $5.00 to $9.00 per student.

The LAQ was first introduced on a pilot basis at UW–SP in the fall of 1977. Sixteen hundred LAQs were given to incoming students as a control/evaluation group. This group also completed the DASH questionnaire. The intent of this initial distribution of the LAQ was to study the mechanism of distribution and the computer programming capabilities of the new system. That group of students was not charged for the LAQ.

FACULTY AND COMMUNITY INVOLVEMENT

Following the development of a referral listing for each of the 27 topics from the personal growth section of the LAQ, copies of these resources were distributed to community agencies and faculty departments. A cover letter instructed interested participants to make improvements or additions to the LAQ referral sources. Thirty responses were received from 200 faculty, staff, and community professionals. The suggestions were reviewed and selectively included in the referral sources.

In the spring of 1978 a proposal was developed to discontinue the DASH system and implement the LAQ as the recommended health assessment instrument for the University of Wisconsin–Stevens Point. (By the time the cost of the DASH system had risen to $12.50 per student.) this proposal was first made to the Student Health Advisory Committee (SHAC). Following unamimous SHAC approval, a formal proposal was made to the full student government. A fee of $7.50 was suggested to cover the cost of the processing of the LAQ and to generate income that could be used to promote wellness. This suggestion received the unanimous support of the student government.

To avoid conflict of interest discussions, the author turned over his copyright interest in the LAQ to the UW–SP Foundation in exchange for $1.00 in cash plus an agreement that the instrument would be offered at cost to UW–SP students as long as it was in use. The Student Life Division established a fee of $7.50—as approved by the student government—which would include the cost of the processing and $5.00 per student to begin developing funds to budget for wellness programming.

FUNCTIONS OF THE LAQ

The LAQ consists of four sections: (1) wellness inventory; (2) personal growth; (3) risk of death (health hazard appraisal); and (4) medical alert sections. Each of these sections has a specific purpose. The students receive an individualized printout based on the responses they make to the questionnaire. (See Figure 3).

The wellness inventory section consists of positive statements in each of the dimensions of wellness. This section encourages a student to recognize his or her strengths in each of the wellness dimensions and also encourages the student to identify areas in which he or she might approve. One purpose of this section is to educate the student as to some of the behaviors or signs of wellness that can be tried and evaluated. This section is immediately followed by the personal growth section.

The topics for the personal growth section consist of 27 different areas. Next to each subject there are three columns for responses. The student can request (1) information, (2) group activities, or (3) confidential personal assistance. Table 5 lists the 27

1

WELLNESS INVENTORY

The following scores indicate your wellness compared with average of people taking this survey with you, and averages of all the people who have taken the survey.

Category	Your Score	Group Average	Total Average
Physical Exercise	68	73	70
Physical Nutritional	52	67	52
Physical Self Care	46	60	48
Physical Vehicle Safety	47	75	49
Physical Drug Usage	72	95	75
Social Environmental	27	56	32
Emotional Awareness Acceptance	20	50	24
Emotional Management	47	69	51
Intellectual	68	82	71
Occupational	73	79	73
Spiritual	65	68	66

2

PERSONAL GROWTH SECTION
AUTOMATED REFERRAL

EXERCISE PROGRAMS
A. Media
1. Movies:Coping With Life On The Run—Sports
      Productions Inc.
      Run Dick, Run Jane—American Heart
      Assocaition
      The Heart: An Attack—CRM
2. Books: Joy of Running—Kostrubala
      Women's Running—Ullyot
      The Complete Runner—Fixx
      Stretching—Anderson
      Sheehan on Running—George Sheehan
      The Ultimate Athlete—Leonard
      Aerobics—Cooper
      Aerobics for Women—Cooper

B. Community Resources
   YMCA or YWCA programs

3

RISK OF DEATH SECTION

Age 40   Height 73
Race White   Weight 222
Sex Male

Life Expectancy Results
      1 5 10 15 20 25 30 35 40 45
Average Years of
Remaining Life in
Your Sex, Age,
Race Group   33 ****************

Your Expected Yrs.
of Remaining Life
Based on your
Answers   25 ***********

You can achieve
this expected yrs.
of remaining life   38 *******************

RISK OF DEATH SECTION (Con't.)

Major Hazards to you
      10 year deaths
Rank Hazard per 100,000   Associated risk factors
1. Cirrhosis
   Average   304   Drinking Habits
   Your   3800
   Achieveable   61

2. Arteriosclerotic Heart Disease
   Average   1861   Systolic Blood Pressure
   Your   2382   Diastolic Blood Pressure
   Achievable   447   Cholesterol Level
                  Smoking Habits
                  Weight

3. Motor Vehicle Accidents
   Average   339   Drinking Habits
   Your   1763   Seat Belt Habits
   Achievable   203

4. Cancer of Lungs
   Average   291   Smoking Habits
   Your   582
   Achievable   58

Suggestions For Increasing Your Expected Years of Remaing Life
1. choosing non-drinking   will add 8.6 exp. years of life
2. choosing non-smoking   will add 2.0 exp. years of life
3. lowering cholesterol
   level   will add 0.7 exp. years of life
4. lowering diastolic
   blood pressure   will add 0.6 exp. years of life
5. lowering systolic blood
   pressure   will add 0.6 exp. years of life
6. losing weight   will add 0.4 exp. years of life
7. always wearing seatbelts will add 0.1 exp. years of life
8. having annual procto
   exam   will add 0.1 exp. years of life
Total   13

Remarks:
We have had to make the following assumptions about you:

You have an average blood cholesterol level.

Hazard Summary

Based on the Lifestyle Assessment Questionnaire you have filled out, you have a health age of 48 years. If you can follow all the suggestions we have given, you can reduce your health age to 35.

4

ALERT SECTION: Medical/Behavioral/Emotional

Significant Past illnesses   Immunizations
1. Diabetic   1. Up-to-date for DPT
2. Physical disability   2. Up-to-date for polio
                  3. Rubella status unknown

Allergies   Emotions
1. Allergic to penicillin   1. History compatible with
                  serious depression

FIGURE 14-3. Sample printouts. University of Wisconsin, Stevens Point, Life-style Assessment Results.

TABLE 5. Student Selected Topics for Personal Growth Section, UW-SP LAQ*

Type of Assistance Required	Information		Group Activities		Confidential Personal Assistance	
	1977-78	1978-79	1977-78	1978-79	1977-78	1978-79
1. Responsible alcohol use	432 (7)	408 (10)	120 (18)	81 (21)	0 (25)	0 (26)
2. Stop smoking programs	280 (20)	285 (20)	120 (18)	96 (16)	24 (19)	18 (14)
3. Sexual dysfunction	272 (23)	285 (20)	104 (23)	42 (24)	32 (13)	36 (4)
4. Contraception	448 (4)	414 (9)	80 (25)	36 (25)	64 (4)	27 (8)
5. Venereal disease	384 (13)	339 (13)	80 (25)	33 (26)	32 (13)	12 (18)
6. Depression	296 (18)	330 (14)	176 (10)	144 (10)	96 (2)	42 (3)
7. Loneliness	280 (20)	261 (24)	224 (5)	177 (6)	80 (3)	21 (10)
8. Exercise programs	544 (3)	594 (2)	554 (1)	507 (1)	32 (13)	3 (24)
9. Weight reduction	376 (14)	453 (5)	304 (2)	201 (5)	56 (8)	6 (23)
10. Breast self-exam	320 (16)	321 (16)	64 (26)	3 (27)	64 (4)	15 (16)
11. Medical emergencies	568 (1)	552 (3)	160 (13)	123 (13)	40 (10)	12 (18)
12. Vegetarian diets	440 (5)	441 (8)	112 (21)	69 (23)	8 (24)	9 (21)
13. Relaxation-stress reduction	424 (8)	540 (4)	192 (8)	213 (3)	40 (10)	15 (16)
14. Mate selection	400 (11)	366 (12)	168 (12)	159 (9)	24 (19)	24 (9)
15. Parenting	280 (20)	282 (22)	176 (10)	138 (11)	0 (25)	0 (26)
16. Marital problems	256 (25)	231 (25)	128 (17)	96 (16)	64 (4)	30 (5)

Item						
17. Assertiveness training ("How to say no without feeling guilty")	440 (5)	453 (5)	232 (4)	168 (7)	32 (13)	30 (5)
18. Biofeedback for tension headaches	424 (8)	327 (15)	104 (23)	87 (19)	16 (21)	18 (14)
19. Overcoming phobias (examples: high places, crowded rooms, etc.)	304 (17)	318 (17)	112 (21)	108 (14)	32 (13)	21 (10)
20. Educational/vocational goal setting/planning	560 (2)	690 (1)	192 (8)	138 (11)	200 (1)	159 (1)
21. Spiritual or philosophical values	272 (23)	312 (19)	216 (16)	168 (7)	32 (13)	21 (10)
22. Interpersonal communication skills	336 (15)	318 (17)	208 (7)	204 (4)	16 (21)	30 (5)
23. Automobile safety	288 (19)	723 (23)	136 (16)	72 (22)	0 (25)	3 (24)
24. Suicide thoughts or attempts	232 (27)	186 (27)	120 (18)	90 (18)	48 (9)	66 (2)
25. Drug abuse	248 (26)	218 (26)	152 (15)	87 (19)	16 (21)	12 (18)
26. Test anxiety reduction	392 (12)	375 (11)	160 (13)	102 (15)	40 (10)	9 (21)
27. Relationships—developing and continuing	424 (8)	447 (7)	288 (3)	243 (2)	64 (4)	21 (10)

*The number of incoming freshman students requesting each item is listed by type of assistance requested. The rank order is listed in parentheses.

topics and the number of student requests from 1977 and 1978 in each of the possible categories. This section of the questionnaire helps the Student Life Division identify the high-interest areas for program planning. This information, which may be of assistance in improving course offerings for academic credit, is also provided to the faculty.

The printout from the personal growth section provides to the student four sources for continued learning in response to any request he or she makes. If the student checks any of the three possible selections next to one of the 27 topics, he or she will be provided by the computer with (1) courses for credit that deal with that subject; (2) people within the university who are competent to deal with that subject and their phone numbers; (3) media resources including books, movies, audio tapes, video tapes, pamphlets, and so on that deal with that subject; and (4) community resources with phone numbers that can provide learning opportunities on that subject. This automated referral puts the responsibility where it appropriately lies—in the hands of the individual student.

An example of the demand for programs related to personal growth occurred when the counseling center developed an anonymous dial-a-tape information system that responded to many of the 27 topics. In the first 2 weeks of operation, this dial-a-tape system received 8,000 phone calls that could not be completed. This was a situation in which overmarketing had occurred. Student Life has since added a second unit for playback.

The risk of death section (health hazard appraisal) elicits information relating to the morbidity and to the mortality of the individual. This information includes family history, current health practices, and certain simple biomedical measurements such as blood pressure, height, and weight. Based on the book *How to Practice Prospective Medicine* by Robbins and Hall[7] and current mortality data from the United States, the individual receives information regarding her or his chances of death in the next 10 years. The computer calculates the probable number of years that the individual would have remaining in her or his life, the leading causes of death for her or him by age, race, and sex, and what behaviors could be changed to improve the chances both of survival and quality of life.

The final section of the LAQ is the medical alert section. This section elicits current potential health problems that would be of interest to the individual for a home self-care record or to any medical or health provider who might see the student in a clinical setting. At UW–SP the entire printout becomes a part of the medical record and a printout of the medical alert section becomes the problem-oriented summary sheet on the inside cover of the chart. This record includes such important information as current status of immunizations, serious medical problems, and allergies.

LAQ AND INCOME GENERATION

It was believed it would be inappropriate to administer a detailed LAQ without developing programs in response to the request that students make after completing such a questionnaire. For this reason the $7.50 fee was established. By using Health Service administrative and secretarial support, the cost per questionnaire to the Student Health Service for processing is $2.50. This leaves a $5.00 per student programming fee that is used to develop wellness-promotion programs. The budget plan for spending this money is developed by the SHAC.

STUDENT HEALTH ADVISORY COMMITTEE

The SHAC was first suggested on the UW–SP campus in the spring of 1972 by a history professor and a health education professor. The original purpose of the committee was (1) to provide students with an opportunity for substantive and procedural involvement in the policies of the Health Service; (2) to improve the Health Center services to regular and continual student evaluation and input; and (3) to aid in the dissemination of health-related information to the student body and to conduct periodic surveys of student opinion regarding the Health Center. The SHAC has existed since 1972. Its activities have fluctuated from year to year, depending on the interest and capabilities of its members. Over the past 2 years, SHAC has developed a strong peer education component. The present membership of 50 was quickly divided into task force groups to develop and to be trained in program delivery. These programs include such topics as physical fitness, nutrition, contraception, and interpersonal relationships, stress management, dental wellness, and blood pressure screening.

The recruitment of new members for SHAC occurs during summer orientation, by word of mouth after school starts, and by presentations in related classes. In addition to running life-style improvement programs in dormitories and in University Center buildings for other students, SHAC sponsors health fairs, lectures, programs for high school, junior high, and grade schools, fun runs, regular blood pressure screening in the University Center, alternative evening activities, and social events for the membership. Each year a number of SHAC student members attend the American College Health Association meeting to gather new ideas and to share their experiences.

INITIAL STUDENT CONTACT

The initial interaction between the Student Life Division and the student occurs during the summer orientation. Approximately 90 per cent of new UW–SP students attend a 2-day, live-in orientation program. Most students attend with one or both parents. The students are given an opportunity to live in the residence halls, to eat the food in the food services, to meet with student leaders of the orientation staff, to be tested for academic programs, to register for their academic courses and to hear presentations by a number of service providers on campus. The initial communication concerning health promotion is provided by one of the SHAC members. An entertaining and informative, 40-minute slide show outlines (1) the dimensions of wellness, (2) the types of services offered by Health and Counseling Services, (3) the activities of SHAC, and (4) the requirement for either the LAQ or the history and physical examination.

During summer orientation, while students are hearing a presentation by the SHAC president, the parents are given an opportunity to have a similar presentation by the director of the Health Service and by the director of the Counseling Service. This presentation outlines the variety of services that are available to the students and encourages the parents to discuss topics of interest to the student during the trip home.

Following the presentation, the student is given a copy of the LAQ with a letter of explanation from the director of Health Services. (See Appendix for LAQ information letter. Copies of the LAQ are available for use through the Institute for Lifestyle Improvements, University of Wisconsin–Stevens Point, Stevens Point, WI 54481.)

At the close of the SHAC presentation on health and counseling services, students are given an opportunity to leave their names and addresses if they are interested in hearing more about SHAC membership. During the summer of 1979, 10 per cent of the 1,800 students who went through orientation walked to the front of the room and left their names and addresses with the SHAC president. These students were contacted during the summer by letter and encouraged to attend the first meeting. (See Appendix for SHAC membership letter.)

The first SHAC meeting was held in the late afternoon on the first day of school, with 50 students attending. The SHAC meetings have continued to experience an average attendance of 50 people who have been assigned to program areas on the basis of their interests. Following training and experience in providing programs in a given area, these students will be given an opportunity to switch to other groups to expand their experience.

The SHAC also provides a social function for interested students. A number of activities have been planned and implemented. (See SHAC membership letter in Appendix for a partial listing of SHAC activities.)

LAQ RESULTS

The Health Service collects the LAQs, codes them, and transfers them to the Data Processing Center for computer processing. One copy of the results is placed in the student's chart. The other copy is sealed in an envelope and sent to the student. An interpretation sheet has been developed that explains the results to the student. In addition to this written explanation, however, the student is encouraged to attend an interpretation session that is run by the director of his or her residence hall. The residence hall directors are master's-level counselors and have been trained to interpret the LAQ. For those students who live off campus, interpretations can be provided by SHAC members or members of the Health Service or Counseling Service staff.

The staff of the University Health Service is encouraged to discuss the LAQ results with the individual students, when appropriate, during a Health Service visit.

EVALUATION OF THE IMPACT OF THE LAQ

A thorough evaluation of the impact of the LAQ and wellness programming is underway. A preliminary evaluation of 268 students was accomplished in the spring of 1979. Twenty-three per cent of these students indicated that the computer printout results led them to change one or more of their life-style factors. The factors listed on the questionnaire include smoking, alcohol consumption, weight, seat belt use, breast self-examination, cholesterol, or blood pressure.

UNIVERSITYWIDE SUPPORT

In addition to the SHAC programs the resident assistants in the residence halls provide a number of programs that address themselves to other dimensions of wellness. Because of the evolving interest in wellness promotion at UW–SP, a number of courses have been added to increase the learning opportunities in this field. During the spring of 1979, a lecture forum entitled "Wellness" was attended weekly by more than 100 participants. The Communications Department has developed courses in health communication and wellness promotion. The Health and Physical Education Department has developed a course entitled "The Healthy American." The Intramural Program has developed wellness clubs. A number of the residence halls have formed wellness, jogging, or nutrition clubs. The Food Service Committee has been working with a SHAC task force to alter the menu provided at UW–SP.

Two hundred faculty and staff members have participated in LAQ seminars and have received individual printouts with interpretations. The Physical Education Department has posted in the faculty newsletter and in the physical education building a schedule of times when the indoor running track, swimming pool, and other facilities are available for open activities by students, faculty or staff. The university has developed dual-purpose trails for running and cross-country skiing in a forest reserve adjacent to the campus. A par course is being developed as one part of that reserve. An active employee assistance program has been established and is growing. There has been top administrative support for the wellness promotion program from the very beginning.

COUNSELING CENTER PROGRAMMING

The Counseling Center offers a number of group activities for self-improvement. Topics such as assertiveness training, reading and study skills, vocational and career planning, stop-smoking programs, "body tune-up," couples' communication, sexuality groups, and individual counseling as required are part of the programming.

THE LIFEGAIN MODEL

The entire UW–SP program has been influenced by the work of Robert Allen of the Human Resources Institute (HRI) of Morristown, New Jersey. The "Lifegain" program developed by HRI focuses on evaluating the cultural norms that exist to support desired changes by the population. A university where the external forces can be modified is an ideal location to attempt a wellness promotion program. The place where the student lives is often supervised by university employees. The selection of the resident assistants is within the control of the university. The food service contract can be modified toward a wellness offering. The university centers can be programmed to offer a number of positive alternatives for evening activities. The health and counseling centers can be supportive, with programs and individual consultation. Another asset is that, at this point in time, most students are at the healthiest stage of their life.

The widespread public support for higher education could support the argument that wellness promotion is a responsibility of the university. If the citizens of tomorrow have more skills in dealing with the forces of society and develop positive health practices during the college years, they will be more productive citizens and decrease the amount of illness care required in future years. As Don Ardell has stated: High level wellness is more rewarding than low level worseness."[8]

DUPLICATING THE UW–SP MODEL IN OTHER SETTINGS

The barriers to implementing such a program on any campus exist in the minds of the people working there. St. Cloud State University in St. Cloud, Minnesota, for instance, has been developing a similar program. St. Cloud or any other institution could purchase the soft ware to provide the LAQ on its own campus or it could have that service provided by the Foundation of UW–SP. The cost to outside user schools in presently $4.00 per appraisal in quantities over 100. A university or community could charge individual clients or students $7.50, or any other reasonable fee, and use the difference between the cost of the processing and its fee to run the programs that would be indicated on the basis of the questionnaire results. The automated referral section of the LAQ can be individualized for different communities. Thus students at another university could be referred to the learning opportunities available on that campus and in that community. Dial-a-tape systems can be purchased or developed locally. Student health advisory committees can be formed and nurtured. Significant student involvement greatly enhances the credibility and capability of the program.

It is difficult to reliably assess the cause-and-effect relationship in the area of behavioral change. Society is changing so rapidly, and there are so many forces that influence the decisions that people make, that it will be difficult to evaluate the true impact of the wellness-promotion program. The preliminary data, however, tend to support the concept that an active, positive approach toward health and wellness can bring about behavioral change. Whether this change will be sustained remains to be proven. For better or worse, however, humans will influence humans. Why not try to make it better? We teach best by example.

REFERENCES

1. Dunn, H., *High Level Wellness*. Arlington, Va.: R. W. Betty Co, 1961.
2. Sorochan, W., *Personal Health Appraisal*. New York: John Wiley & Sons, 1970.
3. Diesendorf, M. and Furnass, B., *The Magic Bullet*. Australia: Society for Social Responsibility and Science, 1976.
4. Travis, J., *Wellness Workbook for Health Professionals*. Mill Valley, Calif.: Wellness Resource Center, 1977.
5. Fuller, R., *Utopia or Oblivion: The Prospects for Humanity*. New York: Bantam Books, 1969, p. 80–94.
6. Blankenbaker, R., "Total Care the Cost-Effective Way." *Thirteenth Annual Meeting of the Society of Prospective Medicine*. Bethesda, Md.: Health and Education Resources, 1977.
7. Robbins, L. and Hall, J., *How to Practice Prospective Medicine*. Indianapolis, Ind.: Methodist Hospital of Indiana, 1970.
8. Ardell, D., *High Level Wellness: An Alternative to Doctors, Drugs, and Disease*. Emmaus, Pa.: Rodale Press, 1977.

APPENDIX A. SAMPLE STUDENT CONTACT LETTERS

LAQ Information

Dear Student:

Welcome to the University of Wisconsin/Stevens Point. We plan to offer you up to date medical care and an opportunity to develop the healthiest life-style possible for you. We expect you to be willing to consider change toward higher levels of wellness during your career here in Stevens Point. We expect you to be a *partner* in helping us provide you with the best care possible. As a first step in forming this *partnership*, we require you to provide us with some information about your current health status, past problems, future risks, and possible areas in which you would like to improve. This partnership is initiated in one of two ways. During the summer orientation/registration program you may elect one of the following:

1. You may fill out a Lifestyle Assessment Questionnaire. This is a self-administered health and wellness assessment instrument. It is the recommended method for providing us with necessary information about you. All new students are billed $7.50 for this service.
2. As an alternative, you may request a standard history and physical form at orientation or from the University Health Service and have your physician fill it out and return it to us. (At an average cost of $25 to $40 per physical.)

We recommend the Lifestyle Assessment Questionnaire because it is less expensive, more convenient, and provides us with the most appropriate information.

The $7.50 charge covers the cost of the computer analysis of your Lifestyle Assessment Questionnaire and programs that will be offered to you for life-style improvement. We believe that out of 27 possible areas of self-improvement offered, all students, will be able to find at least one topic in which they are interested. Any student choosing the standard history and physical will have the $7.50 fee waived on receipt of the physical by the University Health Service. If you enter UW–SP at a time when no formal orientation program is offered, you may pick up a Lifestyle Assessment Questionnaire at the Health Service.

As a University requirement, you must select one of the above two options. We feel the Lifestyle Assessment Questionnaire will give you an accurate measurement of your current level of wellness, current risks, future risks, and will give you an automated referral to sources of information or activities that lead to higher levels of wellness. You may omit any answer you are not sure about or feel is not pertinent. We will process the forms and return the results to you. This material as with all of our medical records is kept confidential. No one can have access to your records without prior written permission from you.

Please stop in and see us when you get to campus. We are located in the lower level of Nelson Hall. We have an active Student Health Advisory Committee and we welcome your input. Thank you for your assistance.

SHAC Membership

Dear Student:

This letter is a follow-up to the health presentation made during the summer orientation program. At that time, you indicated an interest in the Student Health Advisory Committee (SHAC). We hope you will maintain that interest and join us in the fall. We believe there are many advantages to being involved with SHAC. We have listed below some of the reasons that we feel students would benefit from being involved with our organization:

1. An opportunity to practice public speaking.
2. An opportunity to improve your self-confidence.
3. An opportunity to list an important activity on your resumé at the time of graduation.
4. An opportunity to learn about health center–health services administration.
5. Satisfaction of helping other people improve their health practices.
6. An opportunity for direct experience relating to many careers such as health, medicine, nursing, dietetics, and teaching.
7. Academic credit is offered for SHAC participation.
8. An opportunity to practice policy making.

9. A chance to make close friends and develop long-term-relationships.
10. An additional source for social functions.

The Student Health Advisory Committee is planning to have at least one social function each month. These functions will include such activities as:

Picnics
Group outings to Fine Arts and other campus presentations
Iceskating
Winter camping
House parties
Pizza parties
Folk dancing
Swimming parties
Bike trips
Rollerskating
Skiing
Tobogganing
Pot luck dinners
Square dancing
Social dancing
Fun runs
Canoeing

These functions will give SHAC members an opportunity to know each other on a more personal basis and also get to know members of the University Health Service staff.

The first three weeks of the fall semester will be spent in organization and training for new SHAC members. During the fall semester, SHAC will have at least one social function per month. We plan to have a weekly column in *The Pointer* (the school paper). We also have a weekly SHAC meeting. Each member will be encouraged to participate in one or more interest groups. We will be selecting leaders for SHAC which will include treasurer, public relations director, editor, student Government representative, Residence Hall Council representative, and Student Affairs Committee representative. We will also need task force leaders in a number of areas. On the enclosed interest sheet, please indicate your levels of interest by checking the appropriate spaces.

The first meeting for 1979–80 will be held on Monday, August 27, at 4 p.m. in room 125A & B of the University Center. Please try to make this first meeting, if you are interested in participating. At that time we will discuss other possible meeting times.

Please fill in all appropriate information on the enclosed SHAC participation form. This information will be used by us in planning for the first semester's activities.

Carol Weston
SHAC Chairperson 1978–79

John Carini
SHAC Chairperson 1979–80

Joy Amundson
Health Educator
UW–SP Health Service

Bill Hettler, M.D.
Director, University Health Service
and Lifestyle Improvement Program

APPENDIX B. LIFESTYLE ASSESSMENT QUESTIONNAIRE

LIFESTYLE ASSESSMENT QUESTIONNAIRE

2nd Edition

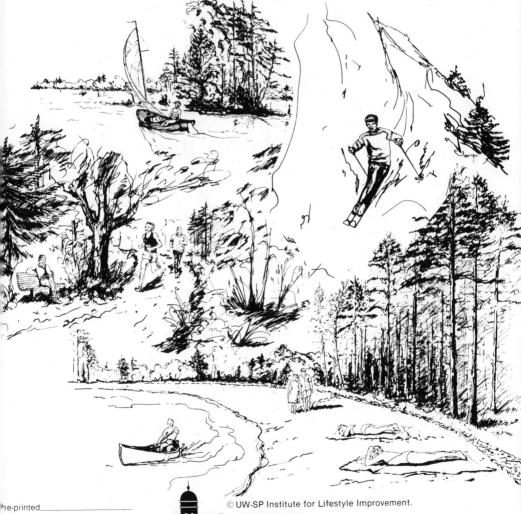

© UW-SP Institute for Lifestyle Improvement.

UW-SP Foundation
Stevens Point, WI 54481
(715) 346-3811

Pre-printed_____

Code # _____

Referral Source _____

purpose

This Lifestyle Assessment Questionnaire is designed to help you assess your current level of wellness and the potential risks or hazards that you choose to face at this point in your life. The printouts that you will receive will reflect your strengths and the possible consequences of risks that you choose to take. The questionnaire will also assess your interest in improving the quality of your life. The printout will indicate sources of information that will help you learn more about gaining higher levels of wellness.

THE MAJOR DETERMINANT FOR JOYFUL LIVING IS YOU AND YOUR LIFESTYLE

The circle graph below indicates the factors that contribute to increasing your enjoyment and quality of life. While it is true that doctors and hospitals have a significant role to play in the quality of our lives, this graph clearly indicates that it is individuals, through the choices that they make each day, that con- tribute the greatest percentage toward maximizing the quality of life and health. We believe this instrument can be a useful adjunct in helping individuals identi- fy the most likely causes of death and disability, but more importantly identify the areas of self-improvement which will lead to higher levels of joy and well- ness. This instrument can be used to begin a positive, wellness approach toward living. It is our belief that this instrument can help people realize that they are the most important provider of health or "illth" care. Many of the common kill- ers in America are the direct result of individual behaviors. We all know that our behaviors can improve our chances for leading a long useful life. Collectively, all of our behaviors can be described as our lifestyle.

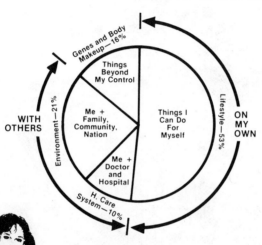

GENERAL INFORMATION CONCERNING THE LIFESTYLE ASSESSMENT QUESTIONNAIRE (LAQ)

The LAQ is organized into four sections: 1. Wellness Inventory; 2. Topics for Per- sonal Growth; 3. Risk of Death Section, and 4. Alert Section: Medical/Behavioral/ Emotional. The Wellness Inventory Section will help you identify your strengths. You will receive a printout that will indicate the percent of possible points that you gained in each topic area. The printout will also provide you with average scores for the people in your group and the total average for all people who have ever used this instrument.

The automated referral or Personal Growth section of this questionnaire will pro- vide a printout indicating resources available for up to six topics.

The Risk of Death section will result in a printout indicating the probable number of years that you have remaining in your life, the leading causes of death for your age, race, and sex, and what behaviors could be changed to improve the chances of survival and the quality of your life.

The final section of this questionnaire entitled the Alert Section: Medical/Be- havorial/Emotional will provide information which can generate a problem list for your home health record. This could also be used as part of a medical chart in a health care delivery system. We feel it will be useful for people to maintain, in their home, a current record of their immunization status and other significant problems.

It is our desire that this questionnaire be used in a positive sense to improve the understanding of self and your role in maintaining a life of high quality.

confidentiality

The Institute for Lifestyle Improvement will maintain the confidentiality of your answers. The Institute will not permit any individually identified information from your questionnaire to be released to any person or organization other than the source from whom the LAQ was received.

Bill Hettler M.D.
Bill Hettler, M.D.

Dennis Elsenrath
Dennis Elsenrath, Ed. D.

Fred Leafgren
Fred Leafgren, Ph.D.

THE UNIVERSITY OF WISCONSIN-STEVENS POINT
INSTITUTE FOR LIFESTYLE IMPROVEMENT
STEVENS POINT, WISCONSIN 54481 (715) 346-3811

The Institute for Lifestyle Improvement, which exists within the structure of the UW-SP Foundation, has three broad missions: 1. To provide health promotion services to public and private agencies; 2. To conduct research on lifestyle improvement activities; and 3. To provide continuing educational and training programs for those interested in wellness promotion strategies.

The Institute offers services in four major areas:

Lifestyle Assessment Questionnaire

—Individual and group needs assessment
—Motivational tool
—Health planning tool to estimate current and future disease care needs
—Self-care tool to provide home health care record

Consultation and Presentation

—Keynote speakers for local and national meetings
—Planning for community forums
—Facilitators for health fairs
—Speakers for corporate wellness programs
—Corporate wellness program planning and evaluation
—Consultation for community health promotion

Continuing Educational and Training Programs

—Annual wellness promotion strategies conference
—Specialized conferences for target groups
—On site training programs for corporations, universities or communities
—In-service training for teachers and other youth workers

Audio-Visual Materials and Self-Care Modules

—Production of movies on wellness promotion topics
—Production of videotapes, audio-tapes and slide/tape presentations on wellness promotion
—Written materials to support wellness promotion activities
—Other assessment instruments for wellness promotion
—Cold self-care module

1 lifestyle assessment questionnaire
WELLNESS INVENTORY SECTION

INSTRUCTIONS:

This section will help determine the current level of wellness that you are experiencing. We hope that it will also give you ideas for areas in which you might improve. If you are uncomfortable in answering any item in this section or following sections, you may leave that item blank. Please respond to these statements using the following choices and circle your response:

A—Almost always (90% or more of the time)
B—Very frequently (approximately 75% of the time)
C—Frequently (approximately 50% of the time)
D—Occasionally (approximately 25% of the time)
E—Almost never (less than 10% of the time)
  —If item does not apply to you do not mark item

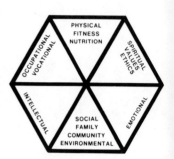

PHYSICAL EXERCISE—Measures one's commitment to maintaining physical fitness.

	Almost always	Very frequently	Frequently	Occasionally	Almost never	If item does not apply to you, do not mark
1. I exercise vigorously for at least 20 minutes three or more times per week	A	B	C	D	E	
2. I determine my activity level by monitoring my heart rate	A	B	C	D	E	
3. I stop exercising before I feel exhausted	A	B	C	D	E	
4. I approach exercise in a relaxed manner	A	B	C	D	E	
5. I stretch before exercising	A	B	C	D	E	
6. I stretch after exercising	A	B	C	D	E	
7. I walk or bike whenever possible	A	B	C	D	E	
8. When feeling tired, I arrange for sufficient sleep	A	B	C	D	E	
9. I participate in a strenuous sport (tennis, running, swimming, handball, basketball, etc.)	A	B	C	D	E	
10. I use foot gear of good quality, designed for the activity in which I participate	A	B	C	D	E	
11. If I am not in shape, I avoid sporadic (once a week or less often) strenuous exercise	A	B	C	D	E	
12. After vigorous exercise, I "cool down" (very light exercise such as walking) for at least five minutes before sitting or lying down	A	B	C	D	E	

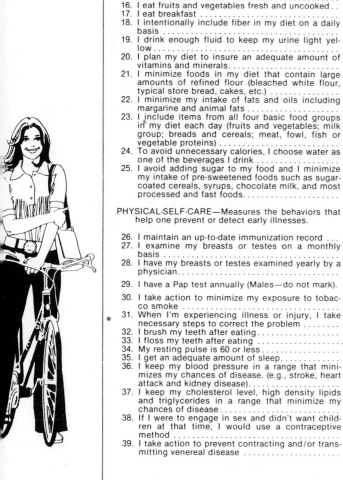

Almost always
  Very frequently
    Frequently
      Occasionally
        Almost never
          If item does not apply to you, do not mark

PHYSICAL-NUTRITIONAL—Measures the degree to which one chooses foods that are consistent with the dietary goals of the United States as published by the Senate Select Committee on Nutrition and Human Needs.

13. When choosing non-vegetable protein, I select lean cuts of meat, poultry and fish. . . . .   A B C D E

14. I maintain an appropriate weight for my height and frame . . . .   A B C D E

15. I minimize salt intake . . . .   A B C D E

16. I eat fruits and vegetables fresh and uncooked . .   A B C D E

17. I eat breakfast . . . .   A B C D E

18. I intentionally include fiber in my diet on a daily basis . . . .   A B C D E

19. I drink enough fluid to keep my urine light yellow . . . .   A B C D E

20. I plan my diet to insure an adequate amount of vitamins and minerals. . . . .   A B C D E

21. I minimize foods in my diet that contain large amounts of refined flour (bleached white flour, typical store bread, cakes, etc.) . . . .   A B C D E

22. I minimize my intake of fats and oils including margarine and animal fats . . . .   A B C D E

23. I include items from all four basic food groups in my diet each day (fruits and vegetables; milk group; breads and cereals; meat, fowl, fish or vegetable proteins) . . . .   A B C D E

24. To avoid unnecessary calories, I choose water as one of the beverages I drink . . . .   A B C D E

25. I avoid adding sugar to my food and I minimize my intake of pre-sweetened foods such as sugar-coated cereals, syrups, chocolate milk, and most processed and fast foods.   A B C D E

PHYSICAL-SELF-CARE—Measures the behaviors that help one prevent or detect early illnesses.

26. I maintain an up-to-date immunization record . . .   A B C D E

27. I examine my breasts or testes on a monthly basis . . . .   A B C D E

28. I have my breasts or testes examined yearly by a physician. . . . .   A B C D E

29. I have a Pap test annually (Males—do not mark).   A B C D E

30. I take action to minimize my exposure to tobacco smoke . . . .   A B C D E

31. When I'm experiencing illness or injury, I take necessary steps to correct the problem . . . .   A B C D E

32. I brush my teeth after eating. . . . .   A B C D E

33. I floss my teeth after eating . . . .   A B C D E

34. My resting pulse is 60 or less . . . .   A B C D E

35. I get an adequate amount of sleep. . . . .   A B C D E

36. I keep my blood pressure in a range that minimizes my chances of disease. (e.g., stroke, heart attack and kidney disease). . . . .   A B C D E

37. I keep my cholesterol level, high density lipids and triglycerides in a range that minimize my chances of disease . . . .   A B C D E

38. If I were to engage in sex and didn't want children at that time, I would use a contraceptive method . . . .   A B C D E

39. I take action to prevent contracting and/or transmitting venereal disease . . . .   A B C D E

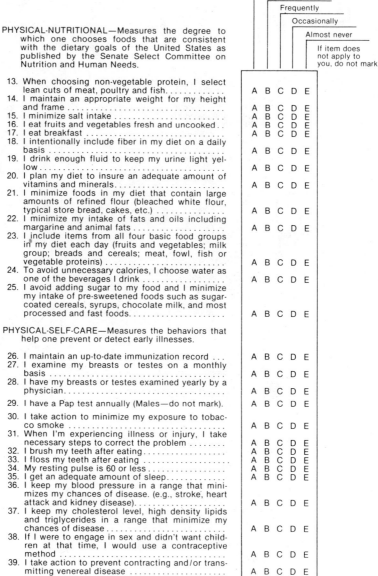

1

	Almost always	Very frequently	Frequently	Occasionally	Almost never	If item does not apply to you, do not mark

PHYSICAL-VEHICLE SAFETY—Measures one's ability to minimize chances of injury or death in a vehicle accident.

40. I do not operate vehicles under the influence of alcohol or other drugs . . . .   A B C D E
41. I do not ride with vehicle operators who are under the influence of alcohol or other drugs . . . . .   A B C D E
42. I stay within the speed limit . . . .   A B C D E
43. I use the information I learned in a driver education or defensive driving course . . . .   A B C D E
44. When traffic lights change from green to yellow, I prepare to stop . . . .   A B C D E
45. I maintain a safe driving distance between cars based on speed and road conditions. . . . .   A B C D E
46. Vehicles which I drive are maintained to assure safety. . . . .   A B C D E
47. Because they are safer, I use radial tires on cars that I drive. . . . .   A B C D E
48. I use caution when riding bicycles or motorcycles (e.g., helmets, adequate lights, etc.) . . . . .   A B C D E

PHYSICAL-DRUG USAGE—Measures the degree to which one is able to function without the unnecessary use of chemicals.

49. I use drugs only when necessary . . . .   A B C D E
50. I avoid the use of tobacco . . . .   A B C D E
51. I do not consume more than two alcoholic drinks per day . . . .   A B C D E
52. Because of the potentially harmful effects of caffeine (e.g., coffee, tea, cola, etc.), I limit my consumption . . . .   A B C D E
53. I avoid using marijuana . . . .   A B C D E
54. I avoid the use of hallucinogens (LSD, PCP, MDA, etc.). . . . .   A B C D E
55. I avoid the use of stimulants ("uppers"—e.g., cocaine, amphetamines, "pep pills", etc.) . . . . . .   A B C D E
56. I avoid the use of depressants ("downers"—e.g., barbiturates, minor tranquilizers, etc.). . . . .   A B C D E
57. I avoid using a combination of drugs unless under medical supervision . . . .   A B C D E
58. I follow the instructions provided with any drug I take . . . .   A B C D E
59. I avoid using drugs obtained from unlicensed sources . . . .   A B C D E
60. I understand the expected effect of drugs I take.   A B C D E
61. I consider alternatives to drugs . . . .   A B C D E

SOCIAL-ENVIRONMENTAL—Measures the degree to which one contributes to the common welfare of the community. This emphasizes the interdependence with others and nature.

62. I take steps to conserve energy in my place of residence . . . .   A B C D E
63. I consider energy conservation when choosing a mode of transportation. . . . .   A B C D E
64. I offer support to members of my family when appropriate . . . .   A B C D E
65. I contribute to the feeling of acceptance within my family . . . .   A B C D E
66. I do my part to promote clean air . . . .   A B C D E
67. When I see a safety hazard, I take action (warn others or correct the problem) . . . .   A B C D E
68. I avoid unnecessary radiation . . . .   A B C D E
69. I report criminal acts I observe . . . .   A B C D E

	Almost always	
	Very frequently	
	Occasionally	
	Almost never	
	If item does not apply to you, do not mark	

70. I contribute time and/or money to community projects.................................... A B C D E
71. I actively seek to become acquainted with individuals in my community .... A B C D E
72. I use my creativity in constructive ways .... A B C D E
73. My behavior reflects fairness and justice....... A B C D E
74. When possible, I choose an environment which is free of noise pollution .... A B C D E
75. When possible, I choose an environment which is free of air pollution...................... A B C D E
76. I participate in volunteer activities benefiting others .... A B C D E
77. I go out of my way to help others.............. A B C D E
78. I beautify those parts of my environment under my control............................... A B C D E

EMOTIONAL AWARENESS & ACCEPTANCE—Measures the degree to which one has an awareness and acceptance of one's feelings. This includes the degree to which one feels positive and enthusiastic about oneself and life.

79. I have a good sense of humor................. A B C D E
80. I feel positive about myself................... A B C D E
81. I feel there is a satisfying amount of excitement in my life.................................... A B C D E
82. My emotional life is stable.................... A B C D E
83. I am aware of my needs..................... A B C D E
84. I trust and value my own judgment............ A B C D E
85. When I make mistakes, I learn from them....... A B C D E
86. I feel comfortable when complimented for jobs well done .... A B C D E
87. It is okay for me to cry....................... A B C D E
88. I have feelings of sensitivity for others......... A B C D E
89. I feel enthusiastic about life .... A B C D E
90. I find it easy to laugh .... A B C D E
91. I am able to give love .... A B C D E
92. I am able to receive love .... A B C D E
93. I enjoy my life .... A B C D E
94. I have plenty of energy...................... A B C D E
95. My sleep is restful.......................... A B C D E
96. I trust others.............................. A B C D E
97. I feel others trust me .... A B C D E
98. I accept my sexual desires................... A B C D E
99. I understand how I create my feelings.......... A B C D E
100. At times I can be both strong and sensitive..... A B C D E
101. I am aware when I feel anger.................. A B C D E
102. I can accept my anger .... A B C D E
103. I am aware when I feel sad .... A B C D E
104. I can accept my sadness .... A B C D E
105. I am aware when I feel happy .... A B C D E
106. I can accept my happiness .... A B C D E
107. I am aware when I feel frightened .... A B C D E
108. I can accept my feelings of fear............... A B C D E

EMOTIONAL MANAGEMENT—Measures the capacity to appropriately control one's feelings and related behaviors including the realistic assessment of one's limitations.

109. I am able to be open with those with whom I am close.................................... A B C D E
110. I can express my feelings of anger .... A B C D E

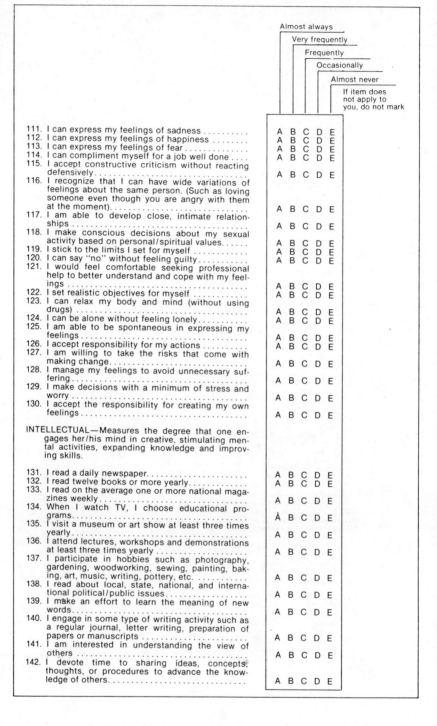

Almost always
Very frequently
Frequently
Occasionally
Almost never
If item does not apply to you, do not mark

111. I can express my feelings of sadness ....   A B C D E
112. I can express my feelings of happiness ....   A B C D E
113. I can express my feelings of fear ....   A B C D E
114. I can compliment myself for a job well done ....   A B C D E
115. I accept constructive criticism without reacting defensively..   A B C D E
116. I recognize that I can have wide variations of feelings about the same person. (Such as loving someone even though you are angry with them at the moment).............................   A B C D E
117. I am able to develop close, intimate relationships ....   A B C D E
118. I make conscious decisions about my sexual activity based on personal/spiritual values......   A B C D E
119. I stick to the limits I set for myself ....   A B C D E
120. I can say "no" without feeling guilty...........   A B C D E
121. I would feel comfortable seeking professional help to better understand and cope with my feelings ....   A B C D E
122. I set realistic objectives for myself ....   A B C D E
123. I can relax my body and mind (without using drugs) ....   A B C D E
124. I can be alone without feeling lonely...........   A B C D E
125. I am able to be spontaneous in expressing my feelings ....   A B C D E
126. I accept responsibility for my actions ....   A B C D E
127. I am willing to take the risks that come with making change..   A B C D E
128. I manage my feelings to avoid unnecessary suffering..   A B C D E
129. I make decisions with a minimum of stress and worry ....   A B C D E
130. I accept the responsibility for creating my own feelings ....   A B C D E

INTELLECTUAL—Measures the degree that one engages her/his mind in creative, stimulating mental activities, expanding knowledge and improving skills.

131. I read a daily newspaper......................   A B C D E
132. I read twelve books or more yearly.............   A B C D E
133. I read on the average one or more national magazines weekly..   A B C D E
134. When I watch TV, I choose educational programs..   À B C D E
135. I visit a museum or art show at least three times yearly..   A B C D E
136. I attend lectures, workshops and demonstrations at least three times yearly ....   A B C D E
137. I participate in hobbies such as photography, gardening, woodworking, sewing, painting, baking, art, music, writing, pottery, etc. ....   A B C D E
138. I read about local, state, national, and international political/public issues.................   A B C D E
139. I make an effort to learn the meaning of new words..   A B C D E
140. I engage in some type of writing activity such as a regular journal, letter writing, preparation of papers or manuscripts ....   A B C D E
141. I am interested in understanding the view of others ....   A B C D E
142. I devote time to sharing ideas, concepts, thoughts, or procedures to advance the knowledge of others.............................   A B C D E

```
                                                    Almost always
                                                      Very frequently
                                                        Frequently
                                                          Occasionally
                                                            Almost never
                                                              If item does
                                                              not apply to
                                                              you, do not mark
```

143. I gather information to enable me to make independent decisions. . . . .   A B C D E
144. I listen to radio and/or TV news . . . .   A B C D E

OCCUPATIONAL—Measures the satisfaction gained from one's work and the degree to which one is enriched by that work.

Please answer these items from your primary frame of reference, (e.g., your job, student, homemaker, etc.) If you are unemployed or retired, do not mark this section.

145. I enjoy my work . . . .   A B C D E
146. My work contributes to my personal needs . . . . .   A B C D E
147. I feel that my job in some way contributes to others and/or society . . . .   A B C D E
148. I interact cooperatively with others in my work . .   A B C D E
149. I take advantage of opportunities to learn new skills in my work . . . .   A B C D E
150. My work is challenging. . . . .   A B C D E
151. I feel my job responsibilities are consistent with my values . . . .   A B C D E
152. I find satisfaction from the work I do. . . . .   A B C D E
153. I find healthy ways of reducing excessive stress when it occurs in my job . . . .   A B C D E
154. I use recommended health and safety precautions . . . .   A B C D E
155. I make recommendations for improving occupational health and safety . . . .   A B C D E
156. I am satisfied with the degree of freedom to exercise independent judgments in my job . . . .   A B C D E
157. I am satisfied with the amount of variety in my work. . . . .   A B C D E
158. I believe I am competent in my job . . . .   A B C D E
159. My co-workers and supervisors respect me as a competent individual . . . .   A B C D E

SPIRITUAL—Measures one's ongoing involvement in seeking meaning and purpose in human existence. It includes an appreciation for the depth and expanse of life and natural forces that exist in the universe.

160. I feel good about my spiritual life. . . . .   A B C D E
161. Prayer, meditation, and/or quiet personal reflection is/are important part(s) of my life. . . . .   A B C D E
162. I contemplate my purpose in life . . . .   A B C D E
163. I reflect on the meaning of events in my life . . . .   A B C D E
164. My values guide my daily life . . . .   A B C D E
165. My values and beliefs help me to meet daily challenges . . . .   A B C D E
166. I recognize that my spiritual growth is a lifelong process. . . . .   A B C D E
167. I am concerned about humanitarian issues . . . . .   A B C D E
168. I enjoy participating in discussions about spiritual values . . . .   A B C D E
169. I feel a sense of compassion to others in need . .   A B C D E
170. I seek spiritual knowledge . . . .   A B C D E
171. My spiritual awareness occurs other than at times of crisis . . . .   A B C D E
172. I believe in something greater or (that I am part of something greater) than myself . . . .   A B C D E
173. I share my spiritual values . . . .   A B C D E

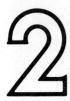

lifestyle assessment questionnaire

TOPICS FOR PERSONAL GROWTH SECTION

INSTRUCTIONS:
This section is intended to help you identify areas in which you would like more information or sources for group activities for continued learning or confidential personal assistance. In response to your selection from the following topics we will provide you with resources or services to meet your requests.

With regard to the following list, I would like:

	Information	Group Activities	Confidential Personal Assistance
1. Responsible alcohol use	1	2	3
2. Stop smoking programs	1	2	3
3. Sexual dysfunction	1	2	3
4. Contraception	1	2	3
5. Venereal disease	1	2	3
6. Depression	1	2	3
7. Loneliness	1	2	3
8. Exercise programs	1	2	3
9. Weight reduction	1	2	3
10. Self breast exam	1	2	3
11. Medical emergencies	1	2	3
12. Vegetarian diets	1	2	3
13. Relaxation - stress reduction	1	2	3
14. Mate selection	1	2	3
15. Parenting skills	1	2	3
16. Marital (or couples) problems	1	2	3
17. Assertive training (How to say no without feeling guilty)	1	2	3
18. Biofeedback for tension headache	1	2	3
19. Overcoming phobias (ex. high places, crowded rooms, etc.)	1	2	3
20. Educational/Career goal setting/planning	1	2	3
21. Spiritual or philosophical values	1	2	3
22. Interpersonal communication skills	1	2	3
23. Automobile safety	1	2	3
24. Suicide thoughts or attempts	1	2	3
25. Drug abuse	1	2	3
26. Test anxiety reduction	1	2	3
27. Enhancing Relationships	1	2	3
28. Time Management Skills	1	2	3
29. Nutrition	1	2	3
30. Death and Dying	1	2	3
31. Learning Skills (Speed reading, comprehension, etc.)	1	2	3

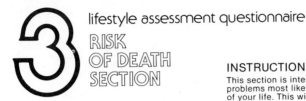

lifestyle assessment questionnaire
RISK OF DEATH SECTION

Age in years _____

Height _____ ft. _____ inches

Weight in pounds _____

INSTRUCTIONS:

This section is intended to help you identify the problems most likely to interfere with the quality of your life. This will give you a statistical assessment of the most likely causes of death facing you for the next ten (10) years. This section will also indicate what impact various personal behavioral choices have on that risk of death. Although this section will give you a printout indicating a statistical measurement of your risk based on national morbidity and mortality data, the printout will be no guarantee. Pre-existing disease or chance occurrence can completely negate the recommendations or suggestions made on this printout. We do feel, however, that it is a fairly accurate assessment of your current state of risk and offers suggestions for improving the quality of life and useful longevity.

1. Sex:
   1. Male
   2. Female

2. Race:
   1. White
   2. Black
   2. Other

3. How would you describe your body build?
   1. Small
   2. Medium
   3. Large

4. What is your systolic (top number) blood pressure?
   1. 190 or more
   2. 170-189
   3. 150-169
   4. 130-149
   5. Less than 130
   Note: If you don't know your blood pressure, we will use the average for your age, race, and sex.

5. What is your diastolic (lower number) blood pressure?
   1. 103 or more
   2. 97-102
   3. 91-96
   4. 85-90
   5. Less than 85

6. What is your blood cholesterol level?
   1. 270 or more
   2. 230-269
   3. 210-229
   4. 190-209
   5. Less than 190
   Note: If you don't know your cholesterol level, we will use the average for your age, race, and sex.

7. Are you
   1. An uncontrolled diabetic
   2. A controlled diabetic
   3. Not a diabetic

8. Which of the following best describes how much physical activity you get per week including work?
   1. Climb less than 5 flights of stairs or walk less than ½ mile 4 times per week (or equivalent activity)
   2. Climb 5-15 flights of stairs or walk ½-1½ miles 4 times per week (or equivalent activity)
   3. Climb 15-20 flights of stairs or walk 1½-2 miles 4 times per week (or equivalent activity)

9. Family history of heart disease:
   1. Both parents died before age 60 of heart disease
   2. One parent died before age 60 of heart disease
   3. Neither parent died before age of 60 of heart disease

10. Do you smoke tobacco?
    1. Yes
    2. No

11. If yes, how much do you smoke per day?
    1. 2 packs of cigarettes or more
    2. 1½-2 packs of cigarettes
    3. 1-1½ packs of cigarettes
    4. ½-1 pack of cigarettes or heavy pipe or cigar
    5. Less than ½-1 pack of cigarettes or light pipe or cigar

12. If 10 is yes, how many years have you been smoking?
    1. Less than 2
    2. 2 - 5
    3. 5 - 10
    4. 11 - 15
    5. 16 or more

13. Are you a former smoker?
    1. Yes
    2. No

14. If yes, how much did you smoke per day?
    1. 2 packs of cigarettes or more
    2. 1½-2 packs of cigarettes
    3. 1-1½ packs of cigarettes
    4. ½-1 pack of cigarettes or heavy pipe or cigar
    5. Less than ½-1 pack of cigarettes or light pipe or cigar

③

15. How many years ago did you quit?
    1. 0-2 years
    2. 3-4
    3. 5-6
    4. 7-8
    5. 9 or more

16. Do you drink alcoholic beverages?
    1. Yes
    2. No

17. If yes to the question above, how many per week?
    1. More than 40 drinks
    2. 25-40
    3. 8-24
    4. 3-7
    5. 1-2

18. When consuming alcohol, I do not consume more than one drink per hour.
    1. Yes
    2. No

19. How many miles a year do you travel in a motor vehicle as a driver or passenger?
    1. Under 10,000
    2. 10,000-20,000
    3. 20,000-30,000
    4. 30,000-40,000
    5. Over 40,000

20. While traveling in a motor vehicle how often do you use seat belts?
    1. 20% or less of the time
    2. 20%-40%
    3. 40%-60%
    4. 60%-80%
    5. 80%-100%

21. Are you depressed much of the time?
    1. Frequently
    2. Seldom
    3. Never

22. Has anyone in your immediate family (parents, brothers, sisters) committed suicide?
    1. Yes
    2. No

23. In regard to your heart, have you had:
    1. A murmur without preventive antibiotics
    2. A murmur with preventive antibiotics
    3. No murmur

24. In regard to your heart, have you had:
    1. Rheumatic fever without preventive antibiotics
    2. Rheumatic fever with preventive antibiotics
    3. No rheumatic fever

25. To the best of your knowledge, do you have any signs or symptoms of rheumatic heart disease?
    1. Yes
    2. No

26. Have you ever been arrested for burglary, robbery, or assault?
    1. Yes
    2. No

27. Do you carry a weapon with you?
    1. Yes
    2. No

28. Have you ever had bacterial pneumonia?
    1. Yes
    2. No

29. Have you ever had emphysema?
    1. Yes
    2. No

30. Has anyone in your family (parents, brother sisters) had diabetes?
    1. Yes
    2. No

31. Have you ever had polyps (growth in the intetines?)
    1. Yes
    2. No

32. Have you ever had undiagnosed rectal bleeding?
    1. Yes
    2. No

33. Have you ever had ulcerative colitis?
    1. Yes, 10 or more years ago
    2. Yes, less than 10 years ago
    3. No

34. Have you had a rectal examination with a lighte instrument within the last year?
    1. Yes
    2. No

IF FEMALE, ANSWER THE FOLLOWING 9 QUESTION

35. Do you perform a regular monthly self-brea examination?
    1. Yes
    2. No

36. Do you have a yearly exam by your physician?
    1. Yes
    2. No

37. How many of your blood relatives (mother, siste aunts) have had breast cancer?
    1. 2 or more
    2. 1
    3. None

38. Have you ever had fibrocystic breast disease other noncancerous disease?
    1. Yes
    2. No

39. Are you Jewish? (Cancer of the cervix is very ra in Jewish women)
    1. Yes
    2. No

40. Age of first intercourse. (Cancer of the cervix more common in females who have first inte course in teens and/or have multiple partners)
    1. Under 20 years old
    2. 20-25 years old
    3. Over 25 years old or never

41. Pertaining to a Pap smear, mark the respons most accurate for you (we assume none were a normal)
    1. Haven't had one in last five (5) years
    2. Had 1 normal within the last five (5) years
    3. Had 1 normal within last year
    4. Had 3 normal within the last five (5) years
    5. Had one normal each of the last five (years

42. Have you experienced undiagnosed vaginal blee ing?
    1. Yes
    2. No

43. Do you now take birth control pills?
    1. Yes
    2. No

lifestyle assessment questionnaire

ALERT
SECTION

medical/behavioral/emotional

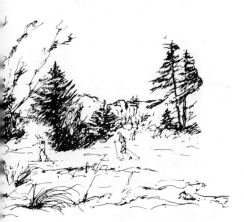
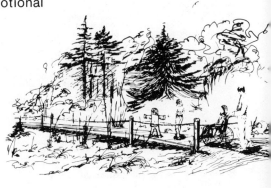

INSTRUCTIONS:

This section is intended to be used to identify high risk problems or past medical problems that we feel are important in establishing one's medical records. This can be used for a personal record by the individual or can be used by professionals as a problem list to be incorporated with the remainder of the individual's medical records. Please circle the number that is most correct in answering each question. Any question that you do not feel comfortable in answering or you think is not pertinent please leave blank.

MEDICAL

Do you have diabetes?	1. Yes 2. No
Do you have a seizure disorder (epilepsy)?	1. Yes 2. No
Do you have known heart **trouble** (acquired or congenital)?	1. Yes 2. No
Did any of your blood relatives die of heart disease under the age of 50?. . . .	1. Yes 2. No
Have you had major surgery?.	1. Yes 2. No
Do you have a physical disability that interferes with routine activities including physical fitness programs?	1. Yes 2. No
Have you had a skin test for TB in the past two (2) years?.	1. Yes 2. No

8. If YES to number 7, which result did you have?.	1. reaction / no 2. reaction
9. Do you take any medication daily or several times per week?	1. Yes 2. No
10. Do you have allergies to drugs?	1. Yes 2. No
11. Are you allergic to penicillin?.	1. Yes 2. No
12. Are you allergic to sulfa?	1. Yes 2. No
13. Are you allergic to aspirin?.	1. Yes 2. No
14. Do you have additional drug allergies not listed above?	1. Yes 2. No
15. Do you have asthma?	1. Yes 2. No

IMMUNIZATIONS

16. Did you have baby shots for DPT (diphtheria, whooping cough, and tetanus)? Ask your parents or doctor. . . . . **1.Yes 2. No**

17. Have you had a booster for tetanus in the last five (5) years? (Recommended interval is 5-10 years.). . . . . **1.Yes 2. No**

18. Have you had a form of polio vaccine? **1.Yes 2. No**

19. With regard to German measles: **1.Yes 2. No**

> 1. **have had a blood test showing immunity or received rubella immunization.**
> 2. **never had a blood test or the blood test showed no immunity to rubella (German measles.)**

20. Have you had a Pap test in the last year?. . . . . **1.Yes 2. No**

21. Have you ever had an abnormal Pap test?. . . . . **1.Yes 2. No**

22. Were you exposed to DES (diethylstilbesterol) while your mother was pregnant with you? (Ask your mother to check with her doctor if you are not sure.). . . . . **1.Yes 2. No**

BEHAVIORAL/EMOTIONAL

NOTE: The leading cause of death among young adults is auto accidents.

23. Do you drive a car, motorcycle, or bike after drinking alcohol?. . . . . **1.Yes 2. No**

24. Do you ride with "drinking" drivers? . . **1.Yes 2. No**

NOTE: The second leading cause of death among young adults is suicide.

25. Have you seriously considered killing yourself within the past year? . . . . **1.Yes 2. No**

26. Have you ever attempted suicide? . . . . **1.Yes 2. No**

27. Have any of your relatives committed suicide?. . . . . **1.Yes 2. No**

28. Do you frequently feel that life is not worth living? . . . . **1.Yes 2. No**

29. Does each day look so dull that you would rather not wake up in the morning?. . . . . **1.Yes 2. No**

30. Do you feel overly tired and without motivation much of the time? . . . . **1.Yes 2. No**

31. Do you feel you have a serious emotional problem?. . . . . **1.Yes 2. No**

32. Do you have a history of/or have you recently experienced hallucinations? (Hearing or seeing things others don't.) **1.Yes 2. No**

33. Do you have difficulty feeling close to people? . . . . **1.Yes 2. No**

34. Do you worry excessively?. . . . . **1.Yes 2. No**

35. Do you feel you've had an excessive number of illnesses in the past year?. . **1.Yes 2. No**

36. Do impulsive behaviors cause you serious problems? . . . . **1.Yes 2. No**

37. Are you unhappy too much of the time?. . . . . **1.Yes 2. No**

38. Do you cry too often? . . . . **1.Yes 2. No**

39. Do you have difficulty controlling your temper?. . . . . **1.Yes 2. No**

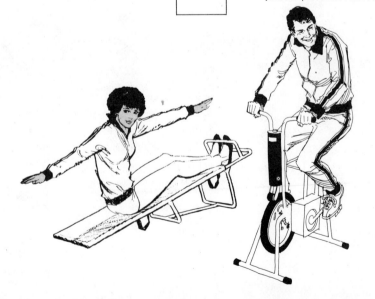

SAMPLE PRINTOUTS

UNIVERSITY OF WISCONSIN-STEVENS POINT
LIFESTYLE ASSESSMENT RESULTS

Prepared for 9002 1 000000000

WELLNESS INVENTORY

The following scores indicate your wellness compared with average of all people taking this survey with you, and averages of all the people who have taken the survey.

Category	Your Score	Group Average	Total Average
Physical Exercise	68	73	70
Physical Nutritional	52	67	52
Physical Self Care	46	60	48
Physical Vehicle Safety	47	75	49
Physical Drug Usage	72	95	75
Social Environmental	27	56	32
Emotional Awareness and Acceptance	20	50	24
Emotional Management	47	69	51
Intellectual	68	82	71
Occupational	73	79	73
Spiritual	65	68	66

2

PERSONAL GROWTH SECTION
AUTOMATED REFERRAL

EXERCISE PROGRAMS

1. Media
   1. Movies: **Coping With Life On The Run**—Sports Productions Inc.
      Run Dick, Run Jane—American Heart Association
      The Heart: An Attack—CRM
   2. Books: **Joy of Running**—Kostrubala
      Women's Running—Ullyot
      The Complete Runner—Fixx
      Stretching—Anderson
      Sheehan on Running—George Sheehan
      The Ultimate Athlete—Leonard
      Aerobics—Cooper
      Aerobics for Women—Cooper

2. Community Resources
   YMCA or YWCA programs

3

RISK OF DEATH SECTION

Age 40	Height 73	
Race White	Weight 222	
Sex Male		

Life Expectancy Results

1 5 10 15 20 25 30 35 40 45

Average Years of Remaining Life in Your Sex, Age, Race Group   33 · · · · · · · · · · · · · · · · · ·

Your Expected Yrs. of Remaining Life Based on your Answers   25 · · · · · · · · · · · · · · ·

You can achieve this expected yrs. of remaining life   38 ·

RISK OF DEATH SECTION (Con't.)

Major Hazards to you

	10 year deaths	
Rank Hazard	per 100,000	Associated risk factors

1. Cirrhosis

Average	304	Drinking Habits
Your	3800	
Achievable	61	

2. Arteriosclerotic Heart Disease

Average	1861	Systolic Blood Pressure
Your	2382	Diastolic Blood Pressure
Achievable	447	Cholesterol Level
		Smoking Habits
		Weight

3. Motor Vehicle Accidents

Average	339	Drinking Habits
Your	1763	Seat Belt Habits
Achievable	203	

4. Cancer of Lungs

Average	291	Smoking Habits
Your	582	
Achievable	58	

Suggestions For Increasing Your Expected Years Of Remaining Life
1. choosing non-drinking   will add 8.6 exp. years of life
2. choosing non-smoking   will add 2.0 exp. years of life
3. lowering cholesterol level   will add 0.7 exp. years of life
4. lowering diastolic blood pressure   will add 0.6 exp. years of life
5. lowering systolic blood pressure   will add 0.6 exp. years of life
6. losing weight   will add 0.4 exp. years of life
7. always wearing seatbelts will add 0.1 exp. years of life
8. having annual procto exam   will add 0.1 exp. years of life
Total   13

Remarks:
We have had to make the following assumptions about you:

You have an average blood cholesterol level.

Hazard Summary

Based on the Lifestyle Assessment Questionnaire you have filled out, you have a health age of 48 years. If you follow all the suggestions we have given, you can reduce your health age to 35.

4

ALERT SECTION: Medical/Behavioral/Emotional

Significant Past Illnesses	Immunizations
1. Diabetic	1. Up-to-date for DPT
2. Physical disability	2. Up-to-date for polio
	3. Rubella status unknown

Allergies	Emotions
1. Allergic to penicillin	1. History compatible with serious depression

WORDS FROM THE PAST

"To ward off disease or recover health, men as a rule find it easier to depend on the healers than to attempt the more difficult task of living wisely."

—Rene Dubos

"It's what you do hour by hour, day by day, that largely determines the state of your health; whether you get sick, what you get sick with, and perhaps when you die."

—Lester Breslow, M.D.

"For many years, while engaged in the practice of medicine, the author of this volume has been more and more impressed with the idea that the causes of the suffering, diseases, and premature deaths, which we witness around us on every hand, lie nearer our own doors... and that the men and women of today, are, at least, equally as responsible for existing suffering, as those who have gone before them, and often much more so. In fact, he feels satisfied that by far the greatest portion of all the suffering, disease, deformity, and premature deaths which occur, are the direct result of either the violation of, or the want of compliance with the laws of our being; calamities, which, were the requisite knowledge possessed by the community, can and should be avoided."

—taken from the Preface to **Avoidable Causes of Disease** by John Ellis, 1859.

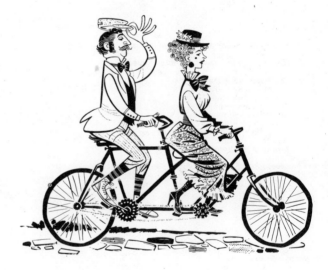

15 / Organizing a Community for Health Promotion

Kenneth L. Rentmeester, M.P.H. / Janet Browne Hall

THE PEOPLE OF PORTAGE COUNTY

Portage County was first settled in 1838. Most of the early settlers were attracted to the area by the timber resources. Stevens Point, the county seat and largest community in Portage County, was incorporated as a city in 1858. Presently, Stevens Point has a population of approximately 23,607.[1] The population of Portage County as a whole is approximately 55,000. Fifty-two per cent of the county population is female. The age distribution represented by the county population shows a markedly higher percentage of the population in the 0 to 19 age group than the statewide population distributions, that is, 41 per cent in Portage County versus 36 per cent statewide. This relative youth of the county population can be attributed to the influence of the University of Wisconsin–Stevens Point with an annual enrollment of approximately 9,000 students.

Several nationalities have influenced and contributed to the life and culture in the Stevens Point area. However, it has been variously estimated that Polish ancestry comprises 60 per cent of the population of the county.[2]

While the name Portage originally applied to the Indian passage between the Fox and Wisconsin rivers, the county retained this name in 1856 not only because it has been applied continuously to the county seat, but probably because one of the most important Indian trails in the central part of the state lay between the Wolf River and Yellow Banks, known as the "Plover Portage," a name which first appears in a government treaty with the Indians in 1837.

The city of Stevens Point was named after lumberman George Stevens who used the point on the Wisconsin River at the foot of the present Main Street to ship supplies by dugout canoe to a sawmill he was building at Wausau.

With a well-established community tradition and the relatively small population base of the community, there exists a strong community spirit in Portage County, represented by the activity of numerous service clubs such as Rotary, Lions, YMCA, Newcomers Club, and numerous women's clubs.

During the last decade, Portage County has experienced a rapid growth rate (second highest in the state of Wisconsin). This growth rate has been due to numerous factors including the rapid expansion of agriculture and agribusiness in the county. The county is a major producer of potatoes, with 54,000 acres in cultivation. Firms such as American Potato and Ore-Ida have established large processing plants in Portage County. The success of agriculture in the county has been greatly aided through the availability of ample supplies of water used to irrigate crops.

In addition to the strong agribusiness component in the county, the paper industry

[1]Central Wisconsin Facts Books, Central Wisconsin Industrial Development Corporation, Stevens Point, Wisconsin.
[2]Pamphlet: Central Wisconsin Chamber of Commerce, "This is Central Wisconsin–Stevens Point and Portage County."

continues to be a large employer represented by Consolidated Papers. In addition, Sentry Insurance has established its world headquarters in Stevens Point and employs several thousand area individuals. The University of Wisconsin–Stevens Point provides the final major factor in the rapidly expanding growth rate of the county. The university has an enrollment of approximately 9,000 students annually and is a major contributor to the economy of Portage County.

Both Sentry Insurance and the University of Wisconsin–Stevens Point have deemed health promotion a top priority within their organizations. Sentry Insurance Company has a well-established and well-integrated employees' fitness program. A complete fitness facility was constructed several years ago with the construction of a new world headquarters building. The fitness facility includes a full-sized gym, 25-meter swimming pool, strength-building equipment, and other aids. Included in this comprehensive health promotion and health education package are the services of physicians and related personnel.

The University of Wisconsin–Stevens Point Student Health Services has been a major innovator of health promotion and risk reduction programs for both university students and the community in general. Under the leadership of Dr. William Hettler, director of the Student Health Services, a life-style assessment questionnaire was first developed and utilized in 1976. This instrument is a health inventory and refers participants to sources of health information and life-style programming. Approximately 90 per cent of the incoming students at the university choose to take the life-style assessment questionnaire instead of a physical examination. The life-style assessment questionnaire has been adopted by several other universities and community groups.[3]

In summary, the Portage County population represents a somewhat ideal base for a community health promotion project. The strong community tradition along with the diversity of industry and the presence of a major university help create an ideal climate for an integrated community-based approach to health promotion.

WHAT IS HEALTH PROMOTION?

Health promotion as applied in the community-based health promotion project can best be defined in terms of providing information, opportunity, and a support environment in which individuals may change life-styles to reflect positive health behaviors. Having stated this, it is important to (1) differentiate health promotion from health education and (2) describe the major components of health promotion.

After working with these two concepts, one finds that the definitions proposed by the Office of Health Information, Health Promotion and Physical Fitness and Sports Medicine are quite realistic. That is, "Health education is any combination of learning opportunities designed to facilitate voluntary adaptations of behavior conducive to health." and "Health promotion is any combination of health education and related organizational, political, and economic interventions designed to facilitate behavioral and environmental adaptations that will improve or protect health."[4]

Thus, health education is a major component of a community-based health promotion program but does not represent the entire activity required to provide for a community-based health promotion program.

[3] Ambly Burfoot, "Eliminating the Need to Be Sick," *Runner's World*, February 1980.
[4] *Focal Points*, Bureau of Health Education, U.S. Department of Health and Human Services, Public Health Service, Center for Disease Control, Atlanta, Georgia, June 1980.

Wellness is another term which is currently used to describe an approach to changing health behavior and life-style. The definition of wellness developed by the Stevens Point Area Wellness Commission (the origin and function of which will be described later in this chapter) is as follows: "Wellness is an active process through which the individual becomes aware of, and makes choices toward, a more successful existence. These choices are greatly influenced by one's self-concept and the parameter of one's cultures and environment. Each individual develops a unique lifestyle which changes daily as a reflection of their intellectual, emotional, physical, social, occupational, and spiritual dimensions." This definition was developed in an effort to recognize the importance of not only the health concepts and life-style changes inherent in health promotion but also the significant role played by the individual's self-concept and the culture and environment of the community. In addition, attempts are made in the definition to broaden the spectrum usually considered by health professionals to include such dimensions as social, intellectual, occupational, and spiritual well-being. This definition allows for the broad-based community involvement of such organizations as churches, education systems, and civic groups, as well as the traditional community health and medical organizations.

A community-based health promotion project must develop approaches to both the individual and institutions within the community. It is important to recognize that a different set of strategies and objectives should be developed for both institutional and individual program initiatives. The cornerstone of the institutional approach to health promotion tends to relate to the fiscal and employee morale advantages of health promotion programming. This approach is quite different from the strategy used to promote individual improvement in life-styles. The approach best suited for the individual tends to provide a personalized scheme which results in a higher level of satisfaction in one's pursuits whether these pursuits are physical, intellectual, or in the other dimensions of wellness described earlier. The individual responds best to personal achievements and a strong support environment whereas institutions respond positively toward dollar savings and improved employee functioning.

GETTING STARTED

Key Community Components

Many community-based health promotion programs tend to be monolithic in both their organizational structure and approaches toward specific health problems. Thus programs may become too narrowly focused with specific medical/model outcomes.

The initial leadership for a community-based Wellness Commission in Stevens Point was spearheaded by Dr. William Hettler of the University of Wisconsin–Stevens Point Student Health Service and the author. The concept was to involve a number of key community leaders in the grass roots development of a community-based health promotion program. The initiative for this movement was precipitated by the realization that in communities of this size an integration of programs, services, and approaches is necessary to have a positive impact on large segments of the community. Thus, in April of 1978, the Stevens Point Area Wellness Commission was first organized. In the beginning, this commission was a loose aggregate of community leaders representing the following key community organizations: the only hospital in the county, St. Michael's Hospital; Sentry Insurance, Health and Fitness Department; the Stevens Point Area YMCA; the University of Wisconsin Student Health Service; the Stevens

Point area Catholic schools; the Stevens Point area public schools; the Better Living Center; the Portage County Health Department; the Portage County Human Services Board; and the Portage County Department of Social Services. These ten representatives from key positions, that is, either the top administrator or his or her designee, formed the original commission. Several meetings of the commission were spent laboriously discussing perspectives on health promotion and the importance or lack of importance of health promotion throughout the community. From this initial discussion, the commission developed a community health promotion goal which was quite general in nature. The goal is "to improve the health and well-being of Stevens Point and Portage County residents through increased awareness of, and participation in, wellness programs directed at the family through a number of public and private community institutions including schools, churches, and employers."

Development of Community Planning Committee

Subsequent to the development of the major focus for the community-based Wellness Commission, the commission developed an area wellness project. This project was funded through the Wisconsin State Department of Health and Social Services through a special allocation of $1 million for health promotion and prevention earmarked by the governor in 1979. Over 300 projects throughout the state applied for funding under this program. Twenty-nine projects, diverse in nature and representative of all areas of the state, were funded. The Stevens Point Area Wellness Project was one of the funded projects and was granted funds for a 2-year period commencing July 1, 1979. This chapter was written after completion of 1 year of that project.

The community-based wellness project is a joint effort by numerous governmental and nongovernmental, educational, health, and social service organizations to improve the health and well-being of area residents pursuant to the general goal established by the Wellness Commission.

The project is focusing primarily on the planning, integrating, and provision of health promotion and wellness programs in a coordinated approach through schools, employers, peer groups, and churches. Through these avenues, the project will attempt to impact positively on the family unit. The development of positive self-concept will form the basis for efforts to assist individuals and families in improving their health awareness and life-style.

Figure 1 highlights graphically the concept of the family unit as the major focal point for the wellness project efforts. Because self-concept was seen by the project authors as a major influence on life-style and eventually health-risk behavior, the major program emphasis would focus upon the improvement of self-concept.

Figure 2 details the critical elements involved in individual life-style, life-style risks, and chronic diseases. One may note the means of intervention for the different levels of individual health or illness, that is, the last level of intervention when a disease is apparent, is through medical treatment and disease screening programs. Prior to this level of intervention, life-style change programs have attempted to address individual life-style risks involved in chronic diseases. Such risks include obesity, smoking, lack of exercise, improper diet, stress, excessive alcohol consumption, and others.

The community wellness project developed in Stevens Point focused on a more essential component of chronic disease development; that is, the perception by the individual of his or her self-worth and the influences upon that perception. This concept

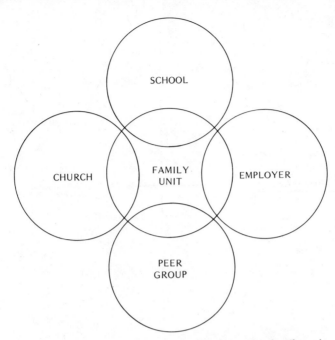

FIGURE 15-1.   Family Lifestyle Model.   The family unit represents the critical lifestyle determinate for individual family members.   The individual within the family unit is impacted upon by one or several groups i.e., school, church, peer group, or employer.   These groups form the individual's behavioral environment.   Self-concept and lifestyle behavior are closely linked for the individual family member as these groups either reinforce or discourage positive lifestyle behavior.

closely parallels the definition of wellness which was developed by the Wellness Commission and which was previously stated.

During the first year of the project, an intense pilot effort involving schools, churches, social groups, and employers was conducted in the suburban area of Plover and Whiting. In the second year of the project, this coordinated effort would be expanded to the entire Portage County area.

This project represents one of the first communitywide efforts in the state of Wisconsin to provide integrated information and programs aimed at the total person and designed to assist the individual in making choices which lead to a more successful existence.

The project was funded for $50,000 over a 2-year period. The Stevens Point Area Wellness Commission formed the governing board for the operation of the project. The grant enabled the project to employ one full-time community health educator and one part-time media specialist. In addition, the services of an additional part-time health educator and several additional experienced media specialists were volunteered by the organizations represented on the commission. One of the most striking advantages of a project which has a broad organizational base of support within the community is

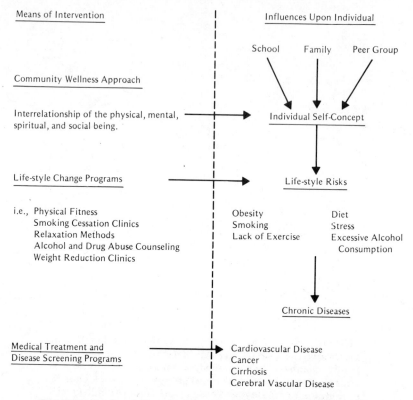

FIGURE 15-2.   Lifestyle diseases process—methods of change.

the ability to utilize resources from a number of these organizations and to combine these efforts to meet the project goals. This joint commitment by the major organizations in a community is essential to promote not only the resources for a project of this nature but also involvement and shared ownership by all organizations involved in the project.

PLANNING FOR COMMUNITY HEALTH NEEDS

Identifying Community Needs

During the preparation of the community-based project, the committee organized, developed, and collected data through a community needs assessment. The purpose of the survey was twofold: (1) to appraise the needs and wants of the citizens-at-large in relation to health promotion and (2) to educate the citizens about their role in maintaining and enhancing their own health and well-being. The survey of the citizens-at-large was coordinated with a survey of health and social service providers throughout the county. This latter survey revealed the availability and current functioning of many health promotion and risk-reduction programs within the community. In review, the major ingredient which appeared to be missing was a system of integrating and coordinating these varied activities. Activities ranged from stop-smoking clinics to weight-reduction clinics to stress-reduction workshops. The other major ingredient which the project would attempt to accomplish would be to increase the impact upon the family unit through working with churches, schools, and several employer groups. This focus was determined by the realization that many efforts aimed at individuals within a family, for example, through the school system, must be complemented by a total program aimed at the family unit. This approach also has the advantage of focusing on a very popular and salable target group. With the completion of the identification of these priorities through the community-based and organization survey, the Wellness Commission was able to develop specific program goals and objectives. The importance of specific measurable, and timely goals and objectives for a community-based project of this nature cannot be overemphasized. It is quite easy without these cleary visible guideposts to lose track of progress and to drift endlessly into numerous community events and endeavors without achieving any great success.

Program Goals and Objectives

The commission established yearly goals and end points with numerous objectives designed to assist in meeting each goal. The third major component of the goals and objectives is a detailed work plan specifying month-by-month activities needed to meet the project objectives. For example, the following two goals were established for the first year of the project: (1) to create an awareness of wellness activities in the Stevens Point metropolitan area by identifying functioning wellness programs, coordinating existing activities, and publicizing wellness efforts; (2) to pilot, in a section of the Stevens Point metropolitan area, a comprehensive wellness model featuring the promotion of a positive self-concept as a means to, and a result of, life-style changes resulting from such activity as proper exercise, improved diet, better relaxation techniques, and spiritual reflection. Each of these major goals had attached to it numerous objectives. For example, one of the objectives to meet the first goal was "by May 31, 1980, the project will have designed and conducted awareness workshops for employers, school personnel, and clergy leaders on project activities and the wellness concept. These workshops will be held intermittently from September 1979 to May 1980. A report will be submitted to the Executive Committee for approval." An example of an objective designed to facilitate the accomplishment of the second goal for the first year was "by December 5, 1979, the project director, through the administrator of curriculum, Stevens Point Public Schools, will have implemented the wellness objectives within the school curriculum among the three elementary schools serving the target area."

In total, there were 28 objectives listed in the project for the 2-year period. Each objective had an identifiable work plan attached to it. Such work plans should be as specific as possible. For example, under an objective for identifying wellness programs in Stevens Point, six work plan elements were listed.

1. Review data from past wellness surveys.
2. Design interview format.
3. Gain approval of executive committee.
4. Identify agencies to be interviewed.
5. Conduct interviews.
6. Report back to executive committee.

With a specific road map such as those previously described, the staff, project committee, and citizens in the community have an accurate understanding of what the community-based project will attempt to accomplish. Often, health promotion projects do a relatively poor job of informing the members of the target population as to the specific goals and objectives of the effort. Unfortunately, this may result in a lack of direction for both project staff and program participants.

MAKING IT HAPPEN

Community Support Groups—Creating Awareness and Involvement

How does one begin to implement a community-based project of this magnitude in a logical fashion? Thus far in this chapter, we have described the important steps of obtaining the support of the leadership of major organizations, coordinating and developing a planning committee from amongst people within these organizations, and developing a specific project with attainable goals and objectives. The next step is the implementation of the program. The key ingredient which should be concomitant with the introduction of the program is the development and establishment of a strong support system with key individuals and decision makers within the community. These key decision makers may be, and likely will be, additions to the individuals and organizations represented on the committee.

This step is especially important and mandatory when working within a rural community because of the close-knit and traditional nature of many components within the community. If the appropriate power figures aren't appraised of the nature of the project and if they are not involved in some way in planning the implementation process, the project is not likely to succeed. The leaders in this community and in many communities are persons in positions such as school board presidents, chairs of county boards and city councils, mayors, school superintendents, chancellors of universities, Lions Club presidents, small and large business owners, directors of health, social, and educational organizations. There also exists a group of nonobvious leaders within every community. It takes time to identify and get to know these local power structures. Project staff must temper their enthusiasm with the realization that this community knowledge is essential to the success of the project. Meetings should be set with these various community leaders and goals and objectives of the projects discussed in detail to enable these individuals to become involved in the program. Special techniques are often required to get these busy people to a meeting for discussion of the project. Techniques used by this project include special luncheons and the use of other influential community leaders for contact purposes in organizing a meeting.

Once you have met and discussed your program with several community leaders, you should be prepared to reformulate some of your specific project objectives. This process is similar to the one described earlier in regard to organizing the Wellness Commission. These objectives include very specific activities that would be carried out within a given time frame. The purpose here is to remain flexible in providing objectives which meet the needs of particular subgroups within the population but ultimately lead to the accomplishment of the overall project goals. For example, one might discover that the director of the YMCA is interested in developing a par course (physical fitness course) or the principal of one of the elementary schools may be interested in organizing a school health fair. Activities such as these could have been overlooked by the entire planning committee as well as other key community leaders but it is now something to be taken into consideration when planning the specifics of a program. In organizing these specific suggestions and activities, one should look for trends and concerns shared by the majority. The importance of including the opinions and concerns of both community leaders as well as "nonleaders" should be emphasized.

Coordination of Community Wide Activity

Once you have met with several community people and you have taken their ideas and concerns into consideration, you are ready to introduce the program to the community and, more specifically, to your initial target group. One of the most effective means of communicating the word about your program is through the media. In small communities, the grapevine can also be quite effective. The local newspaper, television, and radio station should be contacted during the initial phase of your program.

Every health promotion program should have a media specialist or consultant. Both the program director and the media specialist should work closely together. At this time, special consideration should be given to developing a public information action plan.

The following is an example of what one might include in an action plan:

1. Establish your goal. Let's begin by stating that our goal is to communicate a health promotion concept to the Plover–Whiting community (remember this is the target group for the first year of our local program, population approximately 5,000).
2. Develop your overall concept. In this case, we are talking about the fact that everyone has alternatives for creating a positive life-style.
3. Identify the specific target group. Let's consider two target audiences: (a) leadership groups and (b) public-at-large.
4. Determine the approach you will utilize. For example, your approach could involve coordinating and publicizing the existing health promotion activity.

Consider the use of the following communication tools as part of your action plan:

1. Personal contact
   A. Hold meetings to develop and publicize local wellness activities.
   B. Send personal letters and direct mailings.
2. Audio–visual presentation
   A. Develop a theme for a slide program.
   B. Define the health promotion program.
   C. Administer a brief health hazard appraisal or life-style assessment questionnaire. For example, you may wish to ask the following questions:
      (1) Do you keep within 5 per cent of your ideal body weight?
      (2) Do you know how to measure your heart rate?
      (3) Do you get enough sleep to feel good the next day?
   D. Become involved in your organization.
   E. Use community resources.
3. Brochures (theme and summary could be a summary of the slide show presentation)
4. Newsletters
   A. Feature the people involved in a local health promotion event or activity and the benefits they receive as a result.
   B. Provide visibility for as many local health activities as possible.

    C. Give exposure to key organizations and individuals supporting health promotion program.

5. Public service announcements
    A. Proclaim benefits of local activities.
    B. Provide visibility for local activities.
    C. Encourage listeners to attempt or continue positive health activities.

Somewhat different strategies should be employed in approaching the leadership groups versus the public-at-large.

Let's begin by taking a look at the strategies for approaching the leadership groups. Below is a list of steps to follow:

1. Develop a comprehensive target list of community leaders.
    A. Elected officials (county board members, school board members, state representatives, etc.).
    B. Parent-teacher organization members.
    C. Employee clubs and local unions.
    D. Civic and social organizations.
    E. Other appropriate groups.
2. Establish personal contact between your program or commission and each community leader.
    A. Mail newsletter to each leader.
    B. Periodically send a personal letter from the program director or other commission member along with the newsletter encouraging the individual's continued program support and requesting suggestions as to specific program initiatives.
3. Present the slide show and brochures to as many community groups as possible.
    A. Establish a speaking schedule including dates available.
    B. Establish a speaker's bureau.
    C. Develop a list of community resources.
4. Provide direction and support for developing and existing health promotion groups and activities.
    A. Slide show and brochure presentation.
    B. Publicity through existing health communication mechanisms.
    C. Guidance for establishing specific goals and achieving those goals.

The following strategies could be utilized for reaching the public-at-large:

1. Design a health logo to use on:
    A. Letterhead stationery.
    B. Newsletters and brochures.
    C. Slides for slide show and television.
    D. Any other media forms of publicity.
2. Develop a monthly newsletter.
    A. Develop distribution methods.
    B. Establish monthly production schedule.
    C. Design monthly budget.
    D. Explore possibilities for reprints in local publications including an introductory paragraph about the program.
3. Make public service announcements.
    A. Explore possibilities for radio and television spot announcements and talk show interviews.

B. Develop a package of radio and television public service announcements.
4. Establish a communications director in each supporting health activity organization to feed information for public service announcements and newsletters to your advisory committee.

In order for a program to be ongoing, it must develop community support groups. Community support groups can provide your program with necessary strength and commitment from the community to make your program successful. Support groups provide two basic functions. First, they help coordinate the communitywide activity and, second, they provide for ongoing and future direction for your program. This latter point is essential in ensuring "grass roots" involvement and program continuity.

Basically, there are three types of support groups which are appropriate in organizing community health promotion projects: (1) specific health issue groups such as diet, stress, exercise; (2) specific community groups such as schools, businesses, churches; and (3) specific organizational issues groups such as evaluation, program funding, and program coordination. For example, in Portage County there is one support group which is interested in physical and cardiovascular fitness. This group consists of principals, teachers, members of parent-teacher organizations, Lions Club members, and members from the county Parks and Recreation Department. This diverse group is interested in developing a par course[5] within the Plover–Whiting community (the projects's target area during its first year of operation). The group meets once every month and there is a chairperson who is responsible for sending out memoranda and other relevant materials. Another support group is an evaluation committee. This group is responsible for developing evaluation tools, assisting with the data collection process, and making the final analysis of the effects of the program. Still another support group is responsible for planning and conducting a community health day. This group consists of members from the Portage County Commission on Aging, the County Extension Service, Stevens Point Area High Schools, Catholic and Methodist churches, and others.

To reiterate, it is essential that a program involve several community members in the planning process to ensure that the activities that follow are likely to be a success. Remember, support groups are strictly voluntary and members become involved because of their own interest and commitment; support groups will not develop by coercion or manipulation.

Once you have met with various community leaders, developed a public information or action plan, and developed several support groups, it is essential that the program staff coordinate all these components. The term coordinate is rather vague and there are many people who have different ideas as to what a coordinating agency's role is. Your program must differ from, and yet complement, existing and related services within your community. To do this, one must utilize a community approach to health. A community approach to health is a unique and comprehensive approach premised on the need to develop programs which impact on the "total person." This integrated approach to health utilizes services and programs already in existence in the community and attempts to coordinate services. The integrated approach will also identify coordinated objectives for a community health plan in which each involved organization has a defined role.

The following are specific activities from the Stevens Point Area Wellness Commission's project which illustrate what is meant by an integrated approach.

[5]Par course fitness circuit is a series of 18 exercise stations spaced over a 1- to $2\frac{1}{2}$-mile path, depending upon the location and terrain. Each station provides a type of exercise such as walking, stretching, logging. Illustrated signs "coach" participants and explain how to perform each exercise.

During the first month of operation, the need for organizing a nutrition/wellness workshop for the parent-teacher organizations within our target group arose. Several elementary school principals and teachers, nutritionist, parent-teacher organization members, and school nurses formed a planning committee to start the workshop. Five months later, the workshop was held at one of the elementary schools. Over 200 parents from the Plover–Whiting area attended this workshop. Experts in nutrition and wellness presented their ideas on food facts, snacking, supermarket strategies, packing nutritious school lunches, and many other topics. During the breaks, exercise sessions were led by a physical education instructor from the YMCA. Nutritious snacks were prepared by the parent-teacher organization members. Several community organizations had displays which gave parents an opportunity to learn more about local community resources. The evaluation survey demonstrated the success of this workshop; 80 per cent of the participants said the workshop was very worthwhile. Another workshop has been organized for this school year which will focus upon stress management.

One can involve businesses and employer groups by illustrating the rising cost of medical care and talking with the top level administrators about the amount of money that is going into their employee health insurance coverage. In 1975, General Motors spent $825 million on health care benefits for employees—adding $175 to the price of every car and truck built by GM.[6]

Consolidated Papers, Inc., for example, approached the Wellness Commission regarding development of a life-style/safety survey for their employees. A proposal was organized and submitted to the plant manager for approval and discussions. Presently, there is a planning committee designing a life-style/safety survey to assess what type of program to organize for the employees at Consolidated.

One can involve various church groups by approaching members of the clergy and asking them if they are interested in your program. For example, a seminar was held in which several clergy were invited to attend an introductory meeting about our program. An expert in the area of spiritual wellness was asked to participate to answer any specific questions. Since the initial meeting, several clergy from the Catholic, Lutheran, and Methodist churches have been involved in presenting a seminar on spiritual wellness for the general community.

The Wellness Commission was also involved in organizing health fairs for the elementary schools within the Plover–Whiting area. A task force was organized which included principals, teachers, several parent-teacher organization members, the school nurses, and student representatives. The purpose of the fairs was to create an awareness of important health issues to the children and to encourage teachers to begin implementing the K-6 health curriculum. Health experts in the community were called upon to facilitate the sessions at the fair. The topics covered were first aid, stress management, nutritional awareness, environmental sensitivity, alcohol education, and physical fitness. The fairs were organized for a half day. The children were divided into age groups of first-to-second-graders, third-to-fourth-graders, and fifth-to-sixth-graders. Each of these groups spent an hour at the fair. During that hour, the students chose three 20-minute topics of particular interest to them. A flyer was developed to send to parents informing them of the fair. It is important to have as much parent involvement as possible. A pre- and posttest was administered to evaluate what the children learned as a result of attending the fairs. These are just a few examples of what your community can do!

[6]*A Practical Guide for Employee Health Promotion Program.* Madison, Wisc.: The Health Planning Council, Inc., February 1979.

Barriers, Problems, and Adversities

It sounds like everything has been easy, but, to be realistical, one will always encounter barriers and major "road blocks." Any number of barriers can arise while organizing a communitywide project. First, there will be some resistance to change. It is important to remember that one of your goals is to help people help themselves. Second, it takes time for any program to become organized and accepted by the community. Building up one's credibility and establishing rapport takes time and energy. Third, it takes money. Fourth, it requires lots of patience, persistence, and willingness to work with people in any community.

The concept and practice behind health promotion has really picked up momentum. However, many are skeptical of the outcome and effectiveness of health promotion programs. People want to see proof, especially the funding sources! Therefore, the evaluation component is a crucial aspect of your program. Basically, there are two kinds of evaluation. First, there is the annual process evaluation, to identify by the end of each program year the extent to which the program objectives have been met on a timely basis. For example, has a wellness curriculum been implemented in the three target-area elementary schools? Has a public information plan been developed?

The project director's weekly journal, the telephone log, the public service announcements, and other media (newletters and brochures, *Stevens Point Daily Journal* coverage), the number of community presentations, and other kinds of involvement can be compiled and utilized to measure the numbers of participants and their involvement in your program during the first year.

Second, there is the annual outcome evaluation, to determine the extent to which the overall project outcome objectives have been accomplished. For example, was there a 10 per cent or greater reduction in both obesity and smoking among employees at various industrial sites? In order to collect the baseline data for your outcome evaluation, you will need cooperation from several community organizations. For example, have the principals and teachers help design and conduct a pre- and posttest for elementary school children in the district. The pre- and posttests can be utilized to determine health/wellness knowledge improvements resulting from school-based wellness programs.

Absenteeism rates, dietary histories, and percentage of fat-to-body weight testing can be conducted by the school health nurses.

To reiterate, your evaluation component is a very important part of your program; however, bear in mind that life-style changes as a result of health promotion programs are difficult to ascertain because of the diversity and nature of each individual's life-style.

Additionally, behavioral change measusrments may be greatly influenced by the timing and design of the measurement and instrument. An individual's recidivism into past life-style risk patterns increases with increasing time intervals from involvement in a particular program.

YOU CAN DO IT TOO

Following is a six-step community approach to health which will serve as a means of summarizing our chapter on organizing a rural community for health promotion. Remember, you can do it, too!

1. Obtain leadership commitment to the program.
   A. Workshops, seminars, and so on for school boards, school administrators, employers, service agency administrators—outline potential benefits.
   B. Formation of a health promotion committee broadly representative of public and private health and education agencies.
2. Analyze existing health culture and health promotion programs.
   A. Survey community agencies to determine existing health promotion programs.
   B. Conduct community assessment to gather information on consumer knowledge levels and areas of interest.
3. Develop specific task forces.
   A. Organize task forces or advisory committees, such as:
      (1) School health curriculum.
      (2) Individual school committees.
         (a) Staff wellness.
         (b) School nutrition.
         (c) Family-life-style.
      Similar groups can be established in church and employee settings.
4. Encourage high involvement in the process.
   A. Workshops for:
      (1) Teachers.
      (2) Employees.
      (3) Church and civic groups.
   B. Programs for involvement:
      (1) School health days.
      (2) School, employer, and church-based specific programs on nutrition, physical fitness, stress management, and so on.
5. Organize and involve local support groups.
   A. Organize ongoing local committees for continued planning and implementation.
   B. Blend neighborhood committees into a communitywide coordinated wellness program.
6. Evaluate and renew.
   A. Process evaluation—have the objectives been met and the process completed?
   B. Outcome evaluation—measure:
      (1) Participation levels.
      (2) Changes in awareness.
      (3) Life-style changes and health improvement.
      (4) Duration of impact.

REFERENCES

Allen, Robert F., "Changing Lifestyles Through Changing Organizational Cultures." *Proceedings of the Society of Prospective Medicine*. St. Petersburg, Florida, October 1978.

Allen, Robert F. and Kraft, Charlotte, *Changing Community and Organizational Cultures.* New York: McGraw-Hill, 1979.

Ardell, Donald, *High Level Wellness*. Emmaus, Pa.: Rodale Press, 1977.

Harris, Sara and Allen, Robert F., *The Quiet Revolution*. New York: Rawson Associates, 1978.

Human Resource Institute, Tempe Wick Rd., Morristown, N.J. 07960 (201-267-1496).

Collis, Martin, *Employee Fitness*. The Minister of State for Fitness and Amateur Sport, Supply and Services Canada, Ottawa, Canada, K1A OS9, 1977.

Fessler, Donald, *Facilitating Community Change: A Basic Guide*. LaJolla, Calif.: University Associates, 1976.

Abramson, J. H., *Survey Methods in Community Medicine*. London: Churchhill Livingstone, 1974.

Davidson, Park and Davidson, Sheena, *Behavioral Medicine: Changing Health Lifestyles*. New York: Brunner/Mazel, 1980.

16 / The Wisconsin Advisory Committee on Prevention and Wellness

William Blockstein, Ph.D.

Public health efforts, and indeed the rudiments of health promotion, began before Wisconsin became a state. The Wisconsin Territorial Legislature in 1839 required governing bodies of all municipalities to serve as local boards of health and gave these boards a number of powers relating to the control of infectious diseases. After statehood in 1848, there was little organized activity until 1910 when the Legislature designated an-1876-created State Board of Health as *the* State Health Department.

Over the 140-year history, Wisconsin's approach to public health generally reflected the approach taken by the nation as a whole. Nineteenth-century programs dealing with environmental sanitation formed the core of activity. These programs were carried out to prevent and to control communicable diseases.

During the past two decades, environmental issues took on an increasingly higher priority on the public health agenda. Greater attention was given to the workplace environment with emphasis both on hazard reduction and screening programs. Finally, as chronic diseases and accidents replaced communicable diseases as primary causes of morbidity and mortality, health agencies began to increase activity in health promotion, health education, and illness and accident prevention.

Modern efforts in Wisconsin began in May of 1971, when Governor Patrick J. Lucey announced the creation of the Governor's Health Planning and Policy Task Force. The body was composed of health and illness care providers, human services professionals, educators, consumer activists, union leaders, and elected officials from county to state legislative levels. The Health Planning and Policy Task Force was charged with "developing a comprehensive state health policy which would take advantage of the unique possibilities of the state role in the regulation and delivery of health services." That group worked for 18 months, took public testimony at hearings around the state, conducted numerous investigations using task force subgroups with state persons as staff, and met often to hammer out a report that appeared in three volumes—*The Final Report*, a *Summary Report* and a *Supplement* containing public testimony and bibliographic material supportive to the findings and recommendations in the *Final Report*.

The task force's findings and recommendations dealing with, *Informing the Public*, stated:

> In the past health education has never received a high public priority. Little money has been spent on health education. Existing efforts in health education in Wisconsin have not been integrated or coordinated since there is no single agency assuming the responsiblity for comprehensive health education. Health education personnel are often ineffectively used. Furthermore, health professionals are often inappropriately prepared to serve as health educators, nor do they always see themselves in this role.

A STATE HEALTH EDUCATION POLICY COMMITTEE

The task force recommended a state health education policy committee be established by the Health Policy and Program Council.*

This committee will provide the needed leadership at the state level for all consumer health education efforts, including school health education.

The committee will act in a policy-making capacity for all consumer health education matters. It will develop health education plans, establish priorities, recommend allocation of state and federal health education funds and provide general statewide coordination.

This committee will include representatives from the University of Wisconsin system, the Department of Health and Social Services, the Department of Public Instruction, voluntary health organizations, industry, private institutions of higher learning, provider organizations and consumer groups.

The committee will act in an advisory capacity to the Governor and the Legislature on health education policies, priorities and programming. The committee will communicate policy regarding health education to the citizens of the state, to other key policy councils and to provider groups within the health system.

For the consumers of health care in Wisconsin this will mean that their knowledge, beliefs and misinformation will be identified and their health education needs determined. Specific programs will then be developed to address their health education and information needs, using a style and language that the people can understand.

The Task Force concluded this section by declaring:

It is clear that poor, incomplete health education of the public has meant that many individuals have paid a terrible price for their lack of sound information. Education is at the very heart of preventive care, yet curiously health education has not enjoyed any priority in public expenditures. In other areas addressed by the Task Force, where programs have been operating, it was possible to evaluate the results in terms of the dollars spent and services provided and make recommendations. In health education so little has been done to establish programs, however, that the Task Force made a more general recommendation that health education, broadly construed, be given a high public priority and that the process of developing working programs, responsive to the needs of Wisconsin health care consumers, be initiated.

At the same time, in 1971, that Lucey created the Govenor's Task Force on Health Planning and Policy, he created the State of Wisconsin Health Policy Council. The council was to stand at the ready, so to speak, to receive the report and recommendations of the task force and to act on these directly, through assignment, or by the influence of legislation. We will return to the Health Policy Council at a later time because it became our State Health Coordinating Council after President Gerald Ford signed P.L. 93-641, the Health Planning Resource Development Act of 1974.

Another element that bears mention in this brief history relates to federal funds from Health Services and Mental Health Administration, awarded a research group I led in 1970–71. We developed a model showing how land grant universities might engage in consumer health education and health promotion efforts, using the agricultural extension model, by extending the knowledge and research base of the university and its medical and health science schools out to the people.

*Final Report, The Wisconsin Governor's Health Planning and Policy Task Force, Madison, Wisconsin, November, 1972, pp. 79–80.

The Wisconsin research group efforts overlapped the efforts of President Nixon's Committee on Health Education. Created on September 14, 1971, that committee reported almost a year later than was expected because of some internal committee disagreement and the political necessity for a delay in release, both by the White House and by HEW key people, of the *Final Report.*

Selected paragraphs from the President's Committee Report sound much like the Wisconsin Task Force Report:*

- . . . health education has been neglected . . . the whole field of health education is fragmented, uneven in effectivness and lacks any base of operations. No agency inside or outside of government is either responsible for, or even assists in setting goals, maintaing criteria of performance or measuring results.
- School health education in most primary and secondary schools is either not provided at all or is tacked onto other subject matter such as physical education or biology, assigned to teachers whose main interests and qualifications lie elsewhere.
- . . . legislation actually impedes development of effective school health programs.
- The U.S. Office of Education (Department of HEW), in a report prepared for the Committee, could not cite a single program of research or evaluation it is supporting in the area of school health education.
- . . . health education has generally been stereotyped.
- . . . $30-million is for specific programs in health education; $14-million more for general programs. That amounts to less than one-fourth of one percent. Of $7.3-billion allocated for health purposes to all other federal agencies, even a smaller fraction is spent on health education.
- On the state level, heath departments spend less than half of one percent of their budgets for health education.
- . . . needs, problems and opportunities in health education are so large, so urgent and so complex that progress will depend upon a major long-term commitment to it by the nation's leaders.

CREATION OF THE WISCONSIN ADVISORY COMMISSION ON PREVENTION AND WELLNESS

In late 1977 and early 1978, Wisconsin Health and Social Service Secretary Donald E. Percy, working with Acting Governor Martin J. Schrieber (who had assumed his office when Governor Lucey was named Ambassador to Mexico by President Jimmy Carter), developed an item in the Executive Budget request for health promotion to focus more resources on preventing physical, mental and social ills in Wisconsin.

Secretary Percy, in support of the budget item, at one hearing before the Senate Committee on Human Services had, among others, Nobel Prize Winner Howard Temin, discussing cancer prevention; Bill Hettler, M.D. (fellow author in this text), discussing fitness activities and wellness programs, and Norman Jensen, a university physician, who, using a specially installed computer terminal, administered Health Hazard Appraisals, and reported findings instantly to several overweight, florid-faced, cigar chomping state senators.

Secretary Percy's point was made. The executive budget request dealing with prevention and wellness became sections of the laws of 1977 for the state of Wisconsin. (See Appendix A to this chapter.) In essence, the law provided for a prevention and wellness initiative in the Department of Health and Social Services by funding three

*The Report of the President's Committee on Health Education, New York, 1972.

positions; it created the Advisory Commission on Prevention and Wellness; and it provided for a prevention and wellness project fund of $980,000 for demonstration grants. The monies were to be released in a manner that will be described later.

It is fair to say, however, that the legislature, flush with almost a billion-dollar state treasury surplus, was willing to consider the *possibility* of releasing approximately 0.1 per cent of that amount for prevention and wellness. Contrast that amount with the nearly half billion dollars budgeted for treatment, possible cure, rehabilitation, and habilitation following the usual course of disease and its aftermath! A start, modest as it was, had been made. With the potential of a million dollars set aside for a commission and for funding innovative demonstration grants, Wisconsin appeared to be pulling ahead of the pack. What the 1971 Governor's Task Force had talked about, what the 1970-71 Consumer Health Education demonstration model suggested, and what the President's Committee on Health Education had recommended was going to get a trial, finally, in one of the 50 states.*

The governor wrote the secretary on May 23, 1978: Having signed the Annual Budget Review Bill, I am prepared to move forward with the next stages of our wellness initiative. We must help Wisconsin people, local communities, civic groups, labor, business and industry to promote prevention and wellness projects. On our own part we should continue to develop human services that emphasize prevention wellness.

We are seeking to make better health a way of life in Wisconsin. We are seeking to help people help themselves to better health. Our goal is to provide matching and seed money to public and private groups to encourage the development of programs to help people improve their own health through exercise, diet, improved health habits and prevention of illness. Our goal is to help develop projects that can reduce preventable illness or improve physical, mental and social health. I believe that an advisory commission consisting of knowledgeable and committee individuals representing different professions and communities will help plan successful prevention and wellness efforts.

I urge you to announce the selection of members of the Commission on Prevention and Wellness and call their first meeting at the earliest possible date. According to our previous discussions, this commission should be prepared to:

1. Identify areas, projects and target groups that should receive increased attention.
2. Recommend to the secretary of the Department of Health and Social Services a four year plan for prevention and wellness programs.
3. Monitor ongoing and special demonstration efforts for health and wellness programs.
4. Review existing prevention and wellness efforts and relationships in the Department of Health and Social Services and other human service agencies.
5. Make recommendations on legislation which affects prevention and wellness efforts.
6. Ascertain those areas where federal recognition and support should be provided.
7. Undertake special tasks as the secretary deems necessary.

Please convey my support to the commission chair and the commission members. I am very enthusiastic about their efforts and the importance and significance of this effort for the future of Wisconsin people.

Even before the budget had been adopted in March, the secretary had been giving thought to the makeup of the commission. Given political realities, the commission had to be broadly representative of the people of the state. This meant men, women,

*Communication, Governor Schrieber to Secretary Percy, May 23, 1978.

whites, blacks, Native Americans, and Spanish-surnamed persons. It meant advocates for programs for children and youth and for the elderly or other interest areas as well. Given the nature of the responsibility and the commitment of time over a 15-month period that would be involved, persons who could give time would need to be selected. Since the charge was prevention and wellness and not sickness and coping, the spectrum of persons interested in prevention, detection, health promotion, and illness care had to be covered. Given the nature of the state, a large land mass with only one large city—over 650,000 population—and two others approaching, at most, 130,000 to 180,000 each, a mixture of urban and rural people had to be considered.

Finally, a leader for this disparate group of persons from the far left to the far right of the wellness spectrum would need to be chosen—the chairperson, in the secretary's view, ought to be one with some grasp of health-related activities and with a strong tie to the state's State Health Coordinating Council, the group Wisconsin calls the Health Policy Council. As vice chairman of the Health Policy Council, and as one who, nearly 10 years earlier, had done research in the area of health education, I fit Percy's specifications and accepted his invitation.

By June 10, 1978, the commission had its first meeting. Addressed by the governor, the secretary, and the chairman, the commission heard its keynote address from Vernon Wilson, M.D. Dr. Wilson had been administrator of Health Services and Mental Health Administration where the first notion of the "activated patient" and consumer health education had developed. Dr. Wilson closed his keynote address saying "The task undertaken is an absolutely essential step in the direction of a more rational health care plan. It brings you to face with a reality that many of us have tried to avoid—namely, the essential nature of the participation of the consumer public if the effort is to be successful. It has the challenge of demanding the highest type of social planning and engineering which must be carried out in the context of a non-intrusive process."

"The exciting thing about it," Dr. Wilson concluded, "is that, if addressed in digestible quantity, the task is doable, and, perhaps, the most important thing of all, it can never be completed, so there will be plenty for everyone to do."

As proof of the truth of Dr. Wilson's wry comment that "there would be plenty for everyone to do," the commission each day of its existence, created instant history. Establishing a committee on organization and rules, writing a conflict-of-interest statement, abiding by sunshine and ethics rules and regulations for the conduct of business of public bodies were just the first steps. And balancing interests and personalities on the commission's committees was a story in itself.

THE WORK OF THE COMMISSION

In the legislation, the Prevention and Wellness Commission and the Department of Health and Social Services were mandated to begin at once to survey the principal causes of mortality, disability, and absenteeism in the state and to identify existing prevention programs within the department. This was an easy task; the commission used health status indicators and morbidity and mortality data from our comprehensive State Health Plan. The high rankers were cardiovascular ills, car accidents, alcoholism, and pulmonary diseases.

The real work, once organization was completed, began with the writing (and submission for review and comment) of the criteria and guidelines for the Prevention and Wellness Demonstration Grant Program. A special committee worked long and hard between June and November 1978 to produce guidelines for elegibility, funding, project criteria selection, due dates, formats for submission, provision for technical assistance, directions for delineation of project goals and objectives, evaluation protocols, work plans, timetables, and all the one thousand and one details that accompany the seductive rustle of project dollars.

From December 1978 through February 15, 1979, publicity about the grant program, kits for applications, and technical assistance by the core staff were provided to applicants. Applicants came out in droves. Three hundred and one completed applications were received by the postmark deadline. A 3-step review—(1) across the Department of Health and Social Services regions, (2) by Prevention and Wellness Commission review subcommittees, and (3) in a special review and ranking session by the Commission itself—was followed to the letter.

Operating in full public view, commission protocol demanded that each applicant have equity in treatment and judgment. As modest proof, the commission received less than a handful of letters of complaint about the process. No suits, from within either the successful or nonsuccessful applicant pool, were filed.

On April 30, 1979, the commission reviewed, ranked, and recommended 51 proposals out of the 301 received as potentially fundable under the Prevention and Wellness Commission demonstration grant program. The 301 proposals carried a price tag of $16 million. The required 25 per cent proposal match by applicants raised the total to $20 million. The "short list" of 51 proposals had a price tag of $2 million and provided the secretary some leeway in selecting out proposals that he would recommend to the legislature's Joint Finance Committee for funding. On May 14, Secretary Percy reported to the Prevention and Wellness Commission that he had selected 29 proposals for recommended funding of $980,000 from the Joint Finance Committee. Percy and I appeared before that body on June 18, 1979—1 year and 8 days after the formal opening of commission activity!

Recall that the Prevention and Wellness Commission was to address concerns for physical, mental, and social ills. Just three of our recommended projects will demonstrate this. Under *cardiovascular disease prevention,* support was recommended for $13,700 for a fitness program for 292 commissioned officers and 77 civilian employees of the city of Madison Police Department; under *health promotion*, the commission recommended $5,000 to a theater workshop to develop a mime theater medicine show on health promotion for presentation to children. The engaging entertainment format was expected to reach young people often uninterested in being informed about health and wellness issues. Under a *multiple goal format aimed at promoting physical and mental health of women,* such as problem-solving issues related to alcohol and other drug abuse, child abuse, and the potential of reduction in the incidence of sexually transmitted diseases, the commission recommended support of $10,000 for a project aimed at counseling women involved in prostitution.

Our desire to address physical, mental, and social ills through prevention and health promotion was sincere. Our recommended projects ran afoul, however, of political reality! Elected officials, unlike appointed commission members, must stand for reelection in the political arena.

First, at the June 18 hearing of the Joint Finance Committee, the Senator co-chairman moved to refer *all* recommendations back to the commission with the request that Percy and I return, recommending only physical fitness and cardiovascular disease prevention programs. The fiscal year would end on June 30. There was no time (and the senator knew it) for us to react to his motion, if it passed. It failed, on a 8-3 vote. Next, the assembly Joint Finance co-chairman moved that the $980,000 project funding be cut in half and that the committee recess to negotiate specific projects within that funding level with the secretary and with me. This motion would allow "negotiation," in my view, to kill off our socially minded efforts at prevention that might be highly unpopular in the political sense. That motion lost, 8-3, as well.

Finally, the Joint Committee on Finance faced the question, how should it handle this politically hot potato thrown to it by a citizens' advisory body to a cabinet officer? The answer—no debate on the issues, merits, or shortcomings of any of the 29 proposals. The vote to endorse the secretary's list of recommended projects—9-1. The projects were in, and the grant program could get underway!

In addition to the grants program, however, there were other areas of responsibility given over to the Advisory Commission on Prevention and Wellness. We turn next to these.

DEPARTMENT OF HEALTH AND SOCIAL SERVICES INVENTORY AND OTHERS

One of the exciting things that happened to the citizen members of this commission was the rare opportunity to look inside a state agency. The commission had been charged with an inventory of existing programs in prevention in the Department of Health and Social Services. The first responses to our request for inventories were so poorly prepared, so laden with bureaucratic jargon, so self-serving, and so incomplete that we rejected the several divisional and bureau reports totally. Suddenly, that lumbering giant called the Department of Health and Social Services woke up. The advisory commission meant business! The next set of inventories received from the many sections of the department were truly meaningful ones. This response was very important in that, for the first time, a serious examination and public accounting had been accomplished by persons responsible for prevention, wellness, and health promotion. Just as evidence, the department's Division of Corrections examined what it was doing (and what it might do) with imprisoned youthful offenders in the area of health promotion and wellness.

The commission had *no* mandate from the legislature to inventory the Department of Health and Social Services. Things were stretched a little; the commission gained cooperation from the state's Educational Communications Board and modest cooperation from the state's Department of Public Instruction. The materials were useful; a clearer picture of organized health promotion and prevention and wellness activities in the state began to emerge. So, we stretched our mandate just a little more.

Commission staff devised a questionnaire for Wisconsin leaders of business and industry and for union leaders. Commission members wanted to know about health promotion in the private sector; we wanted to know about the extent and kind of employee assistance programs. The response to the commission's survey was far beyond expectations; more information was available for analysis and review.

Once again, the commission stretched its mandate to the fullest. Using official stationery, we queried Wisconsin-based 501(c)(3) tax exempt not-for-profit organizations or disease-oriented organizations to report about activities in health promotion, prevention, and wellness. Much information was supplied. They were, in the main, seriously in the wellness and health promotion business.

The result of all this effort was that the Prevention and Wellness Commission created a health promotion mosaic composed of as many bits and pieces of information as it was possible to get in one state. This process is recommended to other state prevention and wellness or health promotion commissions. Consideration for a broad mandate or stretching limited mandates as far as possible to obtain the data needed to accomplish assigned tasks is strongly urged.

SPECIAL EFFORTS

Recall that the governor's charge to the Prevention and Wellness Commission indicated that we would undertake such special tasks as the secretary deemed necessary. Wisconsin's State Health Coordinating Council was considering the National Academy of Science's Institute of Medicine Report on Primary Care, dealing with essential primary care services. The State Health Coordinating Council wanted a set of definitions and a list of priorities for relevant services not now reimbursed (for example, health education and preventive services) to be studied. What better group to study the question than the Prevention and Wellness Commission?

Given the assignment by the secretary, and bearing in mind that goal No. 10 of P.L. 93-641 calls for "the development of effective methods of educating the general public concerning proper personal (including prevention) health care and methods for effective use of available health care services," we examined the issue.

Out of a special committee of the Prevention and Wellness Commission came the recommendation that new health professionals, specifically nurse practitioners, clinical pharmacists and physician assistants be encouraged to provide patient education and be reimbursed for this effort by third-party payers. The committee suggested that further study be given to the notion of consumer education and its reimbursement. The special study committee was chaired by an attorney; it included physicians, nurses, economists, insurers, and the state commissioner of insurance as members. The political, economic, and professional impacts of this recommendation are yet to be realized. Some pilot efforts to test our suggestions are planned both at state levels and in the private sector.

IMPACT OF THE PREVENTION AND WELLNESS COMMISSION

First, a few general observations about the innovative grant demonstration program:

1. Several projects voluntarily developed cooperative and information-sharing "networks" with each other. For example, the Cooperative Educational Service Agency (CESA) in Green Bay and the Great Lakes Inter Tribal Council in Ashland each received grants to develop youth-oriented educational materials in prevention of alcohol and drug abuse. The CESA produced a television series and teacher-inservice materials. The Tribal Council worked on curriculum and filmstrips geared to a Native American population. Since both projects involved a "positive lifestyle" approach to prevention, including workshops and teacher involvement and media production, the directors voluntarily coordinated their projects to avoid unnecessary duplication of effort and shared ideas for program development.

   Milwaukee Goodwill Industries and the industrial-based Louis Allis project directors exchanged ideas for program development and problem solving as soon as the grants were awarded. Both work-site health promotion projects reported measurable effects in accident reduction and increased activity both in fitness and in employee assisstance programs.

2. A number of projects reported an increased level of recognition and support for their efforts from among local public and private agencies, health and social service providers, and the public. They reported optimism that their prevention and health promotion projects would maintain and increase that support so that the commitment of local funding resources for project continuation beyond the duration of the state grant would be secured.
3. Interest grew in those projects promoting health and fitness programs in the workplace (Louis Allis and Goodwill in Milwaukee; the Association for High Level Wellness in Brown County; the community project in Stevens Point and the Northwoods Wellness Resource Center at the Howard Young Medical Center in Woodruff). The business community's interest in health care cost containment in employee benefit plans and recent publication of *Healthy People: The Surgeon General's Report on Health Promotion and Disease Prevention* have focused attention on potential outcomes of these and similar projects.

In terms of publicity, media coverage of commission meetings was almost nonexistent. The notion of prevention, as opposed to treatment was too new to have captured public attention. And media representatives responded accordingly. Committee meetings went uncovered and unreported. The Joint Finance Committee's hearing, however, on proposal funding was covered. Following the discussion about the kinds of recommended demonstration projects that were funded, the Prevention and Wellness Commission's speaking engagement calendar was expanded; our vice chairperson as well as our two principal staff persons and I spoke at meetings all over the state of Wisconsin. Our local presentations were reported and received both positive and negative editorial comment in state newspapers; and we responded to each type. The responses were accorded good coverage; fairness was the operative rule.

With all the positive tone to this report, the reader must wonder what really happened. After all, the Prevention and Wellness Commission is no longer operative in Wisconsin. Other states (New York and California) now have similar commissions, but not Wisconsin.

POLITICS AND MONEY

Recall, please, that the legislature, with close to a billion-dollar surplus, "went along" with the acting governor and the DHSS secretary on the idea of spending a little on prevention. But a funny thing happened. Acting Governor Schrieber, sitting on his surplus, was challenged by a university professor of communications turned campus chancellor who promised to give back $950 million to the people if elected. He was elected. And he did return the surplus to the people.

Newly elected Governor Lee Sherman Dreyfus asked Donald E. Percy to remain as secretary of the Department of Health and Social Services in his new administration. And, surprise of surprises, the governor included 2-year funding, $980,000 each year, for prevention and wellness innovative demonstration grants in his own executive budget request. But the state's cookie jar was close to empty. OPEC had raised prices three times, inflation cut away at the remaining $35 million surplus, and elected officials ran scared.

The Senate chipped Governor Dreyfus's Prevention and Wellness Commission request in half—$980,000 for the next 2 years. The assembly went in for a zero sum. The $490,000 per year compromise met the Senate's request. By the time that the budget bill reached the governor's desk, he said, "Wellness is an idea whose time has not yet come" and vetoed his own funding request. The commission was dead. What remained was a decent burial service.

In an almost unprecedented move, DHSS Secretary Percy issued a press release blasting the governor's veto of continuation funding for the commission, while at the same time, promising to press forward with the Prevention and Wellness program underway in his own department.

On the political front, and operating from my home, I decided to take on the task of an override of Governor Dreyfus's veto. This, in Wisconsin, requires a two-thirds positive vote in each house. Calling on the president *pro tem* of the Senate, I gained his support and agreement to use his name in the attempt. Letters and calls went to key senators; positive responses were received *in writing*. The State Medical Society agreed to lend its efforts on the override. The SMS president made speeches, petitioned the legislature, and wrote to the newspapers. The Wisconsin Public Health Association's legislative committee made contact with legislators in both houses. Since Wisconsin is an open state, in many meanings of the word, I called the governor's office to tell his communications secretary about the override effort and asked for two Republican votes in the Senate. The response was that "wellness" was tied to the previous (and Democratic) administration. The communications secretary and I discussed, informally, the fact that the effort would stress "health promotion" rather than wellness and that the override forces would push ahead.

When the veto override session was held, we lost by three votes short of our needed 22. These were the two Republicans and only one Democrat who had been a consistent opponent—you recall—this was the senator who served as co-chairman of the Joint Finance Committee.

The commission was not to continue. Its final work came from the efforts of the Long Range Planning Committee. With that, the commission delivered its final report, the recommendations of which were to serve as guide to the secretary and the Department of Health and Social Services in its next 4-year planning. To the degree possible, commission recommendations are being implemented. And, through two initiatives to be described, other recommendations are being given very serious consideration. The Prevention and Wellness Commission 18-month effort, like that of the earlier Governor's Task Force on Health Planning and Policy, was worth the investment.

THE FUTURE: THE STATE HEALTH PLAN AND HEALTH PROMOTION

In Wisconsin, the State Health Plan is built up from the Health Systems Plans and Annual Implementation Plans of our seven Health Systems Agencies.

At the substate regional level, each health systems agency reviews facilities and services which are proposed for development or expansion in its area. All proposed uses of federal funds for development, expansion, or support of health resources by any entity other than the government of a state from any of the following sources must obtain HSA approval: Public Health Services Act, Community Mental Health Services Act, the Drug Abuse Office and Treatment Act of 1972, and the Comprehensive Alcohol Abuse and Alcoholism Prevention, Treatment and Rehabilatation Act of 1970. HSAs nominate members to serve on the Health Policy Council and develop Health Systems Plans and Annual Implementation Plans. In 1979, all seven of the Health Systems Plans gave attention to wellness and health promotion activities.

The Health Policy Council advises the governor on health policy. It develops the State Health Plan from Health Systems Agency Health Systems Plans with staff of the Division of Health and forwards the plan to the governor for approval. It also reviews the plans and the budgets of the Health Systems Agencies. State plans and applications for funds under federal legislation referred to above are subject to its review. Its members are appointed by the governor and include providers, consumers, and members of health systems agencies.

Recently, Wisconsin's Health Policy Council restructured its committees. The new effort at the state level is under the aegis of the Health Policy Council committee on Prevention, Detection and Health Promotion. The charge to the committee is as follows:

• Prepare the Community Health Education, Prevention, Detection and Health Promotion sections of the State Health Plan.
• Advise other committees of the Council on Prevention, Detection and Health Promotion programs.
• Develop policy for state and local public health programs.
• Advise the council on policy for maternal and child health, early and periodic screening, and other programs for health promotion.
• Review and develop state legislation on programs that will promote health, prevent and detect poor health, and make recommendations to the council.

The 1979–1980 Chairman of the Prevention, Detection and Health Promotion Committee was the vice chairman of the State, from 1977 to 1980, Health Coordinating Council. The reader may also recognize that person as the chairman of the former Wisconsin Advisory Commission on Prevention and Wellness, this chapter's author.

THE FUTURE: DHSS ACTIVITIES—HEALTH PROTECTION AND PROMOTION

Earlier, we reported that the Department of Health and Social Services Secretary Percy, in blasting the governor's veto of wellness support, promised to keep the effort alive through departmental initiatives.

The proof for the continuing effort is found in the secretary's July 1980 memo detailing Planning Guidelines for Health Protection and Promotion. Percy said:*

> The earnest pursuit of health promotion among our citizenry is of *crucial* significance in the years immediately ahead simply because the 'costs' in human and financial terms, of not pursuing these goals will be all the more staggering.
> We have begun the process of identifying in our major program areas, opportunities for *preventing*, rather than simply ameliorating, the social, emotional and physical problems which impair our citizens.
> *Prevention shall be the strategy of choice in all of our program and policy development* efforts, to the extent possible within state and federal law and funding provisions. Along with promoting health and preventing avoidable illness of impairment goes the opportunity and the responsibility to contribute positively to the quality of life among Wisconsin's people.
> This Planning Guideline starts with a simple premise: *That an individual should have the opportunity to be born physically healthy, to avoid preventable illness,*

*Planning Guideline No. 5, Mimeograph, Department of Mental and Social Services, Madison, Wisconsin, July 1980.

and to maximize physical and emotional health, mental acuity and life functioning. Whether called wellness or health protection and promotion, this needs to be our ultimate goal; it should inform all of our decision-making, as we review long-standing policies and programs or explore new areas where growth and development are needed.

The goal of wellness for all our citizens is extraordinarily ambitious. Progress toward our goal requires that we develop a full understanding of the context within which we work to inform our sense of priorities and urgency.

Public health services must move beyond the successes of the past. The new era requires us to rethink roles, functions, and service priorities not only for traditional health agencies, but also for programs such as mental health and drug abuse, which relate to our health promotion and protection aims. The victories of recent history— the conquest of certain life threatening communicable and infectious diseases, the control of others through improved sanitation, immunization, diagnostic and early treatment capabilities—provide us with a challenging standard of effectiveness and an example of vigorous systematic effort. *We need both a commitment to sustain those current services proven necessary to protect the public's health and a new resolve to actively PROMOTE better health and to address contemporary public health needs.*

Today we may be healthier than we were, but we are not nearly as healthy as we could be. In Wisconsin as nationwide, degenerative diseases (heart disease, cancer, stroke) and accidents (particularly alcohol-related motor vehicle accidents) are the leading causes of death and disability. We have gained important insights into the negative effects of environmental hazards as well as individual behavior on health. There is, however, growing evidence of the preventability of the incidence or at least the most disabling effects of these leading cripplers and killers, and increasing knowledge about useful prevention strategies.

We have taken the first steps toward making that knowledge effective through the efforts of the Commission of Prevention and Wellness and through Departmental support for community health promotion projects. But, that knowledge and insight will be fruitless in the long run without coordinated planning, sensible and sensitive application of existing resources, and legislative and administrative commitment to state leadership.

Percy detailed four priorities for DHSS in Health Protection and Promotion terms. These are Public Health Delivery Systems; Occupational Health; Health Risk Reduction; and Children's Health.

The reference to the efforts of the Commission on Prevention and Wellness are pointedly made. The findings and recommendations of the commission permeate the departmental priorities and those described earlier as the charge to the Prevention, Detection and Health Promotion Committee of Wisconsin's Policy Council.

Clearly, the initial investment of almost a million dollars of state revenue will continue to provide dividends to Wisconsin citizens for years to come.

SUGGESTED READINGS

Final Report, Madison, Wisc. The Wisconsin Governor's Health Planning and Policy Task Force, November 1972.

Research and Information Supplement, Volume I. Madison, Wisc. The Wisconsin Governor's Health Planning and Policy Task Force, November 1972.

Research and Information Supplement, Volume II. Madison, Wisc. The Wisconsin Governor's Health Planning and Policy Task Force, November 1972.

Blockstein, W. L., "Developing a Model for Consumer Health Education." In *Proceed-*

ings, National Conference on Continuing Education in Nursing, University of Wisconsin-Madison, October 1971.

Blockstein, W. L., Bailey, A., and Hansen, R., "One University's Concept of Its Role in Consumer Health Education." In *Society of Public Health Education Monograph Series,* March 1975.

Blockstein, W. L., Bailey, A., and Hansen, R., "Expanding the Role of a University in Consumer Health Education." In *Health Education Monographs* 3: 1 (Spring 1975).

Blockstein, W. L., "Health and Wellness Strategies." In *Wisconsin Pharmacist and Wisconsin Pharmacy Extension Bulletin,* February 1979.

Percy, D. E., Planning Guideline No. 5—Health Protection and Promotion. Department of Health and Social Services, Madison, Wisconsin, July 1980.

APPENDIX: CHAPTER 418, LAWS OF 1977

Section 923 (18) (am)

Prevention and wellness promotion efforts. 1. The department of health and social services, in consultation with an advisory committee appointed by the secretary of health and social services on prevention and wellness promotion, shall immediately begin a review of principal causes of mortality, disability and absenteeism and identify existing preventative programs.

2. Prior to the release of funds under SECTION 927 (18) (tk) of this act by the joint committee on finance, the department shall submit to the joint committee on finance, the assembly committee on health and social services and the senate committee on human services guidelines concerning the nature of the projects to be funded, the allowable administrative expenses of the projects, the target groups of the projects, the relationship of the projects with existing programs and the goals of the projects and a description of each project, including the location of the project, the group to be served, the services to be provided, the amount of the grant and the goals of the project.

3. Prevention and wellness promotion projects under subd. 2 and SECTION 927 (18) (tk) of this act shall not be funded if funding is available from existing programs.

4. The department shall submit a report to the legislature not later than January 1, 1980. The report shall evaluate the prevention and wellness promotion projects and include recommendations.

Section 927 (18)

(tf) *Prevention and wellness promotion administration* The appropriation under section 20.435 (8) (a) of the statutes, as affected by the laws of 1977, is increased by $80,100 in 1977–78 to provide funding for 3 positions for prevention and wellness promotion efforts of the department of health and social services and to provide funding for the expenses of an advisory commission on prevention and wellness promotion efforts. Funds not spent by June 30, 1978, shall be available during 1978–79.

(tk) *Prevention and wellness promotion project fund.* The appropriation under section 20.435 (8) (a) of the statutes, as affected by the laws of 1977, is increased by $980,000 in 1978–79 for funding of prevention and wellness promotion projects under section 923 (18) (am) of this act. Funds for projects shall not be released until approved by the joint committee on finance.

17 / Background and Perspective on the Centers for Disease Control and It's Bureau of Health Education   *Charles Althafer*

The Centers for Disease Control (CDC) which is headquartered in Atlanta, Georgia, is one of the six major federal health agencies which make up the U.S. Public Health Service.* The CDC originated as a malaria control program during World War II, under the name Malaria Control in War Areas (MCWA). Following the War, it was designated the Communicable Disease Center and soon developed a worldwide reputation for scientific expertise in infectious disease control. The best example of CDC's international work in the infectious disease area is the smallpox eradication program, wherein CDC staff cooperated with the World Health Organization and the governments of most Third World countries to bring about the eradication of one of humanity's most dreaded diseases. Meanwhile, in the United States, other communicable diseases such as tuberculosis and polio were experiencing similar declines as public health programs involving control measures were implemented.

As communicable disease rates responded to the effective application of control measures, the significance of morbidity and mortality from chronic diseases which did not respond to the same control measures became increasingly evident and important. State and local health agencies began shifting their program emphasis to these areas of concern, which created a corresponding demand upon CDC's resources. On July 24, 1970, the Center was renamed the Center for Disease Control, reflecting its expanded scope. In October 1980, the official name became Centers for Disease Control.

A wide variety of factors contributed to the surge of interest in chronic disease prevention programs in the late 1960s and early 1970s. The success of the antismoking programs, initiated by governmental and voluntary health agencies, gave rise to optimism that one of the major risk factors could be controlled. Decline in coronary disease mortality, which started to move downward in 1963 and accelerated by 1968, was accompanied by increased public interest in cessation of cigarette smoking, jogging, polyunsaturated fats, low-cholesterol foods, and weight loss. The National High Blood Pressure Education Program, sponsored by the National Heart, Lung, and Blood Institute and the American Heart Association, screened hundreds of thousands and also created a high volume of media coverage. In the early 1970s, the environmental movement, the concept of self-care, and the women's rights movement (with its accent on health) reinforced a societal trend toward chronic disease prevention and especially toward recognition of the individual's capacity to effect his or her own health.

The beginning of these trends in society, coupled with the growing concern over burgeoning health care costs, led to the establishment of the President's Committee on Health Education in 1971 to examine the nation's needs in this area and make recommendations. One outcome of these recommendations, submitted to the White House

---

*Henceforward, CDC refers to the Centers for Disease Control. The other five agencies of the Public Health Services are: the Alcohol, Drug Abuse, and Mental Health Administration; the Food and Drug Administration; the Health Resources Administration; the Health Services Administration; and the National Institutes of Health.

in 1973, was the establishment of a federal focal point for health education at the CDC in October 1974.

Designated as the Bureau of Health Education (BHE),* this new organization was established with 35 positions and a first-year budget of $3 million. The new bureau's first major activity was to initiate a study to determine the feasibility of a health education center in the private sector in response to another recommendation of the President's Committee. In 2 years the National Center for Health Education became a reality, as a nonprofit corporation. The new bureau also developed a coordinating–liaison system within the federal government, headed by the Intra-Departmental Panel on Health Education, in an attempt to develop a comprehensive understanding of the vast scope of health education activities being conducted by federal agencies, as well as to determine needs and priorities.

At a meeting of this panel in 1976, its Chairman, Dr. Theodore Cooper, assistant secretary for Scientific Affairs of the Department of Health, Education, and Welfare, directed that a health education program for federal employees be developed and implemented. Subsequently, the Director of CDC, William H. Foege, Jr., M.D., determined that the initial program should be first tried on CDC employees. His reasoning was that if CDC could not implement a program, CDC could not work on one for anyone else. The Bureau of Health Education commenced work on a plan of action and was ready to begin by late summer of 1978.

The bureau determined that the health education program for employees needed a catalyst to stimulate interest. The bureau was aware of the Canadian version of Health Hazard Appraisal called "Evalu*Vie" and approached Health and Welfare, Canada, for the use of its computer program. The bureau was impressed with Canada's implementation of the program on a nationwide basis since December 1972 and subsequent expansion of its operational base to three computer centers in British Columbia, Ottawa, and Nova Scotia.

Prior to using the Canadian risk assessment program at CDC, the computer program was subjected to internal scientific review by the Center's Medical Advisory Board. The board considered human subjects' study factors, including privacy, as well as the basic scientific integrity of the data base. The latter issue provoked considerable discussion, as a number of deficiencies were identified in the risk factors and the mortality tables. Provisional approval for use of the Canadian computer program was granted by the board in February 1978, with the understanding that work would proceed on the mortality data in order to provide more current, race-specific tables.

During the time the review process was underway, work on the basic health education plan began. The Board of Directors of the CDC employee's organization SHARE, Inc. (Service to Help All Regular Employees) was approached for primary sponsorship and support. The bureau's staff were convinced that the planned program had the maximum chance for broad workforce participation if it avoided the pitfalls of being perceived as either management or labor controlled. SHARE had a good cross-sectional membership, a successful track record for sponsoring recreational activities—volleyball, softball, bowling—and employee services and was well thought of by employees. Moreover, the organization featured a network of employee representatives throughout CDC's Atlanta workforce of 2,000. The representatives were volunteers, distributed throughout CDC on a ratio of approximately 1 to 25. The SHARE board enthusiastically endorsed the sponsorship in August 1977, with the proviso that the program be conducted as a service project and not as a research study. Evaluation was to be limited to

---

*Effective October 1980, BHE became part of the CDC's new Center for Health Promotion and Education.

"unobtrusive" measurements, such as pre- and postcomparisons of sick leave utilization and participation in behavioral change programs.

Program activities commenced in January 1978 with a symposium on Health Risk Appraisal (HRA), featuring experts on the subject. About 900 employees attended the symposium sessions conducted by Lewis Robbins, M.D., Charles Ross, M.D., and David Thorton, Ph.D. Following the symposium, HRA was offered to CDC employees by SHARE representatives. Over 1,400 employees participated (about 65 per cent of the total work population). Participating employees were provided with a catalog of community resources, listing programs of smoking cessation, weight loss, stress reduction, and exercise and fitness. Employee committees were formed by SHARE to identify and create resources in these four topic areas. The first strategy was to enable employees to find an appropriate program convenient for them—and for their families. Negotiations with a number of commercial facilities resulted in extremely attractive rates for CDC employees and their families.

The second step of the strategy was for the committees to review popular community programs and bring them to the center because for most employees, the greater distance they must travel from their workplace to participate, the less likely they are to take part. Courses in aerobic dance and multilevel fitness were contracted to the YMCA. There were courses also given by Weight Watchers and SmokEnders. In the initial program year, over 440 employees paid between $35 and $60 each to lose weight, become physically fit, and/or to quit smoking. There probably would have been many more participants, but CDC, unfortunately, lacked the physical space to hold them. Many had to be placed on waiting lists or were turned away.

The third strategy was to have employees themselves develop programs, such as a walking program during lunch break and yoga classes. It was obvious that HRA was a useful device to stimulate interest in seeking and utilizing resources for behavioral change. CDC was put in the position of having more demand for health promotion services than its available facilities could provide. A request for adequate and appropriate indoor space was sent to CDC's director by the SHARE Board of Directors. It is anticipated that substantial improvements will be arranged.

DIFFUSION OF THE CDC PROGRAM

Although the CDC Employee Lifestyle Program was not organized on a research basis, and as a result had limited potential for documentation of health education, word about it spread to the public health field. The bureau contributed to the awareness by convening two meetings of about a dozen public sector agencies who were actively using Health Risk Appraisal in 1978 and 1979. The purpose of these meetings was to determine the state of the art and to ascertain areas of technical or program resource need to which CDC would respond. (The areas most urgently needed concerned risk-factor update and improved mortality tables.) These conferences also facilitated a great deal of information exchange and did substantially increase general interest in Health Risk Appraisal from the public health field. At the same time, The W. K. Kellogg Foundation was funding a clinical trial of risk assessment in Arizona, called "Well Aware," which was attracting a great deal of attention in public health publications and the media.

As a result of the rising interest in Health Risk Appraisal, CDC experienced a steadily increasing volume of written and telephone requests for information about Health Risk Appraisal. A mailing package was developed, consisting mostly of materials used in the CDC Lifestyle Program. Also included in the package as sources of information and technology was a listing of all known risk assessment vendors and their range of services.

More recently, CDC has expanded its services to the field. In response to requests for accurate mortality data, CDC developed improved 10-year mortality predictions, which are based upon the 3-year averages from 1975, 1976 and 1977. These are configured into single-year age groups, as well as the previously standard 5-year age groups. CDC also instituted a demonstration program to allow any organization to perform a trial run of Health Risk Appraisal on up to 200 participants with CDC providing data analysis free of charge. This program was initiated because of numerous requests for the computer program which could not be filled because of limitations placed by Health and Welfare, Canada. It was hoped that the opportunity to experience Health Risk Appraisal would provide a positive incentive to continue interest or lead to pursuing negotiations with one of the proprietary organizations. As of August 1980, CDC had batch processed data for over 100 trial runs, with a total volume of over 9,000.

Another major Health Risk Appraisal activity currently being conducted by CDC involves health fairs. In 1979, the National Health Screening Council for Volunteer Organizations, Inc. (NHSCVO) sponsored health fairs in eight major cities. The organizational support for these fairs has been provided by the American Red Cross, Blue Cross/Blue Shield, and the local affiliates of the National Broadcasting Company (NBC). In most instances, NBC has organized promotion, including a large number of public service announcement spots, 5-minute vignettes on the local news broadcasts, and special prime-time public service programs. Also, NHSCVO requested CDC's assistance with the batch processing of Health Risk Appraisal data. In 1979, 1,400 Health Risk Appraisals were processed for the Atlanta health fair and nearly 400 for Chicago's. The results, particularly from DeKalb County in Atlanta, were impressive in terms of the number of participants who returned for interpretation of their computer printouts and the quality of follow-up activities. In 1980, the NHSCVO program was expanded to 16 cities. As of August 1980, 11 cities had participated with a total of nearly 32,000 processed appraisals. The gross data collected is being analyzed prior to future CDC support to determine the usefulness of the procedure.

The Office of Health Information and Health Promotion, and Physical Fitness and Sports Medicine sponsored eight regional conferences on health promotion in 1979–80. CDC, through the Bureau of Health Education, assisted with these conferences by providing staff and Health Risk Appraisals for participants. A summary session was incorporated into the National Forum of the National Health Council.

CDC has engaged in a wide variety of other activities in response to interest or requests from the field for Health Risk Appraisal information or service. These activities have included interviews with the press and media, speaking at public health professional meetings, staff-supporting programs of the American College of Preventive Medicine and the Society of Prospective Medicine, and consulting and providing technical assistance. An informal liaison for Health Risk Appraisal information has developed between CDC and the regional offices of the Department of Health and Human Services. Strong lines of communication exist with most state health agencies who have active Health Risk Appraisal programs.

THE FORMAL COLLABORATIVE RELATIONSHIP WITH HEALTH AND WELFARE, CANADA

In 1979, staff representatives from CDC's Bureau of Health Education and from Health and Welfare, Canada, agreed to negotiate a formal exchange of letters between the two agencies for the purpose of mutually developing a core Health Risk Appraisal program.

It was felt that the agreement would provide a basis for sharing information and technology, including research and development plans, which would enable more efficient utilization of scarce research dollars. The most critically important area in need of mutual development is the issue of risk-factor update. A number of other issues such as predictive validity, reliability, formating, and population targeting are also important. Letters have been exchanged, and negotiations have been concluded. The following represent general features of the collaboration:

1. Participation in the update of precursors/risk factors, with the understanding that CDC will take a strong leadership role;
2. Consolidation and provision of information to facilitate a proposed clearinghouse function;
3. Continuation of the provision of expertise to develop a mutually agreed strategy for the development and evaluation of Health Risk Appraisal;
4. Assuming the availability of funds, the support of research addressing high-priority research and development questions associated with Health Risk Appraisal;
5. Provision of expertise for the development of suitable guidelines and standards on the technical aspects of Health Risk Appraisal and its use.

CURRENT DIRECTIONS OF CDC

Although collaboration with Canada has not been officially formalized, most work underway or planned incorporates and involves mutual cooperation. The centers, through the Bureau of Health Education, have initiated the following research and development projects.

Predictive Validity Study: In cooperation with the National Center for Health Services Research, CDC has undertaken a retrospective study to determine the efficacy of Health Risk Appraisal in determining health outcomes. A final report will be accomplished by the California State Health Department's Human Population Laboratory, utilizing data from the Breslow longevity study in Alameda County, California. Preliminary data, standardized by age and sex, indicate a reasonable degree of accuracy in predicting actual health outcomes.

Risk Factor Update: A project was initiated by the Bureau of Health Education in May 1980, to develop a validated methodology for calculating precursors and risk factors, and then to complete new risk factors on cardiovascular disease and trauma deaths. (Canada has a risk factor update project underway similiar to this.) Other issues addressed by this contract are calculation of composite risks and potential for a comparable data base.

Field Trials: Most current literature indicates HRA has a generally high acceptability among white-collar, middle-class audiences. The Bureau of Health Education is developing a series of four major field trials which will include blacks, Hispanics, Native Americans, and Veterans Administration–eligible veterans. The purpose is to refine or redesign formats of both inputs and outputs and to make them more understandable, acceptable, and maximally useful for priority audiences.

OTHER BHE/CDC ACTIVITIES

In addition to the research and development activity, BHE/CDC is attempting to meet several other critical areas of needs. The following activities are scheduled for implementation in conjunction with Health Risk Appraisal:

Analysis and development of educational materials for use in conjunction with Health Risk Appraisal: This contract is intended to collect and analyze materials and services available from national sources which are useful in support of HRA programs. These materials will be organized into guide manuals for use by public health staff who are planning and conducting HRA programs. This reflects a basic BHE strategy which calls for effective involvement with and utilization of existing community resources, rather than "reinventing the wheel."

Training: There is a lack of useful training and training materials for individuals or organizations who want to understand, plan, and conduct HRA programs. BHE/CDC has commenced work on a specialized package of support materials, designed for use by experienced HRA staff, in training on a local basis. The package is designed to be used in a 2-day, 1-day, or half-day time frame. Materials are targeted for "training trainers." In addition, BHE/CDC is developing several sound/slide packages, which are intended to explain HRA to potential participants, to interpret results to those who have participated, and to assist agencies in understanding the scope of considerations necessary prior to starting a Health Risk Appraisal program.

Development of computer software: BHE/CDC will have a staff-developed HRA computer program available shortly for distribution to requesting agencies. This program is essentially similar to the Evalu*Vie program but has documentation and and an improved format. The bureau has also undertaken development of a microprocessor version which could be used by small health departments or hospitals with relatively inexpensive (approximately $5,000 per unit) tabletop equipment.

Health education-risk reduction grants: BHE/CDC has an active grant program which provided $3.6 million to 46 states, the District of Columbia, and the Virgin Islands in fiscal year 1979. The grant program was expanded in 1980 to almost $15 million, with most of the extra funds directed toward smoking and alcohol prevention programs intended for school-age children and adolescents. Although the school-age smoking and alcohol programs will not involve the use of Health Risk Appraisal, a significant proportion of the risk-reduction project grant funds (nearly $5 million) will utilize Health Risk Appraisal at some point.

COORDINATION WITH OTHER AGENCIES

A great deal of activity has been generated at CDC in recent years related to Health Risk Appraisal. A number of important issues, critical to the successful evolution of Health Risk Appraisal in the federal sector, are not covered in this chapter. Foremost among these is the liaison with other federal agencies, which is imperative as research and development plans are developed and implemented. Three other federal agencies have commenced work on Health Risk Appraisal and at least two more will soon.

At the outset of CDC's program activity, a great deal of information, including drafts of planned contracting activities, was exchanged with a number of other federal organizations. The primary intention of this exchange was to ensure systematic development of Health Risk Appraisal and, in particular, to avoid overlap and duplication of activities. As work on research contracts began, the federal agency project officers held meetings at which research designs, scopes of work, and required deliverable items, such as interim reports were shared. These meetings were expanded to include personnel from the contractors' staffs. The sharing of details of progress on similar content areas enabled savings of cost and effort.

The second in the series of federal liaison meetings was held in Atlanta, Georgia, in August 1980. Convened by the Office of Health Information, Health Promotion, and Physical Fitness and Sports Medicine, it included representatives from the National

Heart, Lung, and Blood Institute, National Center for Health Services Research, U.S. Veterans Administration, Health and Welfare, Canada, and Bureau of Health Education. Seven research projects were discussed by project officers and the contractors. Information was exchanged on several other future contracts. This cooperation has been an example of effective communication and liaison, which has contributed significantly to the establishment of a broad, comprehensive scientific base for Health Risk Appraisal.

Brief summaries of these projects listed by agency are as follows:

National Heart, Lung, and Blood Institute, Lung Division: This agency is developing morbidity data (risk factors) related to chronic obstructive lung disease, which, in turn, is being utilized as a basis for smoking cessation programs.

National Heart, Lung, and Blood Institute, Heart Division: Work is underway on a national survey to determine the extent of HRA usage in occupational settings as an adjunct to cardiovascular disease risk-reduction efforts.

National Center for Health Services Research: Two projects are in the initial work plan. The most extensive effort consists of a national survey to determine the current state of the art of HRA, in terms of who is using it and on what population, including evaluation of effectiveness and changes in preventive medicine practice The first phase of this project also included compilation of an annotated, analytical bibliography, and an assessment of the scientific credibility of the HRA data base. The second field project is aimed at collection of research findings on intervention procedures which support HRA, such as smoking cessation, weight loss, exercise, and stress-reduction activities.

Office of Health Information and Health Promotion, and Physical Fitness and Sports Medicine: A national electronic media campaign is being developed to make the public aware of the importance of health risk factors. The campaign will feature public service spot announcements, which will offer a "paper and pencil," or hand-calculated, risk-assessing instrument. Subsequent expansions of this program are intended to create public awareness of community resources concerning life-style and to gather local support for improving and expanding community facilities and services.

U.S. Veterans Administration: In cooperation with the Bureau of Health Education, a field trial of the Health Risk Appraisal began in late 1980. The major intention of this trial is to develop and test a modified version of the HRA computer program with a typical low-income, high-risk veteran population. (Research for this project is compatible with three other BHE field trials scheduled for black, Hispanic, and Native American populations.)

Health and Welfare, Canada: Work on a major risk factor update will be completed shortly. Although the new data base will include possible Canadian variations in mortality rates, it will be closely compared with similar new data obtained in the CDC/BHE risk-factor update.

SUMMARY

Health Risk Appraisal has potential as a public health tool, particularly as an adjunct to health education. Most experienced HRA advocates believe it demonstrates an important utility in the behavior change process, in which participants are motivated to seek out resources to assist them in making desired health behavior changes. Health Risk Appraisal has the advantage of offering to the participant objective data which are personally relevant. It helps the person to understand the relative importance of health risks and appears to encourage behavior. Improvement in the Health Risk Appraisal process will lie in the direction of simplification, clarification, and a focus on the positive. Hopefully, improvements in the availability and accuracy of morbidity data will provide an even more useful tool.

A LOOK TO THE FUTURE

The long-term plans of CDC/BHE regarding Health Risk Appraisal are linked in large part to collaboration with Health and Welfare, Canada. The collaborative working relationship, if and when formalized, would continue through 1983. Within that time frame, answers for the major questions evident at this time should be largely resolved. Risk appraisal intake questionnaires, computer programs, outputs, and intervention programs will evolve into a variety of new and more effective forms.

The experience of the Bureau of Health Education with Health Risk Appraisal in a variety of settings has been positive and has generated an unexpected volume of interest. The press and electronic media have provided a great deal of coverage, spreading internationally, with a favorable reaction. The research and development plan should enhance the scientific credibility of the data base available to the field. The field trials should result in materials and techniques which will make it educationally useful to a broader audience.

PART IV
Future Directions for
Risk Reduction

What will the future hold for risk reduction and health promotion efforts and for the innovative programs that are being implemented? A second question for this new direction in health maintenance centers on the amount of support the federal government commits to this second "public health revolution."

By 1990, leaders of this effort within the federal government will be able to respond to these questions, as measurable and what are considered to be achievable goals have been clearly set forth in *Healthy People*, Surgeon General's Report on Health Promotion and Disease Prevention.

The following five public health goals have been set forth for achievement between now and 1990 (as delineated in *Healthy People*):

- A 35 per cent reduction in infant mortality by then;
- A 20 per cent reduction in deaths of children aged 1 to 14, to fewer than 34 per 100,000;
- A 20 per cent reduction of deaths among adolescents and young adults to age 24, to fewer than 93 per 100,000;
- A 25 per cent reduction in deaths among the 25 to 64 age group; and
- A major improvement in health, mobility, and independence for older people to be achieved largely by reducing by 20 per cent the average number of days of illness among this age group.[1]

One step that health care professionals, health educators, and community or political leaders might well take is to influence school administrators to include *Healthy People*, Surgeon General's Report on Health Promotion and Disease Prevention, in school health education curricula. Beyond this, programs similar to the "Know Your Body" program should be implemented in both elementary and secondary public schools. If these measures were implemented, students would benefit from gaining knowledge of positive and negative results of life-style behaviors and from knowing that instituting positive behavioral changes and habits can measurably improve their well-being. Students will also benefit from periodic health appraisals and programs designed to provide them with knowledge about healthful nutritional principles, fitness-exercise habits, education for parenthood, genetic counseling, prenatal care and nutrition, available community health resources, dental care, knowledge of how to reduce injuries and accidents (part of driver education), avoidance of smoking and smoking-cessation programs.

A great many positive health maintenance techniques and life-style patterns of behavior can be inculcated in children and youth through education presented in a positive atmosphere by health care professionals and educators who are role models of healthy life-styles.

In Part Four, the editors have included chapters that address the future directions for health promotion.

In Chapter 18, Katharine Bauer addresses a topic central to the future of health promotion. This author describes the policies and activities of the federal government relating to health promotion. This chapter contains essential information for understanding the government's interest in and support of health promotion programs. Bauer illustrates cogently her assertion that "between 1974 and 1980, an astonishing degree of progress was made at the federal level in setting the sights for an intergrated prevention policy, and providing leadership, information, technical assistance, and grant funds. . . ." Bauer wisely concludes her presentation with the caveat that it may be "rash" to predict the future of any federal program not linked to defense.

> In the final analysis, what happens to prevention during the 1980s will depend upon the public's sustained expression of will to make the second revolution in public health a fact, not a dream. For, as Oliver Wendell Holmes observed, policy rests upon "the felt necessities of the time, the prevalent moral and political theories, the intentions of the public, avowed or unconscious."

Chapter 19 addresses the role played by health systems agencies in the planning and implementation of risk-reduction programs. This role is relatively new for health systems agencies. Therefore, the strategies and methods described in this material will suggest directions and foci for other health systems agencies as well as coordination and collaboration between programs within a state.

The senior author, Ernest Schloss, is director of the Health Systems Agency II in Tucson, Arizona.

Although an increasing number of risk-reduction–health promotion programs are presently being developed and implemented, few of these programs have been planned to include an evaluation design. This may be due to the fact that clear, widely accepted standards for evaluation of client outcome have been agreed upon by program planners. However, one outstanding health promotion program is unique in that evaluation has been preplanned into the design of the program, the Well Aware About Health Program, operating in Tucson, Arizona. This project is discussed in Chapter 20 by Sabina Dunton, director of the program.

Much interest is focused on this program by health professionals and planners. Perhaps this is particularly true because of the evaluation phase of the program. As health promotion programs begin to proliferate, often funded by the federal government or state tax dollars, it becomes increasingly important that methods of evaluating outcome of such programs be developed to provide accountability to funding sources at the conclusion of these programs and for supporting "successful outcome" statements and reports. Also, evaluations, whether positive or negative, enable the program planners to learn which methods, strategies, and techniques resulted in positive outcomes and which techniques were not effective.

With these contingencies in mind, the information contained in this chapter is essential for any health professional planning a health promotion program.

Some of the primary requirements upon which the evaluation component of this program is focusing are being derived from analysis of change in physical condition, life-style, health care resource use, individual capacity for self-care, and finally, provider attitudes and practices with regard to patient self-responsibility.

The economic aspects of new preventive and health promotion programs are addressed by Michael Peddecord, Dr. P.H., in Chapter 21. Noting that the health care environment has changed significantly since 1960, Dr. Peddecord cites the growth of health care in terms of America's GNP from 5.2 per cent in 1960 to 8.8 per cent in 1977—impressive as the increase in dollars from $26 to $162 billion during that period.

Why have costs escalated so substantially? Peddecord cites the following reasons:

1. Introduction of new technologies (drugs, surgical treatments, diagnostic tests, medical interventions and devices).
2. The development of a more complex or intense product.
3. The shifting of direct out-of-pocket payment from consumer to third parties, and
4. The establishment of social programs that have increased access to health care in previously underserved population groups.

The author emphasizes that competition for increasingly scarce resources is fast becoming a reality in the health care sector. This fact will force more careful scrutiny, allocation, and accountability concerning those health care programs that are funded in the coming decade.

Due to rapidly escalating costs for acute health care, the potential of *preventing* disease and disability is now viewed as one solution to the problem of providing both cost-effective care and improved health status.

The author points out that as individual risk reduction is continuing in its developmental growth, continued experimentation, innovation, and evaluation of programs are all essential. Peddecord cautions that care should be taken to avoid overselling prevention and health promotion programs as curealls or preventive panaceas. Quality assurance activities need to be integrated into all health promotion and risk reduction programs.

Finally, Peddecord wisely advises that innovative program planners and developers will need to pay a great deal of attention to how to be successful in educating health care providers, third-party payers, and larger purchasers of insurance as well as the public concerning the value and efficacy of risk reduction–health promotion programs.

The final chapter of this volume by editor Marilyn Faber, a health care administrator, and Raymond Faber, M.D., a psychiatrist, focuses on an ingredient essential to the new risk reduction health promotion climate and philosophy, the "new" health care partnership between doctor and patient. One might also characterize this relationship as one in which the "active" or "activated" individual assumes full and increasingly knowledgeable responsibility for his or her own health status. In one sense, the consumer-patient and physician make a "contract," stipulating the responsibilities of each in the task of maintaining and improving the consumer's health status.

The authors illustrate this new behavioral pattern of shared responsibility between physician and patient through descriptions of self-care activities and programs that are occurring nationwide.

The editors conclude with their hope and conviction that during the future decade, risk reduction–health promotion programs, as well as the "activated patient" will become the accepted norm of a healthier America!

REFERENCES

1. U.S. Department of Health, Education, and Welfare, *Healthy People: The Surgeon General's Report on Health Promotion and Disease Prevention*, DHEW (PHS) Pub. No. 79-55071. Washington, D.C.: U.S. Government Printing Office, 1979, pp. ix-x.

18 / Federal Government Policies and Activies in Health Promotion

Katharine G. Bauer

The many as-yet-unrealized opportunities for promoting health and preventing disease in the United States offer challenges to all its citizens and to almost every component of its society. The crucial roles of industry, schools, state and local governments, and voluntary associations, as well as of physicians and other providers of health care in efforts to reduce recognized avoidable risks to the health of children and adults of all ages has been discussed elsewhere in this volume. This chapter reviews the roles and responsibilities of the federal government and its structures for encouraging and assisting this common enterprise, and concludes with speculations about the future.

Under one or another legislative mandate, Congress has over the years authorized a great many different federal agencies to undertake a great many prevention activities designed to accomplish a great many different specific purposes. While in 1980 the sum total of dollar expenditures to support these various activities have amounted to only slightly more than 1 per cent of federal spending for health, and less than 0.002 per cent of the total federal budget, nevertheless, the leverage they provide is significant. Federal activities in health promotion and disease prevention can be categorized as formulating policy goals and objectives; providing leadership; providing information; supporting research; maintaining health surveillance systems; promulgating regulatory standards to protect people from environmental hazards or unsafe food, drugs, and manufactured consumer products; paying for or providing personal preventive health services; giving technical assistance to states and localities; supporting innovative demonstrations in prevention by states and communities as models for wider replication; and, finally, collecting and analyzing data and issuing reports to track the nation's successes and failures in prevention. The overview to follow will touch on many of these forms of federal activity. However, it will not deal with the regulatory functions of government, affording environmental or occupational health protection, or with the direct provision of preventive services to special populations such as veterans, Indians, and members of the armed services and their dependents, or with the surveillance systems to monitor the incidence of reportable diseases.

PROVIDING POLICY LEADERSHIP

The term *policy* is widely used but seldom defined. Webster offers two quite different interpretations. On the one hand, the dictionary defines it as "wisdom in managing affairs," and on the other as "a daily lottery in which participants bet that certain numbers will be drawn from a lottery wheel." Until quite recently, the second interpretation appeared to be the more appropriate characterization of government's policy stance in prevention. In 1977, Philip Lee, after his resignation as Assistant Secretary for Health in the Department of Health, Education, and Welfare (DHEW) observed:

> The lack of a coherent national health policy is nowhere more apparent than in the policies of the federal government in the area of preventive medicine. Indeed,

there are a multiplicity of policies and a maze of programs that affect the health of individuals, families, and communities in the United States. Many of these policies have a favorable impact on health; others, a negative effect.[1]

The most familiar example of contradictory federal policies are the campaigns launched against smoking by the Department of Health and Human Services (HHS)* and the subsidization of tobacco crops by the Department of Agriculture. Even within HHS, however, one finds important contradictions. For example, the Department's Health Services Administration makes grants to states of approximately $20 million annually to conduct hypertension screening programs, and its National High Blood Pressure Education Program at the National Institutes of Health urges people with hypertension to adhere to the drug regimens their physicians prescribe. Yet the department's Medicare program fails to include the costs of the necessary drugs as a reimbursable benefit. Thus, while the federal government pays for the hospital care of elderly heart disease victims, at a possible average of $7,000 an episode, and for their nursing home care when their funds are exhausted, at an average of about $12,000 per year it excludes the less than $400 per year cost of drugs that could prevent a large proportion of these conditions from occurring.

Because most such contradictions stem from the specific provisions of laws enacted to accomplish specific narrowly focused objectives, changes in laws are usually required to resolve them. Such changes are more likely to be rational ones when Congress and voters can relate their particular efforts to combat some particular disease or to assist some special group of the population to some overall guiding health policy. Fortunately, such a policy has been enunciated in the Surgeon General's 1979 report, *Healthy People*. This landmark document established a focal point for informed forward movement toward preventing avoidable illness and death. It sets forth in detail the major causes of premature death and disability among people during the five major stages of the life cycle and establishes the following goals:

For infants—to continue to improve infant health, and by 1990, to reduce infant mortality by at least 35 per cent to fewer than nine deaths per 1,000 live births;

For children—to improve child health, foster optimal childhood development, and, by 1990, reduce deaths among children 1 to 14 years, by at least 20 per cent, to fewer than 34 per 1,000;

For adolescents and young adults—to improve the health and health habits of adolescents and young adults, and by 1990, to reduce deaths among people ages 15 to 24 by at least 20 per cent, to fewer than 400 per 100,000;

For older adults—to improve the health and quality of life for older adults and, by 1990, to reduce the average annual number of days of restricted activity due to acute and chronic conditions by 20 per cent, to fewer than 30 days per year for people age 65 and older.[2]

Besides describing the multifaceted nature of the risks to the population's health today, *Healthy People* identifies a corresponding host of multifaceted approaches that could be undertaken to achieve significant reductions in infant deaths, birth defects, motor vehicle accidents, heart diseases, cancer, strokes, and other diseases whose incidence could be reduced by known prevention measures. Actions that can be taken to advance these goals are grouped into three major categories: health promotion (life-style), health services, and health protection (environment). An accompanying appendix

*Formerly the Department of Health, Education and Welfare (DHEW).

volume to *Healthy People* presents a detailed review of the state of the art, in background papers prepared by the National Academy of Sciences, Institute of Medicine.[3]

A successor report, *Preventing Disease, Promoting Health: Objectives for the Nation*, issued by HHS in December 1980, spells out more than 200 measurable objectives that could be achieved by the nation during the decade of the 1980s in the following areas: hypertension; family planning, pregnancy, and infant health; immunization; sexually transmitted diseases; toxic agent control; occupational safety and health; accident prevention and injury control; misuse of alcohol and drugs; nutrition; physical fitness and exercise; and the management of stress and violent behavior.[4] Thus, in addition to *Healthy People's* comprehensive framework for policy debate, the Department of Health and Human Services has recently provided a specific agenda for health-related government and private agencies and organizations to consider as they formulate their own policies, arrive at their own priorities, and decide on their own plans of action for the 1980s.

All these recent activities within the Office of the Surgeon General represent important steps toward overcoming the pervasive lack of federal policy to guide prevention that had been noted by Lee only a few years earlier.

Healthy People and the national prevention objectives did not spring *de nova* from the Department of Health and Human Services during the Carter administration. They were the fruit of many years of effort by many people both inside and outside of government during antecedent Republican and Democratic administrations who had begun to delineate the nation's major needs and opportunities for prevention and had recognized the need for new structures to encourage greater attention to prevention at the federal level. Thus, the new statements of policy in 1979 drew on the results of several important prior commissions and conferences, as well as on reports from major research projects to identify risk factors that had been going forward since the late 1950s in centers such as Framingham, Massachusetts, and Alameda County, California. The events leading to the current renaissance in prevention are important to understand as background to the current federal activities this chapter will be reviewing.

Since World War II, the Atlanta-based Center for Disease Control (CDC) has been the only agency of HHS dedicated exclusively to prevention. Established in 1946 as the Communicable Disease Center, it was the first Public Health Service agency to coordinate and carry out the national program against many diseases that are spread from person to person, or from insects and animals, or from the environment to humans. During the 1950s and 1960s its mission gradually broadened. Today it is responsible not only for the nation's attack on communicable and vector-borne diseases but also for certain aspects of occupational safety and health, family planning, congenital defects, leukemia epidemiology, sexually transmitted diseases, lead-based paint poisoning, the relationship of smoking and health, and health education. In 1970, while retaining its familiar CDC initials, its name was changed to the Center for Disease Control to reflect this broader mission.

Meanwhile, however, Congress had incrementally given HHS a host of new prevention responsibilities and, in the course of a continuing series of major reorganizations during the 1960s and 1970s, these became assigned to new offices and agencies or to parts of other, preexisting ones. As of 1980, most, but by no means all, prevention programs were centered in the six Public Health Services agencies within the Office of the Assistant Secretary of Health. They were the following:

- Center for Disease Control;
- Health Services Administration;

- Food and Drug Administration;
- National Institutes of Health;
- Alcohol, Drug Abuse, and Mental Health Administration; and
- Health Resources Administration.

As Table 1 illustrates, with the exception of the Center for Disease Control, prevention activities were only a minor part of these agencies' responsibilities. Moreover, because incremental legislation had added their prevention functions in piecemeal fashion over the years, and because the agency reorganizations that seem inevitably to accompany each change in administration interrupt such interagency communication as each successive Surgeon General in turn strives to establish within his office, the separate agencies and their prevention programs tended to coexist rather than to cooperate. Thus, certain common problems, such as the need to develop more effective means of communicating health education and risk reduction messages to the public, whether the subject be nutrition, smoking, or safety, were worked out, if at all, by each program independently. Cross fertilization of ideas and sharing of results was thus the exception rather than the rule.

During the mid-1970s, however, during the Ford administration, a new coordinative structure began to take shape. The creation of a Bureau of Health Education as part of the Center for Disease Control was the first block. Its mission was to support and encourage research and demonstrations in health education at the state and local levels. The bureau was created by a departmental administrative action in response to recommendations made in 1973 by the Presidential National Commission on Health Education appointed by President Nixon. That commission was also responsible for the establishment of the private-sector National Center for Health Education based in San Francisco.

The second block in the new structure was the establishment in 1976 of the Office of Health Information and Health Promotion (OHP) within the Office of the Assistant Secretary for Health. This new office was created for the explicit purpose of coordinating the various facets of federal prevention efforts. Its functions, spelled out in the authorizing legislation, P.L. 94-317, were somewhat expanded in 1978 under the terms of P.L. 95-626. As of 1980, the responsibilities of OHP included the following:

- Coordinating all activities within the federal government and between the government and the private sector which relate to health information, health education,

TABLE 1. Proportion of Public Health Services Agency Budgets Devoted to Prevention, Fiscal Year 1980

Agency	Outlays for Prevention ($000 rounded)	Total Outlays ($000 rounded)
Center for Disease Control	$370,109	$373,960
Health Services Administration	314,547	2,082,452
Food and Drug Administration	282,774	324,936
National Institutes of Health	69,615	3,428,665
Alcohol, Drug Abuse and Mental Health Administration	29,922	1,108,323
Health Resources Administration	10,000	577,485
Office of the Assistant Secretary	5,076	255,046
Total	$1,072,043	$8,150,867

Source: U.S. Office of Management and the Budget.

physical fitness, sports, medicine, preventive health service and education, and the appropriate use of health care—all of which contribute to health promotion.
∘ Developing policies and plans of the Public Health Service related to health promotion, and recommending objectives in the private and federal sectors in general.
∍ Ensuring that aspects of health information, health promotion, and preventive care are integrated into operational-level department programs, guidelines, and regulations.
• Developing a National Health Information Clearinghouse to facilitate access to information relating to health, health promotion, physical fitness, and sports medicine research.

The need for OHP had been first identified under the Ford administration by the Health Protection Section of the Office of Policy Development and Planning. The concept was presented in 1975 as part of the administration's insightful *Forward Plan for Health, 1976–1980.* This document had been able to draw on the fruits of a 2-year effort by eight task forces convened under the joint sponsorship of the Fogerty International Center of the National Institutes of Health and the American College of Preventive Medicine, which had presented their reports in 1975 at the National Conference on Preventive Medicine. The proceedings, published as *Preventive Medicine, U.S.A.*[5] reviewed the history of prevention in the United States, the social determinants of health, and the economic impact of prevention, the goals, opportunities, and state of the art of consumer health education, the theory and practice of prevention and personal health services, and issues in quality control and evaluation.

Subsequently, various members of the task forces worked with the administration and Congress to establish a clear legislative mandate for future prevention strategy and actions. Concerned that the Atlanta location of the Center for Disease Control would block its attempts to provide the necessary leadership and coordinative functions to the many Washington-based federal agencies involved with particular aspects of prevention, they believed that the new office could only fulfill its responsibilities if it were placed directly in the Office of the Assistant Secretary for Health, and had adequate funding.

The resulting law included an authorization of $7 million for the 1977 fiscal year, and stepped up increases to $14 million in 1979. Although this $7 million authorization represented only a small fraction of the almost $40 billion federal health budget in 1977, sponsors of the bill believed that at least a beginning had been made in generating a momentum for prevention. Hopes were dashed when Congress appropriated no funds whatsoever for OHP until fiscal year 1978 and, then, only in the amount of $1.7 million. So, for more than a year, OHP existed in name only. And, in Atlanta, CDC's Bureau of Health Education fared only slightly better, with an appropriation of $3.9 million in 1977 and $3.8 million in 1978.

Even before skeleton funds were in hand to activate the new OHP structure, however, wheels were set in motion within HHS to begin formulating national prevention policies. In December 1977, the Surgeon General appointed a Deputy Assistant Secretary with full-time responsibility to head the new effort. Just a month later, in partnership with the Director of the Center for Disease Control, this official convened a Prevention Task Force composed of representatives of all agencies within the Department, with the charge to review and analyze all federal activities in disease prevention and health promotion. Approximately 60 staff members organized in six work groups produced a report that reviewed both what the department and what other federal agencies were then doing in prevention, outlined what might be feasible to do in the future, and what strategies might be adopted to realize the possibilities.[6] Finally, the task force identified areas of high priority, including childhood immunization and reduction in smoking among children and youth, and presented recommendations for departmental action to address them.

Some notion of the spread of interest represented can be gained by even a partial listing of the agencies serving on the Prevention Task Force: National Institute on Alcoholism and Alcohol Abuse; the Alcohol, Drug Abuse, and Mental Health Administration; the Health Services Administration; the Health Resources Administration; the National Institute for Occupational Safety and Health, Center for Disease Control; Office of Child Health Affairs; Office of Human Development Services; Indian Health Services; Bureau of Drugs, Food and Drug Administration; Office of Research, Health Care Financing Administration; Division of Analysis, National Center for Health Statistics; National Heart, Lung, and Blood Institute; National Institute for Environmental Health Sciences; National Cancer Institute in the National Institutes of Health; Administration on Aging; and President's Council on Physical Fitness and Sports Medicine.

The work of both the 1975 National Conference on Preventive Medicine and the interagency federal task force led directly to the formulation of the national prevention goals and objectives cited earlier. Two other conferences also provided essential contributions. The first of these, in February 1978, was convened by the Institute of Medicine to review the policy options and background state of the art of various prevention intervention approaches subsequently articulated in the two *Healthy People* volumes. The second, held in Atlanta in June 1979, convened by HHS, invited distinguished panels of outside experts to formulate the first drafts of the national disease prevention/health promotion objectives.

Despite a continuing handicap of funding levels far below what had been considered minimum requirements when the OHP legislation was enacted in 1976, the structures developed within the Office of the Assistant Secretary of Health have, so far, also appeared to work reasonably well in providing a locus for leadership and for the expanded prevention activities that will be illustrated in the sections to follow.

LEADERSHIP AND COORDINATION AT THE FEDERAL LEVEL

The Department of Health and Human Services has two major kinds of opportunities for exercising leadership in prevention. First, it can lend its good offices in bringing together the many voluntary agencies, state health agencies, and professional associations throughout the nation that may have a common interest in advancing toward a given prevention objective. Second, it can coordinate the prevention efforts of its own agencies and work with other federal agencies that have overlapping or complementary mandates.

The National High Blood Pressure Education Program of the National Heart, Lung and Blood Institute offers a particularly noteworthy example of a successful federal leadership role in harnessing private and public sector efforts in prevention. Here, since 1972, carefully thought-out strategies for working with health professionals, voluntary associations, and local governments at every level have established a measurably improved understanding of the need to detect and to treat high blood pressure in the population as a major risk factor for cardiovascular disease. The program is also working with Blue Cross plans and employers to help them establish hypertension detection and control programs at the work site.

Meetings focused on special areas of prevention are another way in which the federal government can exercise leadership. A few examples illustrate the diversity of recent efforts in these directions:

- *The Biomedical and Behavioral Basis of Clinical Nutrition: A Project for the 1980s.* (June 19-20, 1978). The National Institutes of Health sponsored a national conference to review the scientific basis for clinical nutrition activities for the last decades and to recommend directions for the 1980s. (Proceedings available from the NIH Nutrition Research Coordinating Committee, National Institutes of Health, Bethesda. Maryland).
- *The National Conference on Health Promotion Programs in Occupational Settings.* (January 17-19, 1979). The Office of Health Information and Health Promotion sponsored the conference to identify ways in which business and industry can improve the health of their employees, a $2\frac{1}{2}$-day conference challenged participants from the business, labor, scientific, and academic communities to identify issues and activities important in developing health promotion programs for the work site. Eight of 11 background papers were published in *Public Health Reports* (April-May 1980).
- *Conference on the Prevention of Alcohol, Drug Abuse, and Mental Health Problems.* (September 12-14, 1979). The Alcohol, Drug Abuse, and Mental Health Administration sponsored a conference to explore ways to strengthen efforts to prevent alcohol abuse, drug abuse, and mental health problems. (Proceedings available through the ADAMHA Division of Prevention.)
- *National Conference on Nutrition Education.* (September 27-28, 1979). In conjunction with the U.S. Department of Agriculture, the Federal Trade Commission, the Office of Science and Technology Policy, and the Society for Nutrition Education, the department sponsored a national conference which focused on the nutrition education needs of the general population, pregnant women, children, adolescents, low-income populations, the elderly, and persons with diet-related diseases. (Proceedings published as supplement to the *Journal of Nutrition Education*, February 1980).
- *National Conference on Physical Fitness and Sports for All.* (February 1-2, 1980). The President's Council on Physical Fitness and Sports and the Office of Education jointly planned the conference to encourage the development of lifetime physical fitness programs and to identify the differences in those programs at different life stages.
- *Regional Forums on Community Health Promotion.* (February-September 1979). The Office of Health Information and Health Promotion sponsored a series of eight meetings on community health promotion in various regions of the country. The forums were convened under the auspices of the National Health Council and drew heavily from its membership. The purpose was to stimulate the development of networks of community organizations committed to health improvement as well as to give the department a clearer understanding of regional differences among existing programs. More than 2,000 people attended the sessions.
- *Workgroups on Prevention Objectives for Minority Populations.* (May-June 1980). The Office of Health Information and Health Promotion convened a series of 1-day meetings with invited representatives of groups representing Hispanic, black, Asian-American, and elderly populations to learn the priorities they assigned to the various prevention objectives developed for the nation under the auspices of the Deputy

Assistant Secretary for Health for Disease Prevention. (Proceedings are available from the Office of Health Information and Health Promotion.)

• *Promoting Health Through the Schools.* (August 25–26, 1980). The Office of Health Information and Health Promotion together with cosponsoring agencies including the American Public Health Association, the American School Health Association, the Association for the Advancement of Health Education, the Bureau of Health Education at CDC, and the National Center for Health Education held a 2-day conference to discuss major factors in the success of school health education programs, strategies used to generate student–faculty administration and community support, training components of such programs, and types of financial program support that are possible. (Proceedings available from the Office of Health Information and Health Promotion.)

During 1979 and 1980, the Deputy Assistant Secretary for Health for Disease Prevention launched a number of specific coordination efforts within the Department. As an outgrowth and continuation of the 1977–78 Prevention Coordinating Committee, in May 1979, he established a 30-member Prevention Coordinating Committee, composed of representatives of each agency of the Department. The intention is to provide a systematic approach to coordinating their prevention programs and to establish a forum for exchanging information about new prevention programs that each agency is considering or is developing. While the importance of such a concept seems obvious, such interagency groups which meet regularly around common concerns are, in fact, rare at both the federal and state levels of the government.

Another mechanism for coordination was the establishment of the Nutrition Coordinating Committee (NCC) in April 1978. The committee is composed of representatives of all HEW agencies with nutrition activities. Standing committees were established to improve Departmental efforts in nutrition research, education, services, status monitoring, and international nutrition activities. A major purpose of the NCC is to improve coordination not only among the organizational components of HHS, such as CDC, NIH, but also between the HHS and other agencies, particularly the Department of Agriculture. A major contribution of this group was to develop the HEW/USDA Dietary Guidelines for the American Consumer, issued in February 1980.

Departmental task forces have also been established around problems of radiation exposure, sexually transmissible diseases, and, together with the Office of Education, comprehensive school health programs.

Finally, following the model developed to launch the national 1972 hypertension control effort, a variety of special initiatives designed to mobilize action in particular areas where prevention activities have lacked focus and drive in the past have been put forward by successive Surgeons General. These include the following:

• The National Childhood Immunization Initiative, announced in April 1977, in response to survey results indicating that childhood immunization levels had dropped to below 65 per cent. The President announced a program to raise those levels to 90 per cent by the fall of 1979 and to establish a follow-up system to ensure provision of immunization services to all newborn children. The 90 per cent goal was achieved for school-aged children by the target date. This childhood immunization program budget initiative increased budget for these purposes from $27.4 million in fiscal year 1978 to $40.4 million in fiscal year 1979. This was stabilized at $30.1 million in fiscal year 1980.

- A Smoking and Health Initiative was announced in January 1978. Based on the findings of a departmental Task Force on Smoking and Health between August and December 1977, the Office of Smoking and Health was established and a program of research and education begun to deter smoking, particularly among children and youth, pregnant women and high-risk occupational groups. One year later, the 1979 Surgeon General's Report on Smoking and Health was released. It summarized the comprehensive range of literature amassed over the last generation on the health consequences of smoking. The Department's budget for smoking research and demonstration programs increased from $19 million in fiscal year 1978 to $29 million in fiscal year 1979. For fiscal year 1980 the level was almost $50 million. (While these amounts seem large, it must be remembered that cigarette manufacturers spend approximately $500 million for advertising their products each year.)
- Adolescent Pregnancy Program—a major national initiative was announced in April 1978, to help reduce teenage pregnancies and to provide comprehensive prenatal, obstetrical, and follow-up health and support services to pregnant adolescents.
- Alcohol Initiative—in May 1979, an initiative was announced to address the serious problems resulting from misuse of alcohol, particularly among women and youth. A program was initiated directed at treatment, research, and prevention of alcoholism. The president's budget for fiscal year 1980 included an additional $16 million over the fiscal 1979 level for community-based alcoholism projects and research.

PROVIDING INFORMATION

The Congress, in establishing the Office of Health Information and Health Promotion, recognized a special need for better provision of information about preventive services to the general public. The response has been to design both a national media campaign and a national health information clearinghouse.

Plans for a national media campaign on a health promotion have been completed and a campaign began in January 1981. Radio and television messages and articles in newspapers and magazines emphasized that health risks differ among individuals and that people can take steps to reduce their risks. Follow-up information is available from the National Health Information Clearinghouse.

The National Health Information Clearinghouse (NHIC) is a major activity of OHP. Although there are many special clearinghouses within the federal government, such as the Office of Cancer Communications within the National Cancer Institute of the National Institutes of Health, too often the layman does not know how to gain access to them. The NHIC was created to answer the public's questions of where to go for health information. It serves the public and the health professionals working with the public through a telephone hotline. The inquiry line (703 522-2590), is open from 9:00 A.M. to 5:00 P.M. Monday through Friday. The NHIC maintains a catalog of relevant information and issues publications. (See, for example, *Health Information Resources in the Department of Health and Human Services*, DHHS (PHS) Publication No. 80-50146), 1980.

TECHNICAL ASSISTANCE TO COMMUNITIES AND STATES

Activities at the federal level to establish national goals and priorities in prevention and to achieve more closely coordinated approaches in implementing health promotion, health services, and health protection activities have, up to now, absorbed the greater part of the department's efforts. While it is clear that actions to translate general policies into specific programs and prevention measures must take place at the local level, within schools, industry, through health insurance efforts and, particularly, local media campaigns, just how this translation takes place is a question that will become more important in the years immediately to come. Beginnings have been made, through meetings such as the conferences on health promotion at the work site and in schools, already referred to, through direct consultant assistance to communities, and through special publications.

Two technical assistance contracts have been administered through OHP. They were designed not only to help specific communities, but to learn what types of help communities want, so as to plan for wider replication. The first contract involved 17 communities, selected from several hundred applicants. In addition to offering expert advisory services for those communities, tailored to their individually expressed needs, meetings of community agency representatives were convened to enable each to learn from the others' experiences and to receive briefings on the latest state of the art in such matters as weight loss, smoking cessation, and other aspects of change toward healthier life-styles. A series of review papers were commissioned as a resource to these and other communities in the following areas: the potential role of community hospitals in health promotion; school health curricula; steps in planning community media campaigns to reduce risks from heart disease and other chronic conditions; and suggestions on how communities can raise funds to support their health promotion activities.

A second contract is providing technical assistance to five communities. It is drawing on their experiences, and those of the other 17 communities to prepare a community guide to implementing health promotion. Particular attention is being devoted to the troubling question of identifying organizational structures that lend themselves both to launching well-coordinated health promotion activities at the local level, and to maintaining these activities over time.

In 1977, under the provisions of P.L. 95-83, Congress required the HHS secretary to "establish model standards with respect to preventive services in communities." To fulfill this mandate, the secretary convened a collaborative work group. Representatives of the Association of State and Territorial Health Officials, the National Association of County Officials, the U.S. Conference of City Health Officers, and the American Public Health Association which, with staff work performed by the Center for Disease Control, developed a report over a 2-year period. The document, *Model Standards for Community Preventive Health Services*, issued in 1979, presents a framework for incremental improvement in the state of any community's state of health through an approach that emphasizes maximum flexibility of programming suited to the community's particular priorities and expressed needs.[7] The standards cover a wide range of prevention activities, including air quality; chronic disease control; communicable disease control; dental health; emergency medical services; family planning; food protection; genetic disease control; health education; injury control; maternal and child health; nutritional services; occupational health; primary care; public health laboratory; radiological health; safe drinking water; sanitation; school health; solid waste management; surveillance/epidemiology and wastewater management. Table 2 reproduces a sample, concerning maternal and child health, to illustrate the format.

RESEARCH

Major research projects launched during the 1970s by the National Heart, Lung, and Blood Institute have been contributing enormously to the nation's understanding of

TABLE 2. Illustration of Model Standards Format (Maternal and Child Health, in part)

Area: Maternal and Child Health (MCH)

Focus	Objectives	Indicators	Population in Need
	PROCESS		
Immunization	P-12. By 19___at least 90 per cent of the 2-year-old population will have completed primary immunization for the officially designated vaccine-preventable diseases, and 90 per cent of 2- to 21-year-olds will have received appropriate immunization boosters.	Percentage of children completely immunized	All children by age 2
	CROSS REFERENCE: COMMUNICABLE DISEASE CONTROL (IMMUNIZATION)		
Screening	P-13. By 19___80 per cent of the children in the community will be screened for disorders of vision and hearing by 3 years of age (gross screening should occur in the first year) and, as appropriate, diagnosed and treated.	(a) Percentage of children screened (b) Percentage of positive screens who are diagnosed and treated	All children by age 3

CROSS REFERENCE: CHRONIC DISEASE CONTROL

P-14. By 19___100 per cent of children in the community will be screened, preferably before entry into school, to determine the existence of any conditions (including speech or perceptual handicaps) which may require special education services, and, as appropriate, be diagnosed and treated.	(a) Percentage of children screened (b) Percentage of positive screens who are diagnosed and treated	All children by age 5

CROSS REFERENCE: SCHOOL HEALTH

P-15. By 19___100 per cent of children who demonstrate school failure, truancy, under-achievement, or discipline problems will receive a comprehensive health evaluation including a psychosocial assessment.	Percentage of children receiving such assessment	School-age children

CROSS-REFERENCE: SCHOOL HEALTH

Poison control	P-16. By 19___the community will have access to a poison control center.	Demonstrable access to such a center	The community (particularly children and youth)

Source: *Models Standards for Community Preventive Health Services.* A Report to the U.S. Congress from the Secretary of Health, Education and Welfare, August 1979, p. 62.

the role of risk factors in cardiovascular disease and the kinds of measures that have proved successful or unsuccessful in enabling people to modify their personal risk factors. These studies include the continued support for the analysis of data from the Framingham heart project, the National Heart, Lung and Blood Institute-sponsored Multiple Risk Factor Intervention Trials, the Hypertension Detection and Followup Program, and major community studies in heart disease prevention conducted at Stanford University and at the Laboratory of Physiological Hygiene at the University of Minnesota.

Other important advances in our understanding of risk reduction have come from evaluating risk-reduction activities of a school health program, "Know Your Body," in New York City, supported by the National Cancer Institute, and from a contract by the U.S. Air Force to the American Health Foundation, designed to reduce risks to Air Force personnel from unhealthy life-styles.

In addition, the Center for Disease Control in Atlanta, through its Bureau of Health Education, has, together with the National Center for Health Education, launched a major project to evaluate school health programs associated with the National School Health Curriculum Project. Most recently, the National Center for Health Services Research, in the summer of 1980, announced the availability of funds for demonstration grants in a broad array of study questions relating to disease prevention and health promotion.

GRANTS AND CONTRACTS

The Congress has been slower to authorize prevention measures through grants and contracts programs than it has to act in some other program areas. Most efforts, so far, have been for particular screening programs, such as grants to states for hypertension screening. However, in 1978 it also authorized grants to the states to encourage them to mount life-style risk reduction programs. This new program, being administered by the CDC's Bureau of Health Education, helps state and local health departments to strengthen their efforts to reduce the prevalence of smoking, heavy drinking, obesity, and hypertension. The initial grants in fiscal year 1979, totaling $3.6 million, were to enable states to gear up their capacity to administer substantive programs planned for succeeding years. Fifty states and jurisdictions received awards. For fiscal year 1980, $16 million in grant funds were awarded after review of more than 600 applications received from states and localities. A major portion of the awards were for activities to reduce smoking and heavy drinking among children and youth.

DATA FOR TRACKING PROGRESS IN HEALTH PROMOTION

The National Center for Health Statistics, under a congressional mandate, is required to furnish a report on prevention every 3 years. The first such report appears in the center's summary volume, *Health United States: 1980* (DHHS Publication No. [PHS] 81-1232.) The national prevention goals and objectives provide a useful framework for such reports.

The 15 work groups that developed the national objectives in 1979 identified the sources of information with which progress toward them could be tracked. The two major sources are National Center for Health Statistics and the Center for Disease Control.

The National Center for Health Statistics collects and analyzes the nation's vital statistics through cooperative agreements with the states and, through its several types of periodic surveys, ascertains the nature and extent of injury and disability in the population, the numbers and types of health facility and health professions workforce resources, and the extent of their use. The Center for Disease Control collects data on particular aspects of health, such as the incidence of communicable diseases, lead-based paint poisoning, and so on. Data from these and from many other federal agencies can monitor future movement toward approximately 112 of the more than 200 objectives set forth in *Promoting Health/Preventing Disease.* The volume contains a comprehensive listing of all these sources.

A major challenge is to make better use of the data already available, not only through analysis within federal agencies but also by helping university researchers obtain better access to data for their own research and to inform planning agencies in the states and HSA areas about health indicators relating to disease prevention and health promotion. Unfortunately, shortages of staff and funding in federal statistical agencies such as the National Center for Health Statistics have up to now seriously limited the realization of such opportunities.

FUTURE PROSPECTS FOR FEDERAL PREVENTION ACTIVITIES

Between 1974 and 1980, an astonishing degree of progress was made at the federal level in setting the sights for an integrated prevention policy and providing leadership, information, technical assistance, and grant funds to states and localities which wanted to implement programs for their populations. Although comparatively few funds were spent for these purposes (in 1980, approximately $1 billion by the Department of Health and Human Services out of a total federal budget of close to $600 billion), a momentum was created that in 1979 led the Surgeon General to observe that we might be entering a second public health revolution to parallel the successful first public health revolution that at the turn of the century launched the conquest of infectious disease.

Yet as we enter the 1980s it would be rash to predict the future of any federal health programs not linked to defense. It is possible that the new push toward prevention by the federal government will be cut short at the pass in efforts to effect short-term reductions in federal spending. But since prevention represents a very low cost investment for improving the health of the population, and since, over the longer term it holds the potential for appreciably reducing federal health expenditures, such approaches may receive renewed commitment. Thus, the Reagan administration might well decide to carry forward the prevention concepts advanced during the Ford administration. On the other hand, many aspects of health risk reduction create political problems. Changes in the population's smoking, eating and drinking habits adversely affect the special interests of multi-billion dollar industries and agribusinesses. And many aspects of reducing health risks, especially to women, such as through venereal disease control efforts, family planning and legal abortions, are perceived by other special interest groups, small but noisy, as being immoral.

In the final analysis, what happens to prevention during the 1980s will depend on the public's sustained expression of will to make the second revolution in public health a fact, not a dream. For, as Oliver Wendell Holmes observed, policy rests upon "the felt necessities of the time, the prevalent moral and political theories, the intentions of the public, avowed or unconscious."

REFERENCES

1. Lee, Philip R. and Franks, Patricia E., "Primary Prevention and the Executive Branch of the Federal Government." *Preventive Medicine* 6 (1977), p. 209.
2. U.S. Department of Health, Education, and Welfare. *Healthy People: The Surgeon General's Report on Health Promotion and Disease Prevention.* DHEW (PHS) Publication No. 79-55071. Washington, D.C.: U.S. Government Printing Office, 1979 (Stock No. 017-001-00416-2).
3. U.S. Department of Health, Education, and Welfare, *Healthy People: Background Papers.* DHEW (PHS) Publication No. 79-55071A. Washington, D.C.: U.S. Government Printing Office, 1979 (Stock No. 017-001-00417-1).
4. U.S. Department of Health and Human Services, Promoting Health/Preventing Disease: Objectives for the Nation. Public Health Service, GPO Superintendent of Documents Fall 1980 (Stock no. 017-001-00435-9).
5. Breslow, Lester, ed., *Preventive Medicine, U.S.A.* New York: Prodist, 1976.
6. U.S. Department of Health, Education, and Welfare, *Disease Prevention and Health Promotion: Federal Programs and Prospects.* Report of Departmental Task Force on Prevention. DHEW (PHS) Publication No. 79-55071B. Washington, D.C.: U.S. Government Printing Office, September 1978 (Stock No. 017-001-00418-9).
7. U.S. Department of Health, Education, and Welfare, *Model Standards for Community Preventive Health Services: A Report to the U.S. Congress from the Secretary of Health, Education, and Welfare.* August 1979. Washington, D.C.: Publication No. 640-185-4430. U.S. Government Printing Office, 1980 (No Stock Number listed).

19 / The Potential Role of Health Systems Agencies in Promoting Health Through Risk Reduction *Ernest Schloss / Susan Evans / Sabina Dunton*

HSAs AND HEALTH PROMOTION

The United States spends more on health care than any other nation on earth: $192.4 billion in 1978, or 9.1 per cent of our gross national product. Of that amount, 38.7 per cent was expended by federal, state, and local governments.[1] Nevertheless, the traditional measures of morbidity and mortality demonstrate that we do not enjoy the highest levels of "health" in the world and despite our unprecedented expenditures, we also experience unequal access to health care by many segments of our population, particularly those who reside in rural and inner-city areas.[2]

In spite of the inequities in service distribution, there are those who maintain that we have reached a point of diminishing returns on health care. Fuchs and others[3,4] have demonstrated that increased expenditures in the traditional areas of crisis-oriented medical care will not bring about corresponding benefits in the health status of our population. Rather it appears it is through changes in our life-style and environment that we will get the greatest return for our investment, as measured by health status.[5,6]

It is within the context of these problems that Congress enacted the National Health Planning and Resources Development Act in 1974. This act addressed a myriad of problems confronting the health care delivery system, but focused on three major issues: the skyrocketing cost of care, problems of accessibility to health care for underserved populations, and the health status of the country's population. The primary purpose of the health planning agencies was to improve "the health of residents of the health service area."

The health planning law established a health planning system with national, state, and local components. The local core of this system is the 204 regional health systems agencies (HSAs) which blanket the nation. These agencies are dependent upon community volunteers, a majority of whom must be consumers, to make decisions concerning the configuration and development of the health care delivery system in their areas. The central idea behind this organizational form is that in order for there to be effective changes in both the health of the American people and in the system that provides their health care, the entire community must be involved in that change process.

The first major responsibility of health systems agencies is planning, or answering, three basic questions: (1) Where are we now? (2) Where do we want to go in the future? and (3) How do we get there? Planning defines the future requirements of our health care system, based upon a systematic examination of the needs of the population. The public law requires that as a first step in this process "the agency shall assemble and analyze data concerning:

A. The status (and its determinants) of the health of the residents of its service area.
B. The status of the health care delivery system in the area and the use of that system by residents of the area.

C. The effect of the area's health care delivery system on the health of the residents of the area.
D. The number, type, and location of the area's health resources, including health services, workforce, and facilities.
E. The patterns of utilization of the area's health resources.
F. The environmental and occupational exposure factors affecting immediate and long-tern health condition.[7]"

Once the agency has developed its plans, the second congressional requirement is that it implement these plans. There are two ways this may be accomplished: through health systems development activities and by means of regulatory powers. Both implementation strategies are to be based on what has been agreed to in the public planning process conducted by the agency and prescribed in the plan documents themselves.

Health systems development refers to proactive efforts designed to correct deficiencies in the current system through the granting of incentives, although no money was ever appropriated by Congress for this activity. In actuality in most HSAs, this takes the form of raising the awareness of appropriate community groups to the deficiencies and providing technical assistance to groups or individuals in the community who wish to move in the areas of needed change.

The HSA activity that receives the most public attention is the second implementation strategy, or the regulatory function of the agency. This is accomplished in most states primarily through certificate of need and grant review. In the former, health care institutions must essentially receive permission from their local HSA, and ultimately the state health planning agency, before being allowed to expand or change significantly the nature of their services. In the latter, the HSA has approval or disapproval power over the use of certain federal grant funds. Both regulatory activities tend to be reactive, but can also be used creatively to help mold the health care system in the direction of the changes outlined in the agencies' plans.

It should be noted at this point that the congressional mandate to HSAs was nothing short of massive social and cultural change. That is to say, HSAs are not only charged with shaping and controlling the expansion of the third largest industry in the country, but also with guiding the development of that industry in order to produce an improved health status in the population served. The latter course, because of the life-style and environmental factors that lead to our current level of health, requires changing the health beliefs and behaviors of the entire population, health providers and consumers alike.

Many health planners have become convinced that it is only through the latter course of action, improving health status, that significant change will occur in the health care industry. In an effort to effect real change, many health systems agencies have turned to the concept of wellness,[8,9] and the vehicles of health promotion and health education in order to influence people's perceptions and beliefs about themselves and the nature of illness.

It is important to recognize that alternatives to our current way of doing things were recognized by Congress. One finding in the public law was that

Large segments of the public are lacking basic knowledge regarding proper personal health care and methods for effective use of available health services.[9]

Accordingly, Congress stated, as one of 16 national priorities;

The development of effective methods of educating the general public concerning proper (including preventive) health care and methods for effective use of available health services.[7]

It is ironic, however, that of all the goals outlined in the health planning law, the most basic—the improved health status of the population—has received the least federal attention.[8] While an improved health status is the unstated, underlying mission of all health care activities, the nation's health planning system for the most part has been directed to concentrate on problems with the process of producing health care such as its cost and its inequitable distribution.

We believe that this national focus on process is a result of the state of the art of health planning and not the unwillingness of the health planning system to respond to improving health status, as Ardell and Robins[9] have suggested. One of the major methodological problems confronted by HSAs is how to evaluate the success of proposed interventions to change the health care system, particularly as they relate to cost, accessibility, and other process criteria, as well as to the health status of the population. We are convinced that the process of producing traditional medical care is relatively easy to measure, when compared with trying to measure the impact of its outcomes, that is, the impact on the health status of the population, as required in the public law. Because there are so many life-style and environmental antecedents to many of our current health problems, any changes in the health levels of the population, as measured by traditional mortality and morbidity indicators, may not be due to actions by the health care delivery system.[10] Another problem is that a payoff in prevention of the antecedents of "post industrial" chronic diseases may not occur for 15 to 20 years. Hence, a method needs to be developed that will measure our progress in slowing the incidence and prevalence of future disease.

PROBLEMS WITH METHODS NOW IN USE TO MEASURE HEALTH STATUS AND THE IMPACT OF HEALTH PROMOTION INTERVENTIONS ON HEALTH STATUS

Many indicators and indexes have been developed in recent years to measure health status. The nature of these techniques has been described elsewhere,[10-13] but most rely on a combination of traditional morbidity, mortality, disability, and socioeconomic variables shown to be associated with illness. A major weakness of these methods is that they do not account for the etiology and antecedent conditions of postindustrial disease, and hence cannot measure effectively the impact of changes in the health care system upon those conditions. G. E. Alan Dever[11,14] has developed a new epidemiological model, based upon previous work by LaLonde and Blum,[6,10] for policy analysis in health, which can be used by health planners to begin redirecting the system to deal with the antecedent conditions to our postindustrial, chronic diseases. Dever has separated the health care system into four subcomponents: (1) the system of medical care organization, (2) life-style, (3) environment, and (4) human biology.

Dever defines the system of medical care organization as the traditional health care system in this country, based upon the medical model of illness, and concentrating on curing illnesses. Life-style, he explains are those individual behaviors, such as exercise, nutrition, stress management, smoking, and drinking, which have been closely associated with chronic disease. The environment is the physical and social condition in which we exist, which also exerts influence on our level of health. Human biology is the subsystem of influences on our health which includes inherited conditions and the vagaries of our biological development and make-up.[14]

Dever asked panels of experts to ascertain the extent to which each of his subsystems influenced mortality in the country. The consensus was that the system of medical care organization could have an impact on mortality in only 11 per cent of all deaths, whereas life-style factors accounted for 43 per cent, the environment was responsible for 19 per cent, and human biology contributed to 27 per cent of all deaths. Nevertheless, from 1974 to 1976, 90.6 per cent of our federal health expenditures were on the subsystem of medical care organization.[14]

There have been recent attempts to identify those illnesses which are amenable to treatment and intervention by the subsystem of medical care organization. Rutstein et al.[15] also have used expert opinion to identify those diseases, as listed in the International Classification of Diseases, which can be treated to prevent unnecessary morbidity, disability, and death.

Recently, however, critics of the ability of traditional medical care to deal with modern illness, have called for a new paradigm of health entitled "wellness."[10,11,16] Prominent among these individuals are health planners who feel that approaching the life-style and environmental subsystems will have more positive benefits for our health status than continuing to concentrate on traditional, curative medicine. Embodied in the concept of wellness is the notion of positive health, whereby an individual, or a community, can have varying degrees of positive health states, as well as negative states, or illnesses. The proponents of wellness maintain that these positive states can be enhanced through improved nutritional balance, stress reduction, exercise, risk avoidance, and environmental awareness.[16]

Unfortunately for health planners, however, the wellness concept, while intellectually and emotionally appealing to many (as we will discuss later), is not measurable; hence, there is no way of documenting changes. Therefore, whereas traditional measures of health status cannot truly measure those factors which will influence disease, the alternative, wellness, has not been operationally defined.

Dever[11] does offer a solution, which we have embraced as well. Health hazard appraisals (HHAs) are the only tool we are aware of that quantitively measures life-style and behavioral antecedents to disease and offers the opportunity to begin measurement of states of health and illness.[17,18] A health hazard appraisal questionnaire determines what, if any are an individual's health hazards. From this a computerized health profile is developed showing "risk age" and "achievable age" compared to the individual's chronological age. The profile displays the probability of death occuring within the next 10 years based on national mortality statistics. This probability is computed from either the absence or the degree of presence of those factors which are actuarially provable health hazards. Since a statistical correlation has been established between the factors measured and the chronic conditions we are trying to ameliorate, the HHA is a good measurement tool both for planning and for evaluating the impact of interventions.

The health hazard appraisal has another important feature. Since it measures the antecedents to chronic disease, one can make the assumption that if the antecedents it measures change, the future health status of the population, as measured by traditional indicators and indexes, will also change. For example, if one is able to change high blood pressure, cholesterol, smoking, and stress levels in the population of an HSA, it can be assumed that 15 to 20 years hence we will see a concomitant reduction in heart disease and lung cancer, as well as a more general level of "wellness" in the population. To date, this approach to population health status has not been used, that is, no one has measured the actual levels of smoking, blood pressure, and so on in a uniform, comprehensive manner in a single geographic area.

The potential value of the health hazard appraisal to health systems agencies is twofold:

1. It provides one means of actually measuring the general health status of the pop-

ulation of the area and in a manner which reflects our current knowledge about the antecedents of modern diseases. It also can be used on a periodic basis to review our progress in the geographic area served by HSA of raising the level of wellness, or at least for the time being, reducing the risks associated with illness.

2. It can also be used as a successful evaluation tool for the individual programs designed to affect the level of health in the community. While health promotion appears to be the best means of changing life-styles and behaviors, evidence must be developed to document that change. We believe that HHAs constitute a good evaluation tool to measure which specific health promotion interventions produce the best results.

There remain, however, two problems that we have with HHAs. First, we are not aware of any HHA instruments that have been developed for children. Since many life-destruction behaviors are encoded early in life, it is logical to begin many health promotion activities in the young child. Therefore, an HHA for children is needed.

Second, the current cost of HHAs is high. We believe, however, that the benefits of HHAs to the health planning system would outweigh the costs. While HSAs are prohibited from collecting most forms of primary data, state-level health planning agencies are not. One approach could be to have states collect this form of health status information on a sample basis in each area served by an HSA.

WHAT HSAs ARE DOING IN HEALTH PROMOTION AND HOW THEY ARE USING HEALTH HAZARD APPRAISALS

Despite emphasis by much of the federal government on cost containment and access issues, many HSAs have a serious commitment to health promotion. Donald Ardell, a nationally recognized proponent of wellness, reported that in 1977, only 20 HSAs had committed themselves to wellness, while 30 per cent of agencies surveyed were interested in becoming involved in wellness.[8] Although Ardell does not include all of health promotion within his definition of wellness, he and Leonard Robins[9] found that by 1979, 53 per cent of HSAs had developed a wellness resource base, 90 per cent of responding HSAs were promoting a definition of wellness to the public, and 80 per cent had sponsored wellness seminars.[9]

Our own agency, the Health Systems Agency of Southeastern Arizona, based in Tucson, has always had a health promotion and wellness orientation. However, we have also been concerned about the difficulties of measuring states of positive health, and in measuring the impact of health promotion activities on the health status of the population.

Staff members and volunteers of our agency and staff members of Well Aware About Health, a University of Arizona-based project had several discussions in early 1977 about evaluating both the results of health promotion activities and the overall health status of the population. Well Aware About Health had been using health hazard appraisals (HHAs) as a means of assessing the overall health status of an individual and then again as an evaluation of the success of specific health promotion activities designed to favorably change that individual's unhealthy behaviors.

What seemed exciting to both groups was the potential of using a health hazard appraisal on a sample basis in order to assess the health status of our five-county area population, and then as an evalution instrument to be applied on a periodic basis to determine how successful we had been in changing the health status of our entire population—our congressional mandate. Our agencies jointly developed a proposal to the then Department of Health, Education and Welfare to do a pilot demonstration project in our area to test this methodology. Unfortunately, our proposal was never funded.

We remained convinced of the value of using HHAs both for overall systems evaluations, and as a tool in individual health promotion; so in April 1980, we surveyed all 204 HSAs in the country to determine the degree of commitment to and involvement in health promotion, and what use, if any, was being made of HHAs. The results, consistent with the previous findings of Ardell and Robins,[9] are surprising in view of the federally and state-mandated burdens placed on HSAs.

Of the 176 responding HSAs (87 per cent of all HSAs), 146 were able to estimate the person-hours per week spent on health promotion. The mean was 21.7 hours per week, the high 130 or more hours, and the low, zero. Thirty-four of these agencies, or 23.8 per cent, devote 40 or more person-hours per week to health promotion.

Table 1 shows HSA commitment to health promotion in the health planning and implementation process. For 65 per cent of the agencies health promotion is a planning priority, for 52 per cent a separate health systems plan chapter. Sixty-five per cent of the respondents have integrated health promotion into other plan compontents, while a surprising 28 per cent maintain a task force or committee devoted to health promotion implementation.

We questioned the use of health promotion in review (certificate of need and grant review), and the results are displayed in Table 2. Forty-eight per cent use health promotion review criteria some or most of the time. Forty-five per cent actively solicit certificate of need and grant applications which address health promotion at least some of the time, although only 10 per cent of the agencies make a practice of it. Sixty-nine per cent of the HSAs favor certificate of need and grant applications which include health promotion, and 83 per cent provide technical assistance in this area.

The agencies indicated a broad commitment of resources to health promotion activities as indicated in Table 3. One hundred agencies had sponsored health promotion seminars or workshops; 98 had been involved in some form of public speaking on health promotion; 77 had utilized the media for that purpose; 138 had provided technical assistance; 93 had been involved in school curricula for health promotion or health education; 82 had participated in fairs; 26 had held conventions and 53, public forums; 80 had produced resource directories for health promotion; 41 had produced other

TABLE 1. HSA Use of Health Promotion in Planning and Health Systems Development

Health Promotion Activity	HSA Involvement*		
	Yes	No	Unknown
Planning priority	115	60	1
	(65.3)	(34.1)	(.6)
Separate plan component	92	83	1
	(52.3)	(47.2)	(.6)
Integrated into other plan components	116	59	1
	(65.9)	(33.5)	(.6)
Separate health promotion implementation committee	49	126	1
	(27.8)	(71.6)	(.6)
Other	30	142	4
	(17.0)	(80.7)	(2.3)

*Figures in parentheses indicate percentages of all 176 reporting HSAs.

TABLE 2. HSA Use of Health Promotion in Certificate of Need and Grant Reviews

Health Promotion Activity	HSA Involvement*			
	Usually	Occasionally	Never	Unknown
Specific review HP criteria	30 (17.0)	55 (31.3)	62 (35.2)	29 (16.5)
Actively solicit HP proposals	18 (10.2)	61 (34.7)	70 (39.8)	27 (15.3)
Favor HP in the review process	65 (36.9)	57 (32.4)	24 (13.6)	30 (17.0)
Provide HP technical assistance	75 (42.6)	71 (40.3)	15 (8.5)	15 (8.5)
Other HP review activities	4 (2.3)	5 (2.8)	6 (3.4)	161 (91.5)

*Figures in parentheses indicate percentages of all 176 reporting HSAs.

types of health promotion publications. In addition the agencies listed a wide range of uncategorized activities.

When agencies were asked about the reasons for their lack of involvement in health promotion activities, 10 per cent of all agencies said their agency had higher priorities, 3 per cent said it was not a staff priority, and 14 per cent cited insufficient staff as the

TABLE 3. Types of Health Promotion Activities Engaged in by HSAs

Health Promotion Activity	HSA Involvement*		
	Yes	No	Unknown
Seminar/workshops	110 (56.8)	69 (39.2)	7 (4.0)
Public speaking	98 (55.7)	71 (40.3)	7 (4.0)
Media public relations	77 (43.8)	92 (52.3)	7 (4.0)
Technical assistance to agencies/groups	138 (78.4)	31 (17.6)	7 (4.0)
School curricula development	93 (52.8)	76 (43.2)	7 (4.6)
Fairs	82 (46.6)	87 (49.4)	7 (4.0)
Conventions	26 (14.8)	143 (81.3)	7 (4.0)
Public forums	53 (30.1)	116 (65.9)	7 (4.0)
Resource directory	80 (45.5)	89 (50.6)	7 (4.0)
Other publications	41 (23.3)	128 (72.7)	7 (4.0)
Other	27 (15.3)	142 (80.7)	7 (4.0)

*Figures in parentheses indicate percentage of all 176 reporting HSAs.

**TABLE 4.   Reported Reason That HSAs Are Not Involved
(or More Involved) in Health Promotion**

Reasons	Number of HSAs	Per Cent of All Reporting HSAs
Higher agency priorities	18	10.2
Not a staff priority	5	2.8
Insufficient staff	25	14.2
Disagree with the concept of HP	2	1.1
Not familiar with HP	0	0.0
Community apathy or antipathy	1	0.6
Other	4	2.3

problem. (See Table 4) Most of these agencies were actually involved in limited health promotion, and cited these reasons for not being more extensively involved; in fact, only five HSAs were totally uninvolved or uninterested in health promotion.

Within the general context of health promotion, we also were interested specifically in the use and awareness of the health hazard appraisal instrument. As indicated in Table 5 we found that 80 per cent of the respondents were familiar with health hazard appraisal, and 35 per cent had promoted the use of HHAs. Only five agencies had ever attempted to use HHAs as a methodology to define health status for planning or evaluation, but others remarked that they had not done so only because of a lack of resources. Thirty-four per cent of reporting HSAs had administered health hazard appraisals to agency staff or volunteers, or both.

Several agencies reported that they had not used HHA at all, or not to the extent they would have liked. (See Table 6) Twenty-eight per cent of all agencies cited insufficient staff as the cause; 15 per cent said they were not familiar with HHAs; 2 per cent disagreed with the idea; and 17 per cent said they planned to use HHAs in the future. Other reasons were listed, including lack of funds, HHAs not being an agency priority, and the unavailability of follow-up health education programs.

TABLE 5.   Awareness and Use of Health Hazard Appraisal by HSAs

| Awareness or Activity | HSA Involvement | | |
	Yes	No	Unknown
Familiar with HHA	140 (79.5)	32 (18.2)	4 (2.3)
Promote use of HHA	61 (34.7)	113 (64.2)	2 (1.1)
Used HHA for measuring health status	5 (2.8)	170 (96.6)	1 (0.6)
Used HHA for staff	34 (19.3)	142 (80.7)	0 (0.0)
Used HHA for volunteers	26 (14.8)	150 (85.2)	0 (0.0)

*Figures in parentheses are the percentages of all 176 reporting HSAs.

TABLE 6. Reasons Given by HSAs for Not Using Health Hazard Appraisals

Reasons	Number of HSAs	Per Cent of All Reporting HSAs
Insufficient staff	50	28.4
Not familiar with concept	26	14.8
Disagree with concept	3	1.7
Plan to use in future	30	17.0
Other reasons	41	23.3

We were interested in finding an explanation for why some HSAs have actively embraced health promotion and HHAs and others have not. We hypothesized that there might be regional differences between HSAs which would account for lack of involvement in health promotion activities and the use of HHAs. We also hypothesized that the population size of an HSA's service area might determine the amount of attention given to these two activities since an agency's budget is a direct function of its service area population.

In the first case, we were told by some respondents that some of the nine U.S. Department of Health and Human Services (DHHS) regional offices, which have administrative control over HSAs, were more supportive of health promotion activities than others. Thus, we felt there might be differences between DHHS regions in the amount of health promotion activity by agencies. We further hypothesized that there might be more health promotion activity in what we termed "sun belt" states, or southern and western states with growing populations, as opposed to northern and eastern states with large cities. Our reasoning was based on the fact that from our own experience, and from that of other HSAs we had talked to, areas with rapidly expanding populations had less concern with restricting and shrinking the supply of health resources (like hospitals beds) and could devote more time to more nontraditional health planning areas like health promotion.

To test these regional hypotheses, we used the response to our questionnaire concerning lack of involvement in health promotion due to insufficient staff as a measure of agency resources available for either health promotion or health hazard appraisal activity. We also examined the response by agencies that they had higher priorities than health promotion, and considered this a measure of agency commitment to health promotion. Unfortunately, we had insufficient responses by DHHS region to draw any meaningful conclusions; however, when responses to these questions were tabulated by the collapsed categories of "sunbelt" and "nonsunbelt" states, we derived the results in Table 7.

A higher percentage (11.1 per cent) of sunbelt states reported they had higher priorities than health promotion (contrary to our expectations). However, as we expected, there was a lower proportion of sunbelt agencies which cited insufficient staff as a reason for noninvolvement in health promotion or health hazard appraisal than of nonsunbelt agencies.*

*Since we surveyed the entire population of HSAs and got an 87 per cent return rate, we assumed the remaining agencies were distributed as the respondents, and we performed no tests of statistical significance.

TABLE 7. Reasons Cited for Not Being Involved in Health Promotion and Health Hazard Appraisal by Region*

| | Reasons for Noninvolvement | | |
| | Health Promotion | | Health Hazard Appraisal |
Region*	Higher Priorities	Insufficient Staff	Insufficient Staff
Sun belt N = 63	7 (11.1)†	7 (11.1)	15 (23.8)
Nonsun belt N = 113	11 (9.7)	18 (15.9)	35 (31.0)

*Sunbelt states are Alabama, Arizona, Arkansas, California, Florida, Georgia, Guam, Hawaii, Louisiana, Mississippi, Nevada, New Mexico, North Carolina, Oklahoma, South Carolina, Tennessee, Texas, American Somoa, Trust Territories (DHHS Regions IV, VI, XI).

†Figures in parentheses are percentages for all responding HSAs in the category.

Our second hypothesis concerning population size we believe was more conclusive. We divided HSAs into small agencies (500,000 people or fewer in the service area), medium agencies (500,001 to 1 million people), and large agencies (over 1 million people). Table 8 shows the same responses by agency size. In this case there was no clear relationship between agency size and agency priorities; however, there was a marked difference between small, medium, and large agencies in the amount of staff resources they felt they could devote to health promotion and health hazard appraisals.

Therefore, we believe that if agencies had the liberty to choose their activities, more would become involved both with health promotion and with the use of health hazard appraisals. Larger agencies have greater staff resources, hence greater flexibility, in pursuing health-promoting activities, while smaller agencies must perform DHHS and

TABLE 8. Reasons Cited for Not Being Involved in Health Promotion and Health Hazard Appraisal by Population Size*

| | Reasons for HSA Noninvolvement | | |
| | Health Promotion | | Health Hazard Appraisal |
Population Size*	Higher Priorities	Insufficient Staff	Insufficient Staff
Small N = 42	6 (14.3)†	10 (23.8)	16 (38.1)
Medium N = 74	5 (6.8)	11 (14.9)	25 (33.8)
Large N = 60	7 (11.7)	4 (6.7)	9 (15.0)

*Small agency population size = 0 to 500,000; medium agency population size = 500,001 to 1,000,000; large agency population size = 1,000,000 and over.

†Figures in parentheses are percentages for all responding HSAs in the category.

Congressionally mandated functions which leave little room for innovation in health promotion.

IV. POTENTIAL USES OF HHAs IN HSAs

Our conclusion, then, is that most agencies are involved in health promotion, and a large number advocate the use of HHAs as a tool in health promotion. Unlike Ardell and Robins,[9] however, we are not disheartened by the fact that there is not universal enthusiasm for wellness and health promotion. Rather, given the massive nature of a culture change program such as this, we are encouraged that so many agencies have embraced these concepts, and are trying to do something about them.

We were also not surprised to find that so few agencies were thinking along similar lines to us—using HHAs as a tool for evaluating the health status of the area's population—given the cost of the survey and the prohibition by Congress of large data-collection activities by HSAs.

We are as troubled as Ardell and Robins,[9] however, that many HSAs are feeling frustrated in their attempts to implement significant wellness and health promotion activities. Results from our survey show that there has been an increasing interest by HSAs in health promotion since Ardell's first survey in 1977. However, many HSAs sent us unsolicited comments which indicated that they were feeling constrained to reduce their commitment to health promotion because of stronger federal emphasis on cost containment, and upon accessibility to traditional services.

We operate in an era of increased accountability wherein both HSAs and their community agencies who are involved in health promotion must demonstrate cost-effectiveness. We are convinced that health promotion is the ultimate method to lower medical care costs. HHAs are a powerful tool that can be used to evaluate the success of change at the individual, program, and community level,[17-19] and as such we would urge their use.

REFERENCES

1. U.S. Department of Health, Education, and Welfare, *Health United States: 1979.* Washington, D.C.: U.S. Department of Health, Education, and Welfare, 1980.
2. U.S. Department of Health, Education, and Welfare, *Health United States: 1975.* Washington, D.C.: U.S. Department of Health, Education, and Welfare, 1976.
3. Fuchs, V. R., *Who Shall Live? Health, Economics, and Social Choice.* New York: Basic Books, 1974.
4. Feldstein, P. J., *Health Care Economics.* New York, John Wiley & Sons, 1979.
5. U.S. Department of Health, Education, and Welfare, *Healthy People: The Surgeon General's Report on Health Promotion and Disease Prevention.* Washington, D.C.: U.S. Government Printing Office, 1979.
6. LaLonde, M., *A New Perspective on the Health of Canadians.* Ottawa: Office of the Canadian Minister of National Health and Welfare, 1974.
7. U.S. Congress, National Health Planning and Resources Development Act 1973, as amended.
8. Ardell, D. B., "High Level Wellness and the HSAs: A Health Planning Success Story. *American Journal of Health Planning* 3 (July 1978), pp. 1–18.
9. Ardell, D. B. and Robins, L., "High Level Wellness and the HSAs: The Failure to Move from Advocacy to Action." *Journal of Health and Human Resources Administration* 24: (May 1980), pp. 429–450.

10. Blum, H. K., *Planning for Health: Development and Application of Social Change Theory.* New York: Human Science Press, 1974.
11. Dever, G. E. A., *Community Health Analysis.* Germantown, Md.: Aspen Systems Corporation, 1980.
12. U.S. Department of Health, Education, and Welfare, *Guide to Data for Health Systems Planners.* Washington, D.C., U.S. Government Printing Office, 1976.
13. Donnabedien, A., *Aspects of Medical Care Administration.* Cambridge: Harvard University Press, 1973.
14. Dever, G. E. A., "An Epidemiological Model for Health Policy Analysis." *Social Indicators Research* 2 (1976), pp. 453–466.
15. Rutstein, D. D., et al., "Measuring the Quality of Medical Care." *New England Journal of Medicine* 294 (1976), pp. 582–588.
16. Ardell, D. B., *High Level Wellness, An Alternative to Doctors, Drugs, and Disease.* Emmaus, Pa. Rodale Press, 1977.
17. Robbins, Lewis C. and Hall, Jack H., *How to Practice Prospective Medicine.* Indianapolis: Methodist Hospital, 1970.
18. Faber, Marilyn M., ed., *Family and Community Health, Risk Reduction for Health Maintenance* 3:1 (May 1980).
19. Goetz, A. A., Duff, Jean F., and Bernstein, J. E., "Health Risk Estimation: The Estimation of Risk." *Public Health Reports* 95:2 (March–April 1980), pp. 119–126.

20 / Evaluating a Risk Reduction Program: Well Aware About Health, A Controlled Clinical Trial of Health Assessment and Behavior Modification   *Sabina Dunton, M.P.H.*

Health risk reduction as a result of systematic health hazard appraisal is a relatively new approach to the improvement of health and life-style. Springing from the efforts of Dr. Lewis C. Robbins and Dr. Jack H. Hall in the late 1960s, health risk reduction through the practice of prospective medicine is quickly becoming a medical specialty of its own. To date not much has been reported on the evaluation of the efficacy of this approach. In the summer of 1977, the W. K. Kellogg Foundation funded a 4-year study at the University of Arizona's Well Aware About Health program as a means of systematically evaluating the concepts of health risk reduction. Although the findings of the study are not in, reported here are the evaluation design and hypotheses for the possible outcomes of the study.

ABOUT WELL AWARE, IN GENERAL

Well Aware About Health is an ongoing program developed and administered at the University of Arizona aimed at *Educating* and *Motivating* people to change those personal habits and conditions which, if they remain unchanged, are likely to lead to premature death, from disease or accidental injury. The program, which began 7 years ago as community service of the Arizona Cooperative Extension Service,[1,2] is based on the actuarially epidemiologically documentable links between such health hazards as smoking, drinking, high blood pressure, high cholesterol, obesity, depression, lack of exercise, poor eating habits, nonuse of seat belts, and numerous other life-style behaviors which result in disease, injury, and death from heart disease, cancer, stroke, motor vehicle accidents, and so on.

Currently operating as a component of the University of Arizona Health Sciences Center, the overall service goals of Well Aware are

- To help individuals *understand* the major causes of disease, accidental injury, and death.
- To make individuals *aware* of those factors which are hazardous to their health.
- To help individuals *make the choices* they should make to eliminate—at least to reduce—those hazards.
- To show individuals *how to use* the health care system properly so they can become informed, *active partners* in their own health care and maintenance.

Well Aware's philosophies and practices derive from a relatively recently organized specialty known as prospective medicine.[3-5] Prospective medicine deals with a person's—or a population's—health in the context of what is likely to come about (hence, prospective). In contrast, and with noteworthy exceptions such as pediatrics, the practice of conventional curative medicine deals with a person in the context of what has already happened to impair that person's health.

Well Aware puts its clients through a screening program (it is not a complete physical examination) and reports back each individual's health hazard profile. The profile displays before the client the probability of death occurring within the next 10 years. The probability is computed from either the absence or the degree of presence of those factors which are actuarially proven health hazards. This process is called health hazard appraisal (HHA).

Well Aware's uniquely developed version of the health hazard appraisal questionnaire and health hazard profile are central to the program's evaluative and educational goals. With these the staff hopes to assist individuals in understanding their health (both *quantified* and *nonquantified*) and to begin the reflective process of the way they live each day and learn that their behaviors may influence their overall health status—for now and for the future.

Process

Well Aware places participants in its regular, nonresearch service program of health hazard appraisal through the following process:

1. Health Assessment:
   a. Orientation and health hazard appraisal questionnaire
   b. Physical and laboratory measurements
2. Results session:
   a. Health hazard profile (explained in group setting)
   b. Individual counseling
3. General education programs
4. Risk reduction seminars
5. Well Aware "booster shots" (newsletters and health "events")
6. Rescreening (at later date)

The health hazard profile is a computer printout displaying for each participant the following:

- Risk and achievable ages.
- Ten leading causes of death for those with the individual's risk factors.
- Physical measurements.
- Laboratory results.
- New evidence (nonquantitated risk information).
- Summarization.

Education

Nothwithstanding the great visibility and, occasionally, the drama of the HHA process, the heart of the Well Aware Program is its education component.

The nature of the educational offerings to clients is dependent on the risk classifications they receive as part of their health hazard profile. Although participation in education programs is entirely voluntary, every client classified as either "high" or "medium risk" is urged to take part in the risk-related educational offerings applicable to that person. Education is not recommended for "low-risk" clients. However, they are advised of the subjects offered an may attend—most often out of interest for a friend or family member.

As a practical matter, education begins with seeing the slide-tape orientation, "Focus on Wellness." This program was produced in-house and discusses how life-style decisions affect health. It also explains the crucial concepts of risk age and achievable age for participants and overviews the Well Aware HHA process.[6]

Awareness increased by the *content* of the health hazard appraisal questionnaire is yet another informal education device. Specifically, the questionnaire was designed to elicit accurate, honest responses. But it was formatted into specific health categories to stimulate thinking and awareness about the factors that affect health.

Formal education is conducted by Well Aware's health education staff, physicians, other health professionals, staff of relevant community agencies, and other qualified individuals. Educational follow-up occurs along two main tracks:

1. General education programs:
   Heart disease
   Cancer
   Diabetes
   Motor vehicle accidents/violent death
   Lung disease
2. Risk reduction seminars:
   Smoking
   Eating
   Exercise
   Drinking and drugs
   Stress

As a reinforcement to the formal education component, participants willing to do so sign a Health Improvement Plan "contract" in which they

- Identify at least one negative health behavior they want to change,
- Set goals for changing that behavior, and
- List the education sessions they will attend to help them achieve their goals.

Formal education is followed by "educational booster shots" in the form of letters and events such as "fun runs."

Every phase of the Well Aware program process has been designed and refined over the past 7 years to maximize the *educational*, not just informational, potential of the process. From the orientation and responding to the questionnaire through screening, results, and counseling to the formal disease-specific education sessions and structured risk reduction behavior change seminars, Well Aware materials and methods amplify and reinforce the educational goals. A great deal of time and creative energy were taken to make these products self-explanatory, simple to understand, easy to use, and graphically appealing.

Once gained, knowledge becomes part of an individual—to be used or not, now, later, or never. Knowledge is cumulative and decisions, choices, behaviors, attitudes, and skills are its demonstrable products.[7] The observation and belief at Well Aware is that individuals informed with personally relevant, usable information respond and react to their greater awareness in an appropriate, healthful fashion.

FROM SERVICE TO RESEARCH

The seven years of development of the Well Aware approach to HHA has created a degree of zealous faith in the process among the staff. However, perhaps indicative of the "coming of age" of the program, *evaluation* to substantiate Well Aware's faith in this concept has become a major thrust in recent years. Skepticism of the HHA concept created a need for fundamental research.[8-11] Specifically, the HHA approach seems to be a very effective educational and motivational device. Yet, to date no one has formally tested this. Nor is it known the amount and kind of additional educational and support an individual may need to actually apply this new knowledge, to adapt healthier behaviors, or, most important, to maintain them. Skeptics, some friendly, some not so friendly, asked some very hard, very valid questions about the HHA tool itself.[12-14]

Specifically, the questions were concerned with the following:

1. The validity of the HHA statistical base.
2. The value of HHA as a predictor of health status.
3. The effectiveness of the motivational and educational attributes of HHA.

Also, some skeptics saw grave dangers in the anxiety that might be produced when giving an individual too much "bad news" about himself or herself. Would the individual know how to handle that? Would he or she know what to do, where to turn for help or more information?

The criticisms and concerns of the skeptics served as thought provokers. Through subjective observation and some "quick and dirty" evaluation during 3 years with the Arizona Cooperative Extension Service doing rural and urban HHA service programs, the decision was made to test some of these questions in a sound scientific manner. Specifically, health care groups, as well as business and industry, need to know the following:

- Can behavior be changed using variations of this approach?
- Does HHA help motivate people to make informed, healthier choices?
- Is it a good educational tool? a good health self-monitoring device?
- What educational materials (tools) and methods[15] work? don't work?
- How much does it cost to start such a program? to keep it going?
- Is it a complement to clinical practice? fee-for-service (FFS) versus health maintenance organization (HMO)?

The most profound stimulus for initiating research in this area was the belief in the concept of health education combined with risk appraisal and the desire to contribute sound, scientific proof about the efficacy of each, separately or in combination, and to establish their place in the health promotion and disease prevention field. Stimulated by the inflationary medical economic realities, staying well is going to become a necessity—for individuals and for business. Maybe this risk appraisal/education approach will ultimately contribute to healthier people and a resulting healthier economy.

In 1977, Well Aware received a 4-year, $480,000 research and development grant from the W. K. Kellogg Foundation to begin exploring these questions.

RESEARCH GOALS

The Kellogg-funded research at Well Aware was the first randomized controlled clinical trial in the United States in the area of health education using a health hazard appraisal/ life-style modification approach.

Briefly, the objective of the study, which consists of a main sample of 1,800 from the eligible population at risk, is to test the effects (including costs and benefits) of four health promotion–disease prevention intervention strategies on health behaviors, health and other attitudes, medical care use, and the level of risk factors.

The sample population was selected in 1978 and early 1979. The eligible population included all adults, ages 25 through 55, who were active patients (patients who made an office visit since January 1, 1977) in PrimaCare, a prepaid multispecialty group practice (a health maintenance organization [HMO]) in Tucson, Arizona, and the Tucson Clinic, a *fee-for-service* multispecialty group practice.

The following were the four interventions to be tested:

1. Health hazard appraisal *plus* health education (HHA plus Ed.).
2. Health hazard appraisal *without* follow-up health education (HHA no H. Ed.).
3. Standard assessment (no health hazard appraisal) *plus* health education (HHA plus H. Ed.).
4. Standard assessment *without* health education (no HHA no H. Ed.).

Figure 1 compares the components of health hazard appraisal with those of standard assessment. Health education consists of a coordinated set of small group meetings in which disease, risk factors, and risk factor reduction are discussed. Those sessions recommended to a subject will be dependent on the individual's risk factors and priorities. The groups under study not receiving health education obtain their results separately from those receiving education to avoid contamination. They have no further contact from the Well Aware staff except for rescreening at 1-year and 2-year intervals. The effects being evaluated in each group include health and illness behaviors, health attitudes, risk factor levels, and morbidity and mortality.

RESEARCH PRELIMINARIES

Before beginning the main study of the four groups, a number of matters needed further investigation and refinement. In particular, there was a need to

1. Verify the statistical base of health hazard appraisal;
2. Determine the reliability of the data collection instrument; and

COMPARISON

Health Hazard Appraisal (HHA)	Standard Assessment (SA)
Specific for the Individual	General Health Information
Quantified 10 Year Probability of Death	— — — — —
Computed Risk and Achievable Ages	— — — — —
Ten Ranked Causes of Death	— — — — —
Physical and Laboratory Values	Physical and Laboratory Values
Results Interpreted in Both Group and Individual Counseling Sessions	Results Mailed with No Personal Contact

FIGURE 20-1.

3. Administer a preliminary study to field test many of the procedures and materials needed in the main study.

Verify the Statistical Base

The statistical base upon which the entire concept of health hazard appraisal is based was developed in the mid-1960s, largely through the pioneering work of Harvey Geller, who at that time was chief statistician for the U.S. Public Health Service Cancer Control Program. The important product of Geller's work was a series of 10-year probability tables of death from specific causes for various age, sex, and ethnic groups.[3,16] Geller's probability tables were supplemented by the efforts of Norman Gesner, a prominent life actuary, by the addition of weighted numeric risk factors. The resulting Geller/Gesner tables were the basis for the first attempts at health hazard appraisal.[3] Upon receipt of the Kellogg grant in August 1977, Well Aware invited the participation of Dr. Lewis Robbins, founder of the concept of prospective medicine and health hazard appraisal, in exploring the validity of using these tables as the basis for the main study. In particular, there was review of the means that were used to establish the numeric factors of risk, how each cause-of-death was computed, and how the overall risk and achievable age calculations were determined. Though some questions remained unanswered and there was a consensus that many of the numeric factors and weighted averages needed to be updated in light of new evidence (primarily gained through recent morbidity, not mortality, studies since the inception of HHA), it was decided that the update issues were beyond the scope and funding capabilities of this project. Acknowledging these flaws, Well Aware determined that the Geller/Gesner tables were the best that existed, and, though only a beginning in need of improvement, were a sound base and a valiant attempt to apply the latest epidemiological evidence gleaned from population studies to the whole individual. The Well Aware staff made a commitment to lobby for the need for updated mortality tables and the development of a method to integrate morbidity data into the data base, but these issues were beyond the scope of the Kellogg study. The best tables that existed in 1977 when the study began were those developed by Geller in 1972 with the help of Greg Steele, at that time a premedical student assisting Dr. Jack Hall at the Methodist Hospital in Indianapolis. If the Well Aware study was going to be ongoing for the next few years, there was concern about making mortality predictions in the 1980s against a 1972 mortality base. Consequently Well Aware began to work with the Center for Disease Control (CDC) in Atlanta to update the tables. CDC sought the help of Greg Steele and produced updated 1976 tables. These were entered into the Well Aware data base in July 1979.

Determining the Reliability of the Data Collection Instrument

Before beginning the main study, it was crucial to ensure that the instrument to be used, the health hazard appraisal questionnaire, was field tested and reviewed by experts in the various fields the questionnaire addresses. This was particularly important because of the expanded nature of the Well Aware questionnaire over those of other programs. In recognition of the numerous discoveries in the biomedical sciences since the formation of the basic health hazard appraisal data base, Well Aware elected to include items in its questionnaire that would allow for evaluation and feedback to clients in areas such as nutrition, stress, and some areas of cancer. Also included were questions regarding attitudes, beliefs, and values about health and the use of health services. Although much of this information was not quantifiable in terms of specific risk factors, Well Aware felt it was important to provide participating clients with information in narrative form about these areas in which there exists "new evidence" of potential risk.

Field testing the questionnaire sought answers to such questions as

- Will the instrument provide all of the needed information for risk factor calculations?
- Are certain words or questions redundant or misleading?
- Is the instrument functionally designed? (e.g., Will it be possible to administer, collect, and report information using written directions, coding instructions, and procedures?)
- How consistent (how reliable) is the information obtained by the instrument?

At Well Aware, field testing meant trying out the instrument under conditions similar to those expected for the main study. Therefore, a mini-sample of people who were to participate in the field test were selected by using the same sampling plan to be used for the main study.

This method of establishing reliability was to determine whether someone filling out the same questionnaire responded about the same on more than one occasion. People do change, of course. They become more tired, angry, and tense today than they were yesterday. People also change because of their experiences or because they learn something new, but *meaningful changes* are not subject to fluctuations. A reliable instrument will, or should, provide consistent measures of important characteristics despite background fluctuations.

The stability of the questionnaire was computed by administering the instrument to the same mini-sample on two different occasions, 3 weeks apart, and then correlating the scores from one time to the next.

Reliability for each question was determined using the following method. If a question did not meet a criterion of 90 per cent or more reliability, it was rewritten and retested until it did. The example in Figure 2 is one of the questions regarding exercise in any early version of the questionnaire.

Reliability analysis indicated that there was a problem with this question (Figure 3).

The diagonal of the cross-tab indicates those individuals whose responses were identical after two administrations of the instrument. In this case, out of 168 individuals 46, or 27.4 per cent changed their answers. The reliability score was relatively low, 72.6 per cent; therefore, the question was revised and tested ten more times. Additional information on the reliability of this question was obtained by comparing individual answers with the actual scores on the fitness test administered as part of the appraisal

In your work and/or your recreational activities, do you consider that you get:

- [1] Practically no exercise
- [2] Very little exercise
- [3] A medium amount of exercise
- [4] A great deal of exercise

FIGURE 20-2.

Exercise Level

	Practically No	Very Little	Medium Amount	Great Deal	
Practically No	3	1	0	0	4
Very Little	3	36	7	1	47
Medium Amount	1	17	60	8	86
Great Amount	0	0	8	23	31
	7	54	75	32	168

$$\frac{\text{Same response}}{\text{Total}} \quad \frac{122}{168} = 72.6\% \text{ identity}$$

FIGURE 20-3.

screening process. The revised question which met the 90 per cent criterion is shown in Figure 4.

Specifically, it was discovered that people define and perceive amount of exercise *very* differently. In this self-admitted type of question, it was necessary to give the standard by which one should measure oneself if the question is to be reliable.

Apparently, this study has been one of the few systematic assessments to date of the reliability of health hazard appraisal questionnaire information.[17, 18]

Administering a Preliminary Study

Concurrent with efforts to verify the health hazard appraisal data base and determine the reliability of the questionnaire, an effort was made to conduct a preliminary study using the health hazard appraisal method with health education offerings. It was felt that such a study would provide the best opportunity to field test many of the procedures and materials for the main study.

A. We want to know how physically active you are. Physical activity includes either or both of these:

1) Work activity, if it involves strenuous physical labor such as construction work, yard work, restaurant work, nursing, heavy housework, etc.
2) Exercise such as walking, jogging, bicycle riding, calisthenics, sports, and other similar recreation activities.

Now, on a scale of 1 to 10, mark the number that best describes how physically active you are.

NOTE: Do not mark above 5 unless you do your physical activities at least 3 times a week and for 15 minutes or more each time.

Practically no physical activity	Very little physical activity	A medium amount of physical activity	A great deal of physical activity
1—2	3—4—5	6—7—8	9—10

FIGURE 20-4.

Specifically, the preliminary study allowed for

- Projecting the scope of the participant recruitment effort needed for a 2,000-person research study.
- Perfecting methods of improving participant response rate.
- Field testing and revising newly developed educational programs and materials.
- Debugging the myriad of details involved in organizing and running such a large study.

This preliminary study of a total of 200 persons from the two sites (FFS and HMO) served as an excellent training exercise for the entire Well Aware staff. Without it, many major procedural problems that could possibly jeopardize the main study would have gone undetected.

THE EVALUATION RESEARCH FOR THE MAIN STUDY

Objectives

Well Aware's research objectives for the main study are

1. Test health hazard appraisal (questionnaire, physical/lab measurements, profile) as an education tool *per se*.
2. Assess effectiveness of educational interventions (counseling, education/risk reduction programs, follow-up reinforcement).

To accomplish these objectives, the evaluation research design shown in Figure 5 is being implemented.

Essentially, all of the participants are put through identical health assessment (HA) sessions using identical questionnaire items and physical measurements. This will allow for the determination of change in the following outcome measures:

- Physical condition (lowered BP, weight, cholesterol, fitness, and so on).
- Life-style (smoking, drinking, exercise, diet, and so on).
- Capacity for self-care (due to improved health awareness, knowledge, motivation).
- Health care resource utilization.
- Provider attitudes and practices (vis-à -vis patient self-responsibility).

Health care resource utilization will also be monitored through medical records or special observations by clinic staff.

Provider attitude and practices will be measured by comparing responses from a preliminary and postprogram questionnaire, administered to clinic staff, through observations of changes in clinical programs or personnel with health education responsibilities, and through interviews with the physicians, nurse practitioners, and administrators.

Sample Selection and Eligibility Criteria

The "eligible" population at risk for the main study included all adults, ages 25 through 55 who were active patients at the time of sample selection in PrimaCare, a prepaid multispecialty group practice (a health maintenance organization (HMO), in Tucson,

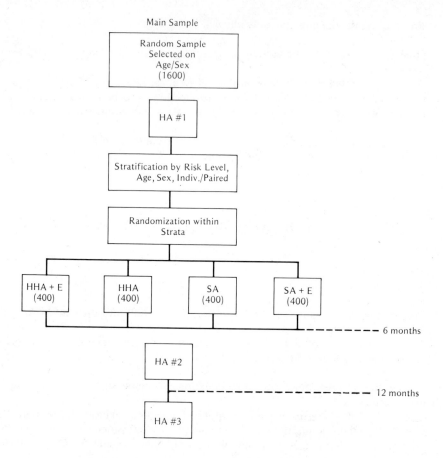

Main Sample

FIGURE 20-5. **Evolution research design.**

HA   = Health assessment (questionnaire and physical/lab screening)
SA   = Standard assessment results (physical measurements & lab results only)
HHA = Health hazard appraisal results (printout, group results session, counseling)
E   = Education and risk reduction

Arizona, and the Tucson Clinic, a fee-for-service (FFS) multispecialty group practice in the same city. (Refer to Figure 6.) Potential subjects were identified from patient registries maintained by each clinic. Numbers were assigned to all registered patients from the two clinics: 15,000 numbers were randomly drawn from the universe of potential subjects at Tucson Clinic and 6,000 at PrimaCare.

The individuals who were randomly selected as candidates for the study were screened for several criteria, whether they

1. Were between the ages of 25 and 55 years;
2. Had visited the clinics since 1977 as a regular practice patient (not just for a preemployment physical, for example); and
3. Live within the Tucson urban area.

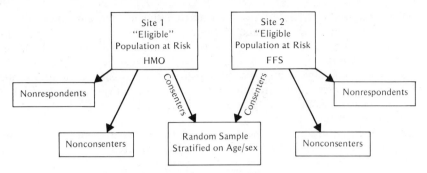

FIGURE 20-6.   Site and sample selection.

These criteria were applied by manually reviewing a total of 21,000 medical charts from both clinics.

Thirty-five per cent of Tucson Clinic patients and 73 per cent of PimaCare patients met these criteria and were mailed a recruitment letter and a short eligibility questionnaire.

Listed here are all the eligibility criteria that each subject had to meet:

1. Year-round resident.
2. No plans to move from area.
3. Not former Well Aware participant.
4. Not employed by the HMO or FFS sites (self or family).
5. Not pregnant.
6. Willing to attend education sessions.
7. Literate in English.

As responses to the recruitment letter were received, they were separated into two groups—"consenters" and "nonconsenters." The affirmative responses were reviewed by Well Aware staff to determine whether a respondent met all of the eligibility criteria. Then, the consenters were divided into "eligibles" and "ineligibles." The ineligibles were sent "We're sorry..., thank you for your interest" letters.

A sample of early consenters was randomly selected for inclusion in the study. That portion of all eligible consenters, to equal 840 or 80 per cent of the targeted sample per site, was drawn from the pool of early respondents from each clinic.

Two weeks after the first recruitment mailing, a second mailing was made to all non-respondents. This mailing consisted of a xeroxed copy of the initial recruitment letter, an additional letter soliciting the individual's cooperation, the eligibility questionnaire, and a stamped, addressed envelope. Approximately 20 per cent of the total study sample was derived from the pool of late respondents, making a total of approximately 1,050 per site. In order to correct a deficit of males in the sample of early consentors, all late responding males were included in the total. Late responding females were selected at random to complete the sample.

Treatment Groups and Stratification Variables to Be Used

The research design is a randomized controlled clinical trial with 12-month and 24-month periods of follow-up. (Please refer again to Figure 5.) Subjects are stratified by important characteristics thought to influence the outcomes prior to randomization, such as age, sex, and risk level. Each stratum was individually randomized using block randomization to ensure an adequate number of subjects in each intervention group.

To review, the objective of the study is to test the effects of the four health promotion–disease prevention intervention strategies on health behavior, health attitudes and knowledge, health care utilization, and the level of risk factors. (Note the four cells near the bottom of Figure 5.)

After the first health assessment, HA No. 1 (questionnaire and screening), subjects were stratified by the following variables which are believed to influence the outcomes of the study.

Variable	Strata
Practice	PrimaCare (HMO)
	The Tucson Clinic
Age	Under 40
	Over 40
Sex	Male
	Female
Risk	Low
	High and medium
Participants	Individuals
	Couples

Risk status (high, medium, or low) is defined according to the following set of criteria.

	High		Medium	Low
One of these:	OR	*Two of these:*	*One of these:*	
DBP 105		DBP 90–104	DBP 90–104	
Smokes 2 packs		Smokes cigarettes	Smokes cigarettes	None
Cholesterol 280 mg%		Cholesterol 260–270 mg%	Cholesterol 260–279 mg%	
Overweight 50%+		Overweight 25–49%	Overweight 25–49%	
		Alcoholic Drinks 15+/week	Alcoholic Drinks 15+/week	
		Exercises–seldom or never	Exercises–seldom or never	
		Depressed–often	Depressed–often	

Couples are organized into strata by mean age of the pair, practice, and risk level. They are randomized within strata as described for individuals.

Since a significant number of couples enrolled in the study, "couple status" became an additional stratification variable. Couples are treated distinctively throughout the study for two reasons:

1. To see whether cohabitant support has any effect on outcome measures, and
2. To prevent contamination when one person is in a certain treatment group and they share information with their spouse or partner.

Subsampling of Nonresponders and Nonconsenters

Two other random samples will be studied from the "eligible" population at risk. People who did not respond at all and to whom mail delivery was made and the nonconsenters, those who express a lack of interest in participating in the study were contacted by telephone. (Refer to Figure 6.) If the contacted individual was willing, a short questionnaire was administered over the telephone. The questionnaire solicits information about key health behaviors, demographic characteristics, attitudes and reasons for nonresponse or nonparticipation. Where applicable, comparisons will be made with main sample participants.

FACTORIAL DESIGN HYPOTHESES AND POSSIBLE OUTCOMES

Factorial Design

Figure 7 shows a factorial representation of the four intervention groups into which the subjects are randomized. These groups represent all possible combinations of the two specific interventions, health hazard appraisal and health education. An additional explanation of each intervention follows.

HEd (Health Education)

Health education or health improvement programs are offered to two of the four treatment groups, one that gets the HHA and one that does not. Though the feedback each group receives about their results is different (refer to Figure l), the educational offerings and information about them is identical. In fact, both HHA and non-HHA participants attend the same class sessions.

Health education consists of a coordinated set of small group meetings for specific health improvements such as weight reduction, smoking cessation, stress management, increasing aerobic exercise, and others. These sessions require 4 to 10 weeks of regular weekly or biweekly attendance. After the weekly sessions end, monthly support, progress sharing, and reporting sessions are held for those participants interested in continuing to meet. The curricula of these courses is designed to maximize active participation and practice and opportunities for participants to talk with each other about health concerns. The sessions are never straight, didactic lectures. They utilize the most effective behavior modification techniques available. The goal is to have each individual identify his or her own habit patterns and discover what it is in oneself or one's en-

Factorial Design

	HEd	No HEd
HHA	I	II
no HHA	III	IV

Interpetation

IF ...	THEN ...
I = II = III = IV	no HHA or HEd effect
I = II > III = IV	pos. HHA effect & no HEd effect
I > II = III = IV	pos. effect of HHA plus HEd (no effect of either alone)
I = III ≧ II = IV	pos. HEd effect, no HHA effect

FIGURE 20-7.

vironment that controls one's habit behaviors—and what reinforces the improvements .
chosen to be made.

The health education programs are based on the fact that each individual is unique
and has a particular combination of problems and also capabilities to deal with those
problems. As an educator, Well Aware seeks to help people find their problems and use
their unique capabilities for sustained self-improvement reinforced by their own choice
for change, increased awareness, learned skill, and self-knowledge.[19,20] The study
hopes to determine the differences, if any, in participation, course completion, and,
most important, desired behavior change in the group that initially received the HHA
or the Standard Assessment (SA).

No HEd (No Health Education)

These two groups will not be invited to the HEd sessions and will receive their results
separately from the HEd groups to avoid contamination. After their initial intervention (HHA or non-HHA) is complete, they will have no further contact except for rescreening at 1-year and 2-year intervals.

HHA and No HHA

The same data collection instruments and methods are used for both HHA and non-HHA
groups, the primary difference is in the content and manner in which feedback is given.
Refer to Figure 1 for a comparison of the information that is provided to the HHA
and non-HHA (Standard Assessment) groups, respectively.

Important to note is that the report to the non-HHA groups consists only of their
values on various nonbehavioral, physical, and laboratory measurements and general
descriptions of the meaning of the measurements. Measurements are not linked with
risks of disease or death and there is no mention of the individual's risk of death.

Reports to non-HHA participants are mailed or distributed to each individual at a
follow-up meeting. No individual counseling about the report is done.

Hypotheses

Very simply, this is a diagram of the hypothesis of how changes occur that will affect
the measured outcomes of the study:

Increased Awareness/Knowledge

↓

Behavior Change

↓

Risk Factor/COD Risk Change

The general categories to be tested are client participation and program effectiveness. Specifically, a look for differences, if any, among program participants and non-
participants will be made.

Client participation will be studied in terms of those who consent to participate in
the study versus those who refused or those who did not respond to the invitation.

The following variables will be analyzed:

1. Educational achievement.
2. Income level.
3. Level of health/wellness.
4. Experience or action to reduce risk factors.
5. Perceived self-control and illness resistance.
6. Social connectedness.
7. Source of medical care.

Those persons who remain as participants will be compared with program dropouts for

1. All of above.
2. Depression, anxiety, and stress levels.

Among the four treatment groups, analysis of differences, if any, will be made to test *Program effectiveness* using the following variables:

1. Awareness of personal risks.
2. Knowledge of disease and prevention.
3. Practice of health maintenance and prevention.
4. Physiological and laboratory measures within "acceptable range."
5. Risk to achievable age scores.
6. Adoption of healthy behaviors.
7. Reduction of health-damaging habits.
8. Attempts to change.
9. Improvements in mental wellness.
10. Attitude change (self-control, resistance, beliefs).

Possible Outcomes

The factorial design of this trial permits the effects of the two interventions (HHA and Health Education) to be evaluated singly and in combination. The possible interpretations of various findings are shown in the lower part of Figure 7.

Using the exercise sample described in Figure 4 and relating possible outcomes to the above general interpretation, the expectation would be that:

1. If all four groups show the same amount of change in exercise habits, whether statistically significant or not there is no effect of either HHA and HEd.
2. If Groups I and II both showed significant changes in exercise habits, whereas in groups III and IV, there was insignificant or no change, then a positive effect of health hazard appraisal and no effect of health education can be concluded.
3. If the amount of change in exercise habits is significantly greater in group I than in groups II, III, or IV, then a positive effect of health hazard appraisal with education but without any effect of these interventions taken alone be concluded.
4. If those individuals in the health education groups show a greater change in exercise habits than those in the noneducation groups, then a positive effect for health education but no effect of health hazard appraisal is shown.

SUMMARY

Certainly, the Well Aware study is expected to uncover more questions than it answers. However, there is the hope that some substantial efficacy information will be contributed to the field in which there is a great swelling of interest.

The collective goal of those working in the prospective medicine field is wellness. This includes helping individuals become more responsible for their own health, make healthier choices about their daily living, and to find the healing power within themselves.

In closing, a quote by the great humanist and physician, Dr. Albert Schweitzer, seems very appropos. He said:

> Each patient (each person) carries his own doctor inside him. They come to us not knowing that truth. We are at our best when we give the doctor who resides within each patient a chance to go to work.

That's Well Aware's challenge; that's certainly the goal of the entire prospective medicine field.

REFERENCES

1. Brown, Sabina Dunton and Ivey, William L., "Project Well Aware About Health," *Extension Service Review*. U.S. Department of Agriculture (March and April 1976), pp. 7–9.
2. Brown, Sabina Dunton and Ivey, William L., "Preventive Medicine for Farm Families." *Arizona Farmer-Ranchman* 54:9 (September 1975), pp. 24–27.
3. Robbins, Lewis C. and Hall, Jack H., *How to Practice Prospective Medicine*. Indianapolis: Methodist Hospital, 1970.
4. Hall, Jack H. and Zwemer, J. D., *Prospective Medicine*. Indianapolis: Methodist Hospital, 1979.
5. Robbins, Lewis C., "A System for Indications for Preventive Medicine in the Behavioral Sciences and Preventive Medicine: Opportunities and Dilemmas." In *Teaching of Preventive Medicine*, Fourth in a Series Kane, R. L., ed., Sponsored by John E. Fogerty International Center for Advanced Study in Health Sciences, Washington, D. C.: National Institutes of Health, 1974, pp. 63–76.
6. Ramsay, Deborah K. and Dunton, Sabina, "Prospective Medicine: 'Focus on Wellness': A Short Course for the Lay Public." *Proceedings of the Fourteenth Annual Meeting of the Society of Prospective Medicine*. Bethesda, Md.: Health and Education Resources, 1978, pp. 58–60.
7. Brown, Sabina Dunton and Sennott, L. Lee, "Issues Related to Developing Criteria for the Evaluation of Risk Reduction." *Proceedings of the Twelfth Annual Meeting of the Society of Prospective Medicine*. Bethesda, Md.: Health and Education Resources, 1976, pp. 66–70.
8. Lauzon, Richard R. J., " A Randomized Controlled Trial on the Ability of Health Hazard Appraisal to Stimulate Appropriate Risk Reduction Behavior." Ph.D. diss. Department of Health Education, Graduate School of the University of Oregon, Corvallis, Oreg., 1977.
9. Dunton, Sabina and Rasmussen, W., "Comparative Data on Risk Reduction." *Proceedings of the Thirteenth Annual Meeting of the Society of Prospective Medicine*. Bethesda, Md.: Health and Education Resources, 1977, pp. 111–119.
10. Goetz, A. A., Duff, Jean F., and Bernstein, J. E., "Health Risk Estimation:The Estimation of Risk." *Public Health Reports* 95:2 (March–April 1980), pp. 119–126.

11. Johns, Richard E., "Health Hazard Appraisal—A Useful Tool in Health Education." *Proceedings of the Twelfth Annual Meeting of the Society of Prospective Medicine*. Bethesda, Md.: Health and Education Resources, 1976, pp. 61–65.
12. Fullarton, Jane E., "Health Hazard Appraisal, Its Limitations and New Directions for Risk Assessment." *Proceedings of the Thirteenth Annual Meeting of the Society of Prospective Medicine*. Bethesda, Md.: Health and Education Resources, 1977, pp. 6–10.
13. Imrey, Peter B. and Williams, B. T., "Statistical Hazards of Health Hazard Appraisal." *Proceedings of the Thirteenth Annual Meeting of the Society of Prospective Medicine*. Bethesda, Md.: Health and Education Resources, 1977, pp. 31–35.
14. Hsu, David H. S. and Milsum, J. H., "Implementation of Health Hazard Appraisal and Its Impediments." *Canadian Journal of Public Health* 69, 1978, pp. 227–232.
15. Best, Allen J. and Milsum, J. H., "HHA and the Evaluation of Lifestyle Change Programs: Methodological Issues." *Proceedings of the Thirteenth Annual Meeting of the Society of Prospective Medicine*. Bethesda, Md.: Health and Education Resources, 1977, pp. 95–97.
16. Robbins, Lewis C., *Probability Tables of Deaths in the Next Ten Years from Specific Causes*. Indianapolis: Methodist Hospital, 1972.
17. Elias, Walter and Dunton, Sabina., "Effect of Reliability on Risk Factor Estimation by a Health Hazard Appraisal." *Proceedings of the Sixteenth Annual Meeting of the Society of Prospective Medicine*. Bethesda, Md.: Health and Education Resources, 1980.
18. Sacks, Jeffrey J., Krushat, W. Mark, and Newman, Jeffrey, "Reliability of the Health Hazard Appraisal." *American Journal of Public Health* 70:7 (July 1980), pp. 730–732.
19. Warner, Lynn H., "Health Hazard Appraisal—An Instrument for Change." *Proceedings of the Thirteenth Annual Meeting of the Society of Prospective Medicine*. Bethesda, Md.: Health and Education Resources, 1977, pp. 120–123.
20. Milsum, John H., "Health, Risk Factor Reduction and Life Style Change." *Family and Community Health* 3:1 (May 1980), pp. 1–13.

21 / Competing for Acute Care Dollars: The Economics of Risk Reduction*

K. Michael Peddecord, Dr. P.H.

During an era of accountability and increasingly limited resources, it is essential to consider the economic aspects of new preventive and health promotion programs.

While risk reduction, like other innovations in the health field, is not a unitarian concept or program, there is a unifying conceptual basis for these interventions which allows discussion of this concept in general. Despite the fact that each program is somewhat unique, all deal with primary or secondary prevention and are grouped together for this discussion and identified as individual risk reduction (IRR) programs.

For the purpose of this article, IRR will be considered a developing technology which is, as yet, relatively untested in the general population. Its potentials, in terms of applicability, acceptability, and long-term benefits and costs, must be demonstrated prior to a conclusive evaluation and widespread implementation. Since IRR is an emerging technology whose widespread adoption might have a significant impact, not only on health care services but on health status as well, it merits critical discussion, as does any other unproven acute health care technology or preventive intervention.

HEALTH CARE ENVIRONMENT OF THE 1980s: A RATIONALE FOR PREVENTION

The success of the United States medical-industrial complex in amassing an increasing proportion of goods and services is well known. The growth of health care in terms of America's GNP—from 5.3 per cent in 1960 to 9.1 per cent in 1978—is as impressive as the growth in dollars from $27 to $194 billion during this same period.[1] The most often-cited causes of this growth are: (1) the introduction of new technologies (drugs, surgical treatments, diagnostic tests, medical interventions, and devices), many with the promising aura of immortality; (2) the development of a more complex or intense product; (3) the shifting of direct out-of-pocket payment choices from consumers to third parties; and (4) the establishment of social programs that have increased access in previously underserved segments of the population.

Despite its unique nature and size, the health care sector is susceptible to the economic pressures that affect society as a whole, and the nation now appears to be approaching a point of the slowed growth and limited resources that have long been forecast by economists.[2] Competition for increasingly scarce resources among various interests is fast becoming a reality in the health care sector. Keener competition and stricter accountability will undoubtedly force more careful attention to the way in which resources are allocated in the decade ahead.

As the slowed-growth or no-expansion environment of the 1980s nears, there is widespread recognition that increases or decreases in care expenditures will have little

*Reprinted from *Family and Community Health* 3:1 (May 1980) by Permission of Aspen Systems Corporation, Germantown, MD © 1980.

impact on life expectancy.[2,3] Accumulating epidemiologic evidence suggests that prevention of at least a portion of premature morbidities and mortalities may be possible.[4,5] The potential of prevention is now widely viewed as one solution to the problem of providing both cost-effective health care and improved health status.[6,7] Whether the approach involves (1) more traditional public health measures (environmental management, occupational product safety, and so on), (2) early detection and treatment, or (3) approaches that emphasize epidemiological-based programs of individual risk reduction such as IRR, all new programs must enter and develop in a health care environment that is more competitive and more apt to critically evaluate the costs and benefits of new health care technologies.[8]

Current Health Status and the Potential for Improvement

There are considerable data suggesting that health status in the United States can be improved. Evidence for this is easily observed from evaluation of life expectancies among various sex and racial segments of the United States and among western industrialized nations. HEW reports that life expectancy in the United States ranked eleventh for males and seventh for females among Western industrialized nations during 1976.[9] Studies of mortality from the major causes of death provide additional information. Gori and Richter examined the 1973 five major causes of death and compared these rates with those of other industrialized countries.[10] The potential per cent of prevention in the United States was then calculated by comparing the United States rate with the next-to-lowest and lowest rates for these nations. As may be clearly seen in Table 1, evidence suggests that a significant number of deaths within the United States are preventable. Within the United States, comparison of the general population with Mormon

TABLE 1. Major Causes of Mortality and Prevention Potential Based on Lowest and Next-to-Lowest Rates Among Industrialized Nations

| | | | Deaths Preventable, Based on Use of Rates from Industrialized Countries | |
Cause of Death	No. of Deaths— U.S., 1973	% of Mortality	Next-to-Lowest Rate No. (%)	Lowest Rate No. (%)
Major cardiovascular and renal disease	1,012,341	51	394,813 (39)	779,503 (77)
Malignant neoplasms	351,055	18	87,763 (25)	270,312 (77)
Accidents—motor vehicle, other	115,821	6	44,012 (38)	45,170 (39)
Disease of respiratory system	92,267	5	15,685 (17)	35,062 (38)
Diabetes mellitus	38,208	2	24,071 (63)	28,274 (74)
All other causes (all other categories each less than 1.7% of total)	363,311	18	N/A	N/A

Source: Gori, G. and Richter, B., "Macroeconomics of Disease Prevention in the United States." *Science* 200 (June 9, 1978), p. 1126.

TABLE 2. Estimated Costs of Illness and Potential Savings for Selected Preventive Interventions in United States (1975)

Disease or Condition	Magnitude of Problem	Intervention	No. of Cases Preventable	Condition or Disease ($ Billion)	Cost of Preventive Intervention ($)	Potential Savings as a Result of Intervention ($)	Benefit-to-Cost Ratio
Hypertension	Prevalence 20 + million Largely unknown to victims	Detection, drugs	10 million	15.9	4–6 billion	4–6 billion	4:1 to 2:1
Cancer of colon	Incidence approximately 100,000/year	Diet	17,000	3.5	Unknown	1.23 billion	Unknown
Heavy cigarette smoking	Incidence 22 million heavy smokers	Cessation (25% success)	5.5 million	20.3	2.75 billion	5.1 billion	1.8:1
Alcohol abuse	9 million alcoholics + 4.8 million male (target population)	Intensive program + follow-up (60% success)	60% of 4.8 million	33.6	6 billion	14 billion	2.3:1
Screening for cancer of colon among all over 55	Incidence approximately 3/100 over 55	Screen for stool guaiac	20% improved survival, reduced costs 50% in 1/3 of cases	0.47	80 million screening	670 million	8.38:1

Source: Kristein, M., "Economic Issues in Prevention." *Preventive Medicine* 6:2 (June 1977), pp. 252–264.

and Seventh Day Adventist religious groups, as well as comparisons of cross-state groups, provides additional evidence that there is significant potential for reduction of morbidity and mortality.[11]

Cost of Disease and Potential for Prevention

In addition to the human costs of suffering and reduction in life quality and expectancy, the economic costs of diseases that have a high potential for prevention are significant. Methods to quantify and compare the costs of disease and the benefits of various interventions have been employed for some time.[12] While these methods attempt to measure only tangible direct and indirect costs, the economic estimates are available for many preventable diseases. These estimates provide an insight into the magnitude of the problem and the potential benefits that could be realized by investment in prevention. Kristein and others have examined not only the costs of disease but also the evidence that preventive interventions exist which could be effectively applied to reduce morbidity and mortality.[13,14] Table 2 summarizes some estimates of cost, interventions, and estimated savings for a number of preventable diseases and conditions. No single preventive intervention provides a total solution; however, IRR and other preventive interventions do provide significant savings in human as well as economic terms.

Although there is a widely recognized potential for cost savings from prevention, the nature of savings is unclear. Before selling prevention as a panacea for health care cost problems, cautions concerning the macroeconomics of prevention must be considered.[15] While there exists considerable potential for improved health status and longevity gains through prevention, it is not clear that prevention of today's major causes of morbidity and mortality will reduce the costs of disease care in the long run. It must be recognized that a surge of other competing morbid conditions is likely as the population becomes older. These new morbid factors in larger "very old" populations may increase rather than mitigate total sickness and maintenance care costs.[16,17] Indeed, improved status of health may truly be a mirage.[18]

The axiom that "an ounce of prevention is worth a pound of cure" (or "abuse") has rarely been taken literally in the community health field.[19] Development of explicit cost-benefit and cost-effectiveness analysis techniques within the public health field is witness to early recognition that, under some circumstances, prevention is not always cheaper than cure. Lest it be believed that cost is all-important—a bottom line in these considerations—Roemer notes that the crucial question to ask when one is interested in human welfare is whether prevention is better than cure.[20] The economic effectiveness question is clearly secondary to the ethical value question.

INVESTMENT IN PREVENTION: MAGNITUDE AND TRENDS

Expenditures for Prevention

Expenditures for health promotion activities such as IRR may be considered within the broader general category of preventive health services. While the expenditures for prevention are significant, they should be kept in perspective. Total expenditures for all health services grew from $66.2 billion in 1969 to $115.6 billion in 1974 (amounting to an increase of almost $225 per capita). The 1978 fiscal year estimates of $192.4 billion, or $863 per capita, continued this trend.[21,22] Estimates for total expenditures for prevention may vary considerably depending on the definition.[23] A widely quoted figure is from 2 to 2.5 per cent (about $16.00 per capita) in 1977 of public and private health care dollars devoted to prevention with one-half of 1 per cent of that total devoted to health education.[24] Federal program expenditures in fiscal year 1976 were estimated to range from $900 million (a figure that includes more traditional public health expenditures) to a ceiling estimate of $7 billion when grants for environmental projects such as air and water pollution control are included.

In an examination of federal policy on prevention, Lee and Franks reviewed the growth of federal prevention expenditures between 1969 and 1974.[25] Total expenditures, in constant dollars, grew from $644 to $830 million (from $694 million to $1.129 billion in real dollars). Disease prevention and control outlays in constant dollars rose only from $241 to $242 million. The large percentage of growth in the period from 1969 to 1974 was in environmental control and consumer protection categories. Lee and Franks also highlight the problems of accountability and effectiveness, reminding us that the magnitude of expenditure for prevention (as with acute care expenditures) is not a reliable indicator of effectiveness or impact on health status.[26]

Prevention in Personal Health Services

It is difficult to accurately tabulate expenditures for preventive services that are incorporated into direct personal health care expenditures. Significant resources are devoted to annual checkups, immunizations, Pap smears, multiphasic screening, well-baby care, and so forth. The extent and efficiency of services, however, are largely unknown. The inability to estimate from the 1973 National Ambulatory Health Care Survey the number of visits to physicians' offices with a high degree of confidence is compounded by coding and classification problems of disease classifications for nonsymptomatic problems. Selecting categories that would be most likely to include preventive care, it can be expected that 11 per cent, or more than 69 million, of the estimated 644 million visits to physicians' offices in 1973 were devoted to some type of preventive care.[27] Despite the magnitude of that number, it should not be believed that these visits are evenly distributed across all segments of the consuming public. Other studies have also documented that a number of social, organizational, and payment factors have a significant impact on utilization of preventive services.[28]

While 11 per cent of personal health care visits devoted to prevention is impressive in magnitude and recognizes the contribution of personal health care services to prevention, it may overstate the impact of prevention which takes place within the personal health services. In his examination of the literature on organization and process in medical practice, Weinerman suggests that preventive activities are one area of client-provider relationships in need of serious investigation.[29] Breslow and Somers have also suggested that much prevention (such as the annual checkup) is imprecise and ill-defined, consisting of vague procedures with nonspecific goals.[30] In fact, it has been suggested that this may be one reason for the poor image of "prevention" among practitioners and public.[31-33]

Logic would also dictate that these suboptimal preventive resources could be redesigned to include more specific approaches such as IRR, the Lifetime Health Monitoring Program and other more effective promotion activities.[34] The methods required to achieve this improvement of prevention within the context of personnel are complex and largely beyond the scope of this article. Indeed, going from identification of the problem to designing a program for its resolution is a large step.[35]

ALLOCATING RESOURCES FOR ACUTE AND PREVENTIVE HEALTH ACTIVITIES

Although there was a time when any discussion of cost seemed secondary to the ingrained imperative of "whatever it takes," today's environment clearly requires more explicit attention to cost and effectiveness. As with other technologies, IRR is being developed at a time when the demand for efficacy and accountability has never been higher.[36] It is also being developed during a time when the recognized potential and need for health promotion and disease prevention through individual life-style and modification of risks is well recognized.[37] Even with this recognition of importance it should be realized that the United States lacks a consistent and national policy on prevention and promotion and a national system of resource allocation. New or expanded prevention and promotion interventions must enter the quasi-free marketplace and compete for dollars now dedicated to acute disease care services.[38]

Evaluation of Acute Care and Preventive Interventions: A Double Standard

It has been suggested that both therapeutic and preventive techniques should be evaluated using equally critical techniques and the same set of criteria.[39] This ideal approach to evaluation of technology has not been applied to most therapeutic interventions in the past.[40] On November 9, 1978, the president signed into law a bill creating a National Center for Health Technology (Public Law 95-623). This legislation is in fact designed to stimulate evaluation of medical technologies—an endeavor that had been largely lacking in the past.[41]

The reality of health technologies evaluation may be observed by a cursory examination of the innovations which reveals that preventive technologies are most always rigorously evaluated prior to and during their introduction. This is in sharp contrast to the vigorous evaluation and rapid promotion of most acute care technologies.

Evidence of rigorous evaluation in the community health field may be seen for such activities as cervical cancer screening, multiphasic health testing, community-based heart disease programs and multiple risk factor intervention trials.[42–45] The trend in acute care technology evaluation is most often evaluation following introduction and spread with initial publications consisting largely of case studies which are quick to extoll the benefits of the latest computerized tomography (CT) scanner, new esoteric diagnostic tests, coronary bypass operation, or monitoring equipment. The development and introduction of drugs is an important exception to this general observation. While there are other exceptions, acute care technologies are more apt to be widely used prior to explicit consideration of costs and benefits to the consumer or to the community as a whole.

The acute care treatment-oriented environment that now exists, as well as the diverse philosophical viewpoints of acute care and preventive health care practitioners, has led to a subtle double standard in evaluation and development of health technologies. The origin of this dichotomy in evaluation practice appears to be deeply rooted in the varied social perspectives, the uncertainty of both preventive and acute care interventions, and our inability to understand and quantify health or economic gains that are gained or lost from a given technology. One important contrast between acute and preventive philosophies is that in prevention the "uncertain call to action" is in the open, without an immediate crisis, while the equally uncertain call to action in acute care is concealed by the immediate and often life-and-death crisis.[46]

Although a subtle double standard may exist, it should not be viewed as a significant handicap to obtaining funds for IRR programs. There is no merit in abandoning vigorous evaluation simply for the sake of expanding IRR programs. In fact, as the call for public accountability and technology reevaluation has increased, much of the prior investment in evaluation of preventive activities will undoubtedly be viewed as wise and far-sighted action.[47] Continued investment in rigorous evaluation must be undertaken within the context of investment in experimentation. As with any innovative health care technology, considerable resources must be devoted to development and evaluation of IRR. Without adequate investment in early development and pilot testing, IRR, like any other product, may not receive a fair evaluation in the marketplace.

It is possible that failing to invest resources to identify populations where IRR will most likely be successful or an adequate investment in behavioral change and follow-up activities could lead to poor results and a premature conclusion that IRR is not widely useful. Given the lack of potentially useful innovations in preventive medicine, every opportunity for the success of IRR should be assured. Aggressive leadership will be required to make certain that IRR is adequately funded during developmental and evaluation stages.

Third-Party Payers and Resource Allocation for Risk Reduction

Within this competitive environment, preventive interventions—for which there is some tentative evidence of positive benefits—should be treated no differently from existing acute care activities for which there is little or no evidence of efficacy. There is no more rationale for third-party payers to exclude IRR from plans that cover preventive services than there is rationale to exclude reimbursement for selected new drugs or therapy from acute care coverage plans. In fact, third-party reimbursement now appears more favorable toward restructuring benefit packages that include "preventive packages."[48,49]

The significance of this third-party recognition of the importance of prevention and promotion activities is as yet unknown. While national organizations such as the Health Insurance Association of America and the Blue Cross Association recognize the importance of preventive services and the diminishing returns on additional acute care expenditures, they can provide little more than policy statements.[50]

The insurance industry is heterogeneous, composed of many smaller companies and state or regional associations (such as Blue Cross and Blue Shield). Even if there is a national organization policy supporting preventive services, each company or association must restructure its own benefit packages according to the demands made from the thousands of group and individual purchasers who buy health insurance plans. Insurance officials also point out that prevention orientation varies greatly across insurers. In addition, some insurers—such as Blue Cross/Blue Shield—are nonprofit and often have a history of provider participation in development of innovative benefit packages. Although there is no empirical work in this area, alteration in benefit structures for preventive services may follow the pattern that was observed for prepaid health care plans.

While some insurers are innovative—taking the leadership in development and marketing of health maintenance organizations in their regions—other insurers are content to change their benefit package structures in reaction to consumer or provider demand. It is possible that this innovative nature of some insurers is due largely to a special interest in prevention on the part of upper-level executives and influential board of director members. And there is also the possibility that leaders in the local health care community could exert a significant influence on insurer attitudes toward prevention.

The trend toward reimbursement of preventive services over the past 4 years may be viewed as significant but not massive. The extent to which insurers are restructuring benefit packages, as well as the cost and benefits of restructuring, is unknown. The only way to assess these trends among third parties appears to be through insurer-by-insurer, group-by-group case studies. Although national associations point to many cases where preventive services are being provided under traditional and innovative arrangements, they are somewhat skeptical about the effects of new services and the responsible use of new benefits.[51]

It appears that restructuring of benefit packages in the short term may be accomplished at the local rather than national level. If IRR programs can demonstrate the efficiency of their activities to large purchasers of insurance coverage (e.g., industry, unions, and other groups), third parties are likely to include preventive services in their packages in order to keep themselves competitive. The problem that could arise here is, of course how to define "covered preventive services." Will IRR be covered or will all vaguely defined preventive services be covered? The education of purchasers, consumers, and insurers is a crucial activity. Individual risk reduction programs should ensure that their activities do not go uncovered at the expense of more traditional and potentially ineffective annual "checkups."

THE FUTURE: OPTIONS FOR GROWTH AND FUNDING OF RISK REDUCTION

The majority of health care innovations are most clearly classifiable into either personal health care or public health activities. This classification is not always clear-cut for some preventive activities, including IRR. Classification of these activities as (1) community health, (2) personal health care services, or (3) a combination of community and personal services may be appropriate for developing IRR programs. Developers and directors of IRR programs may wish to market their activities to one or both sectors—or to a combination—and should do so with the knowledge that program operation within either sector has its own merits and risks.

IRR as a Community Health Program

As more traditional public health prevention interventions have ceased to produce additional reductions in morbidity and mortality, and as the definition of prevention has expanded to encompass social and behavioral determinants of health and illness, it is tempting to conclude that IRR preventive interventions exemplify, to some degree, the economic notion of a positive externality. And to an extent, activities or programs that are characterized by positive externalities benefit the community both directly and indirectly.

One can argue that IRR programs—like many other preventive activities and to a lesser degree acute care interventions—benefit both individual and community and that therefore their costs should not be totally assigned to the IRR participant. While the extent of this externality may be limited and difficult to document, the argument for public funding of IRR programs is as convincing as, or stronger than, many other programs (e.g., well-baby clinics and hypertension screenings) which now benefit from public funding. Casting IRR into the public sector also makes it easier to consider within the governmental health policy arena.[52]

In addition to the economic rationale and tradition appeal, there are several other factors that might favor a community-based approach (not exclusively in an existing health department but also in other community-based agencies). Since IRR will seek to modify personal behavior within the social context of the community, the community approach has both initiative and empirical merit. Many community agencies would also be expected to have a more programmatic approach and expertise in disciplines such as epidemiology, community relations, program development, grantsmanship, health education, and program evaluation. Such agencies might also have well-developed referral patterns for treatment follow-up and other services that would not be available in IRR programs with limited resources.

Some community agencies, such as public health departments, may be willing to develop these programs in an effort to bring themselves into the community spotlight. Health system agencies (HSAs), which have initially been preoccupied with plan development and certificates of need, may now be able and ready to move into implementation and development of their stated health promotion activities.[53] Superficially at least, these broadly representative agencies would appear to be logical foci of efforts, with ability to span personal health care, public health, and voluntary agencies.

Funding would appear to be one of the major limitations of community agencies. If financial support is limited to traditional public funding, the competition of other public programs (such as consumer protection, immunization, environment, maternal and child health, and medical care for the underserved) might leave few resources and little expertise for IRR or other new programs. Traditional perspectives of agency personnel, the consumers' view of these agencies, and existing reward systems may also limit community agencies. A large number of agencies operating in the spotlight of public accountability might also tend to shun innovative and high-risk programs such as IRR in favor of their traditional roles.

IRR as a Personal Health Care Service

Many factors argue for inclusion of IRR within existing personal health care settings. Promotion of continuity of care and improvement of the provider-client relationship are perhaps the two major rationales for implementation of IRR within the context of existing delivery settings. Economically, it may also be argued that IRR has only limited externality and that the primary beneficiary of improved health status accruing from investment in an IRR program is the individual.

There are also those who contend that any new health care development should seek to strengthen greater acceptance of the notion of individual responsibility for health and who might argue for IRR as a personal health service. Current levels of funding for the ambulatory segment of acute care might also suggest IRR initiatives within the existing personal ambulatory care framework. Where reimbursement under existing third-party arrangements is concerned, it may be argued that since it is very much like other covered services, and is consumed on an individual basis, it should be treated no differently from other covered services.

There may be additional systemwide merits of IRR as a preventive component of personal ambulatory health care services. Promotion and prevention activities currently suffer from an image that they consist largely of a group of vague, poorly defined, and usually ineffective activities and procedures. There is also a concern that most interventions that could improve health status are beyond the limited scope of the individual consumer-physician relationship. It might be hoped that IRR (as well as similarly structured programs, such as the Lifetime Health Monitoring Program) would provide a framework for strengthening other preventive practices within the personal health services sector.

' There are many limitations to the personal health service approach. The anticipation that IRR would be adopted enthusiastically by a significant proportion of primary care practitioners may also be viewed as somewhat naive. Although some preventive activities (such as pediatric immunizations and Pap smears) have been successfully implemented through the personal health care sector, other interventions (such as weight control, annual checkups, and smoking reduction) have not been particularly effective within this sector. Overmedicalization may also be a risk of those IRR programs operating in the personal health care sector because it might well place too much emphasis on the role of the practitioner at the expense of minimizing the primary role of the client in prevention.[54]

In evaluating the best method of implementing IRR on a larger scale (should it continue to prove to be effective), consideration must be given to the training and attitudes of those who will be responsible for that implementation. It should also be noted that many of the providers of personal ambulatory care service (both physician and nonphysician) may not possess the knowledge or the conceptual orientation toward IRR that would allow the best chance for success. Most fee-for-service delivery centers lack necessary counseling, education, and supportive services which would be critical to the success of IRR. Viewing past experience with other preventive services, and given no major change in incentives or attitudes, it might be expected that widespread implementation would continue to be slow and haphazard.

IRR and National Health Insurance

For some time, many practitioners hoped that national health insurance (NHI) would bring quick solutions to complex problems. It is not reasonable to believe that NHI will be a panacea that brings about sweeping changes and a preventive orientation and rationalization of the nation's health care system. Such a sudden change in the system is unlikely; it is, rather, likely that any NHI will be implemented incrementally. Accordingly, rationalization of policies and changes in resource allocation priorities are also likely to be incremental and unlikely to remold the orientation of the existing personal care nonsystem within a short period of time.

At best, prevention (and new preventive technologies) will be given an equal chance to compete for resources with acute care interventions. It is important to remember that, depending on the form of NHI, consumers and providers will change slowly, if at all. Even in many prepaid health care plans, which identify themselves as health maintenance organizations, where there is rhetoric and in many cases incentives to practice promotion, there has not been widespread utilization of preventive services.[55] Perhaps this is an indication that prevention in general, and IRR in particular, will be successful on a wide scale only after there have been significant changes in health care and in the larger social systems as well.

The Best Chance of IRR Success

To ensure lasting success, providers involved with IRR must maintain their objectivity. It is still a developing technology. It may have only limited usefulness and should be used very selectively for the present. Practitioners should be realistic in developing definitions of success. It is expected that vaccine effectiveness will approach 100 per cent. However, an IRR program may be cost effective with success rates of 25 per cent since these programs attempt to bring about significant behavioral changes, such as smoking or diet modification.[56,57]

A number of other potential problems relating to future development of IRR have been outlined by Fullarton.[58] A significant problem looming ahead is what might be called "preventive elitism." It should be kept in mind that most IRR and preventive services are more often used by the better motivated, better educated, and the well-to-do who have the option of devoting resources to health promotion.[59] Among those socioeconomic groups with other unmet immediate social and personal needs, including minimum medical care requirements, IRR will have no appeal. Implementation of preventive programs for a minority of the population should never be viewed as a substitute for a rational system that provides an appropriate mix of all health care services for everyone, regardless of ability to pay. Short-run incentives and increased resources for prevention, along with some reallocation for acute care resources, without a comprehensive restructuring of the entire health care system, will be of limited long-term benefit—especially to those who could potentially benefit the most from individual risk reduction.

As IRR is continuing in its developmental growth, continued experimentation, innovation, and evaluation are essential. Care should be taken to avoid overselling it as a cureall or preventive panacea. Creating unusual incentives might also compel practitioners and organizations who are not qualified or who do not accept the fundamental value of prevention to begin establishing IRR programs. Another danger attendant to any innovation that appears to have potential for widespread adoption within our free-market environment is overcommercialization. There should be concern about both potential overcommercialization and overselling by profit-oriented firms whose bottom line may not be improved health status. Just as professionals and health organizations seek to maintain and recognize a minimal level of quality through certification or accreditation, it is not too soon to be concerned with IRR program quality assurance.

Given society's tendency to generalize and lump programs together, if "poor results" or "rip-off" becomes synonymous with the public perception of the "risk reduction movement" (because of the misapplication by a few programs, be they profit or not, well meaning or otherwise), a tremendous potential for effective programs will be made more difficult or lost. Some mechanism to identify programs with demonstrated success or model practices (call it accreditation) is not an unrealistic goal to strive for in the near future. Clearly this is of concern to many members of the Society of Prospective Medicine.[60]

Irrespective of the potential for disease prevention by the use of IRR, no single rational system for allocation of health care dollars between acute care and preventive health services presently exists. Even if reports from well-conducted evaluations and clinical trials continue to show IRR to be associated with favorable outcomes, this preventive intervention will probably be characterized by slow acceptance within the health care community as a whole. Even in light of the importance of and potential for prevention, no sudden windfall of resources should be expected. Improved program funding and willingness of third-party payers to reimburse for health promotion services, such as IRR, will probably be incremental.

If they are to succeed, innovative program developers will probably have to be successful in educating health care providers, third-party payers, and larger purchasers of insurance, as well as the consuming public concerning the efficacy and value of IRR. Given support for programs by consumers and large purchasers of group insurance, restructuring of benefit packages by payers at the local levels is likely to include preventive benefits. Failing to develop this demand for their services, IRR programs will find it difficult to compete with existing services and other new technologies for resources.

Recognition of the competitive nature of the health care field, origin of the demand for services and an understanding of factors that regulate the development of new technologies will aid IRR program directors in securing resources and tailoring their programs to those segments of the population who are likely to benefit from them.

REFERENCES

1. U.S. Department of Health, Education, and Welfare, *Health: United States 1979.* HEW Pub. NO PHS 80-1232, Washington, D.C.: U.S. Government Printing Office, 1980, p. 184.
2. Fuchs, V., *Who Shall Live: Health Economics and Social Choice.* New York: Basic Books, 1974.
3. Gori, G. and Richter, B., "Macroeconomics of Disease Prevention in the United States. *Science* 200 (June 9, 1978), pp. 1124–1130.
4. Kristein, M., "Economic Issues in Prevention." *Preventive Medicine* 6 (June 1977), pp. 252–264.
5. Kristein, M., Arnold, C., Wynden, E., "Health Economics and Preventive Care." *Science* 200 (February 4, 1977), pp. 457–462.
6. Saward, E. and Sorenson, A., "The Current Emphasis on Preventive Medicine." *Science* 200 (May 26, 1978), pp. 889–894.
7. LaLonde, M., *New Perspective on the Health of Canadians: A Working Document.* Ottawa: Minister of Supply and Services of Canada, 1977.
8. Public Law 95-623. The Health Services Research, Health Statistics, and Health Care Technology Act of 1978. Conference Report (S. 2466). October 13, 1978.
9. U.S. Department of Health, Education, and Welfare, *Health: United States 1978.* DHEW Pub. No (PHS) 78-1232, Washington, D.C.: U.S. Government Printing Office, 1978, p. 487.
10. Gori and Richter, *Science*, p. 1126.
11. Kristein, Arnold, and Wynden, *Science*, p. 461.
12. Cooper, B. and Rice, D., "The Economic Cost of Illness Revisited." *Social Security Bulletin* 39 (February 1976), pp. 21–36.
13. Kristein, *Preventive Medicine.*
14. Gori and Richter, *Science.* pp. 1124–1130.
15. Ibid., p. 1129.
16. Rice, D. "Projection and Analysis of Health Status Trends." Presented at Annual Meeting of the American Public Health Association, Los Angeles, Calif., October 17, 1978.
17. Tsai, S., Lee, E., and Hardey, K., "The Effect of a Reduction in Leading Causes of Death: Potential Gains in Life Expectancies." *American Journal of Public Health* 68 (October 1978), pp. 966–971.
18. Dubos R., *The Mirage of Health: Utopias, Progress, and Biological Change.* Garden City, N.Y.: Anchor Books, 1959.

19. Page, I., "Is an Ounce of Prevention Worth a Pound of Abuse." *Modern Medicine* 44 (July 1, 1976), pp. 10–11.
20. Roemer, M., *Social Medicine: The Advance of Organized Health Services in America.* New York: Springer Verlag, 1978.
21. U.S. Department of Health, Education, and Welfare, *Health: United States 1979,* p. 194.
22. Gibson, R. and Fisher, C., "National Health Expenditures, Fiscal Year 1977." *Social Security Bulletin* 41 (July 1978), pp. 3–20.
23. Bauman, P. and Banta, H., "The Congress and Policy Making for Prevention." *Preventive Medicine* 6 (June 1977), pp. 227–241.
24. Breslow, L. and Somers, A. R.: "The Lifetime Health-Monitoring Program, A Practical Approach to Preventive Medicine." *New England Journal of Medicine* 296 (March 17, 1977), pp. 601–608.
25. Lee, P. and Franks, P., "Primary Prevention and the Executive Branch of Government." *Preventive Medicine* 6 (June 1978), pp. 209–226.
26. Ibid., p. 225.
27. DeLozien, J., *National Ambulatory Medical Care Survey, 1973 Summary, May 1973–April, 1974.* '(*Vital and Health Statistics: Series 13, Data from the National Health Survey: No. 21*) DHEW Publication (HRA) 76-1772. Washington, D.C.: U.S. Government Printing Office, 1976, pp. 23–24. Note: To estimate the number of physician office visits which were preventive visits during the National Ambulatory Medical Care Survey, cases with nonsymptomatic codes 900, 904, 997, 906, and residual nonsymptomatic visits were used (p. 23).
28. Hetherington, R., Hopkins, C., and Roemer, M., *Health Insurance Plans: Promise and Performance.* New York: John Wiley & Sons, 1975.
29. Weinerman, E., "Research into the organization of Medical Practice." In *Organizational Issues in the Delivery of Health Services*, I. Zola, and J. McKinley, eds. New York: Prodist, 1974, pp. 29–65.
30. Breslow and Somers, *New England Journal of Medicine,* p. 607.
31. Ibid., p. 601.
32. Blackburn, H., "Medical Economics, Professional Attitudes and Chronic Disease Prevention." *Minnesota Medicine* 60 (November 1977), pp. 821–823.
33. Page, *Modern Medicine.*
34. Breslow and Somers, *New England Journal of Medicine*, pp. 601–608.
35. Lave, J. and Lave, L., "Measuring the Effectiveness of Prevention: I." *Milbank Memorial Fund Quarterly* 55 (Spring 1977), pp. 263–289.
36. Public Law 95–623.
37. J. E. Fogarty International Center of the National Institutes of Health, *Preventive Medicine U.S.A.* New York: Prodist, 1976.
38. Somers, A. R. and Somers, H. M., "A Proposed Framework for Health and Health Care Policies." *Inquiry* 14 (June 1977), pp. 115–170.
39. Lave, J. and Lave, L., "Measuring the Effectiveness of Prevention: I." *Milbank Memorial Fund Quarterly* 55 (Spring 1977), pp. 263–289.
40. U.S. Congress Office of Technology Assessment, *Assessing the Efficacy and Safety of Medical Technologies.* Washington, D.C.: U.S. Government Printing Office, 1978.
41. Public Law 95–623.
42. Schweitzer, S., "Cost Effectiveness of Early Disease Detection." *Health Service Research* 9 (Spring 1974), pp. 22–32.
43. Collen, M. et al., "Multiphasic Check-up Evaluation Study: 4, Preliminary Cost Benefit Analysis for Middle Aged Member." *Preventive Medicine* 2 (Spring 1973), pp. 236–246.
44. Farquhar, J. et al., "Community Education for Cardiovascular Health." *Lancet* I (June 1977), pp. 1192–1195.
45. Breslow, L., "Risk Factor Intervention for Health Maintenance." *Science* 200 (May 1978), pp. 908–912.

46. Kristein, *Preventive Medicine*, p. 281.
47. Shapiro, S., "Measuring the Effectiveness of Prevention: I." *Milbank Memorial Fund Quarterly* 55 (Spring 1977), pp. 291–306.
48. Breslow and Somers, *New England Journal of Medicine.*
49. Tresnowski, B., "To Pay or Not to Pay." Presentation Before the American Public Health Association, Session 4038, Los Angeles, Calif., October 18, 1978.
50. Health Insurance Association of America, *Health Care in the 1980's.* Washington, D.C.: Health Insurance Institute, 1978.
51. Ehrenfried, D., Blue Cross and Blue Shield Association, telephone conversation, October 3, 1979.
52. Bauman and Banta *Preventive Medicine.*
53. Ardell, D., "High Level Wellness and the HSA: A Health Planning Success Story." *American Journal of Health Planning* 3 (July 1978), pp. 1–18.
54. Fullarton, J., "Health Hazard Appraisal: Its Limitations and Directions for Risk Assessment." In *Proceedings of the 13th Annual Meeting of the Society of Prospective Medicine.* Bethesda, Md.: Health Education Resources, October 1–3, 1976, pp. 6–10.
55. Axelrod, S. et al., *Medical Care Chartbook*, 6th ed. Ann Arbor: University of Michigan Bureau of Public Health Economics, Department of Medical Care Organizations, 1976.
56. Kristein, *Preventive Medicine.*
57. Cohen, C. and Cohen, E., "Health Education: Panacea, Pernicious, or Pointless (editorial). *New England Journal of Medicine* 299 (September 28, 1978), pp. 718–720.
58. Fullarton, *Proceedings of the 13th Annual Meeting of the Society of Prospective Medicine.*
59. Eisenber, L., "The Perils of Prevention: A Cautionary Note" (editorial). *New England Journal of Medicine* 297 (December 1, 1977), pp. 1230–1232.
60. Hettler, W., Janty, C., and Moffat, C., "A Comparison of Seven Methods of Health Hazard Appraisal." In *Proceedings of the 13th Annual Meeting of the Society of Prospective Medicine* Bethesda, Md.: October 1–3, 1976, Health Education Resources, pp. 36–39.

22 / Sharing Responsibility:
The New Health Care Partnership

Marilyn M. Faber, M.A., M.H.A.

THE CONCEPT OF SHARING RESPONSIBILITY

Currently in this country, many individuals are beginning to approach health from a changed perspective. In the recent past, responsibility for health had been given over primarily to professionals, with very little prescribed to the persons receiving the health care. In many quarters, medical care is dramatically changing its direction as individuals are beginning to question the heretofore inalienable authority of health professionals and are now asking to share some of the responsibility.

One of the most noteworthy of these changes has been the self-care movement, the name given to the increase in lay health initiatives, which has soared dramatically during the last 10 years. Levin[1] defines self-care as "the self-initiated and self-controlled application of knowledge necessary to the promotion of health, reduction of undesired risk, self-diagnosis and treatment of disease, and where appropriate, the effective and self-protected use of professional health and medical resources." Many health workers see the widespread adoption of this focus on the individual as absolutely crucial to health promotion and risk reduction for the future. Increased participation by the individual is equally important during illness as it can affect in many ways the progress of the illness and aid in restoration to a healthful state. It can also help reduce the risk of iatrogenesis.

Increased participation by the patient (now increasingly called client or consumer) is seen by most as a positive phenomenon rather than a negative reaction to doctors. People are beginning to realize the essential role they have to play in their own health and are desirous of acquiring independence, dignity, and a feeling of self-control. This change in attitudes has come about as a result of a number of developments in our society. It was after World War II that the years of medical "miracles" began. Vaccines, antibiotics, surgical techniques, and complex diagnostic technologies were developed and had such a profound impact on the health care system that people placed all their confidence in the medical establishment.[2] This golden age began to fade with the realization that these marvels could not wipe out viral infection, cancer, or heart disease. Whereas in the past most diseases were of the acute kind (scarlet fever, polio, diphtheria), these have been superseded by the chronic diseases (arthritis, diabetes, hypertension, heart disease) which now make up 80 per cent of all diseases. Such chronic conditions are more amenable to responsible individual interventions.

The changes in the social structure of society (civil rights and women's movements)[3] and the disillusionment with institutions, governmental and otherwise, along with trends toward depersonalization have helped provide the impetus toward individual self-determinism in many areas including health. Additionally, there has been the gradual recognition that there is a great deal wrong with doctors and medicine as Illich[4] and Carlson[5] have summarized in their landmark books. Illich cites the unsettling statistic that one of every five patients admitted to a typical research hospital acquires an iatrogenic disease, which is usually trivial, but in one case in 30 leads to death. Half of these episodes result from complications of drug therapy; and, amazingly, one in ten is caused by diagnostic procedures. Carlson urges us to learn to care for ourselves using providers as resources without becoming dependent on them and to realize that medicine has very little to do with health. We have been allowing organized medicine to define "quality" of care without reference to patient outcomes. The patients should now provide input into the evaluation of the quality of care they receive. Carlson defines an "emerging zeitgeist," as our society changes in a direction complementary to self-care and people become willing and eager to deliver their own care.

Although many health professionals do not share the extreme views of these authors, most will acknowledge that there are at least some tasks in which patients can share. It is often reported that about 70 per cent of all first visits to primary care physicians waste the time of the physician and the patient because they concern self-limiting diseases, such as the common cold, that will go away with no physician intervention. Sometimes these illnesses are actually mistreated with antibiotics which are ineffective for viral infections. Patients themselves can treat many of these (more than one half, some believe) common ailments and injuries as well as doctors can, thus reducing their medical visits and costs significantly. In some cases, though, self-care might cause appropriate doctor visits where they would have been neglected in the past. Thirty per sent of patients seen should have visited the doctor sooner. Thus it is not avoidance of doctors that is necessary, but proper use of them. This reduced and more efficient use of professional resources will contribute to lowering runaway health care costs and, indeed, it is this latter impetus which may provide the most significant motivation toward increased consumer responsibility and participation. Consumer interest in health care has exploded as witness the myriad self-care books now on the market as well as the popularity of jogging, yoga, and natural foods.[6]

HISTORICAL ANTECEDENTS TO THE MODERN SELF-CARE MOVEMENT

The self-care movement appears to be a radical concept to many at this time but it is actually a recurrence of a similar happening in the nineteenth century. Physicians in the early 1800s had no concept of infection and subjected ill people to drastic procedures such as bloodletting, blistering, mercury purgatives, and arsenic tonics; whose purpose was to cleanse the system of the illness. Many people succumbed to these treatments and those who recovered did so in spite of them.[7] Eventually, an aroused public rebelled and began to support a farmer-turned-root-and-herb-doctor. Samuel Thomson eschewed the use of all harmful materials, and advocated gentle remedies such as herbs and teas, and espoused many commonsense ideas for the treatment and prevention of illness. He wrote a book, the *New Guide to Health*,[8] which was published in 1832 and eventually sold over 100,000 copies and went through 13 editions. The success of the book was due to its exploitation of the publics' concern over rising medical expenses as well as their fear of harmful medical practices by traditional physicians. Thomson's solution to the problem was for patients to "depend more upon themselves, and less upon the doctors," especially in cases of "trifling sickness," by purchasing his book and using it for self-instruction. The Thomsonian movement spread rapidly as herbal medical societies were established and his method soon represented not only a therapeutic system but a social movement, a popular revolt against the medicine of the day.

A few years later, in 1858, W. A. Alcott, M.D., published *The Home Book of Life and Health*,[9] which contained ideas that might have been written today: "But another right use of physicians consists in requiring them to give public instruction . . . on the best means of promoting . . . health." However, he acknowledged the unlikelihood of this occurring as "physicians are not taught . . . the laws of health" and it is not part of the course of study in medical schools. This is certainly a present-day criticism of the medical profession by those in the self-care movement.

It is also worth emphasizing that those of us who recoil in horror at the barbaric nineteenth century medical practices need only think for a moment of present-day medical care and certain parallels become obvious: the occasional excess use of antibiotics, X-rays, surgical, and diagnostic procedures, often with ill effects show us that even in this modern age we have not come as far as we might have in reducing our own harmful medical practices.

Similar themes can also be found in the high cost of medical care, its elitist nature, the trend toward the application of commonsense remedies, the restoration of personal autonomy, and the value of shared participation. The flavor of the Thomsonian movement is surprisingly contemporary and provides some perspective for the current self-care literature and the self-care movement in general.

Resistance by some health professionals to increased development of self-care may, of course, be expected for many reasons.[10] In the first place, professionals may resist the perceived invasion of their areas of expertise. They may feel that if self-care practices include functions which had formerly been in their exclusive domain, there will be nothing left for them to do and their economic position will be threatened. This is unrealistic. Primary care providers may indeed be called upon to transfer some of their present functions to patients, but they will then undertake alternative or supplementary functions including education. They will also have more time to devote to serious cases. In addition, many might perceive self-care as an opportunity to enhance their professional status, by transferring many routine tasks which carry only modest economic or social rewards. If properly designed, self-care should be beneficial to physicians as well as to patients since the former will be more comfortable in the knowledge that self-care educated patients will be more self-protective and more able to share responsibility for the outcomes of medical care.

Levin[11] says that professionals must recognize assumptions that are new to their education and previous experience, mainly that people have the intelligence to make many of their health decisions themselves. Indeed, on a quite elementary level, some type of self-care is commonly practiced by the majority of people. The next task is to expand this. An extensive study of existing research conducted by the Center for Health Administration Studies at the University of Chicago[12] found some growth in consumer self-confidence regarding health matters and a growing criticism of professional motivation and the quality of health care. There is "apparently ample public interest in programs where people learn to take responsibility for more of their own care, and generally the results—the ability of people to apply the learning successfully—are believed to be positive." It was noted that the most likely followers of the movement are those who are young, white, suburban, educated, and financially secure.

As to whether individuals are capable of performing functions usually done by the doctor, one can note the diabetics who have been trained to give themselves insulin injections, the kidney patients who have learned to operate complex dialysis machines, and the hypertension patients who have been taught to monitor their own blood pressures at home. Opportunity is much greater now for individual involvement in diagnostic tests with the recent availability of home pregnancy tests, nitrate dipsticks, and dip-culture slides for home detection of urinary tract infections, and portable blood glucose meters for diabetics.

Self-care and increased self-responsibility can be the focus of various groups as well as of the individual. One location for learning of self-care techniques is within the family itself. Pratt[13] discusses the "energized family structure" which describes a family which actively seeks information, makes discriminating choices, and negotiates assertively with the health care system. The importance of teaching self-care practices to the urban poor, who are among the most disadvantaged in functioning within the present health care system, has been discussed by Milio.[14] This area presents some of the greatest challenges.

Other target groups for increasing participation are children and the elderly, sample programs for whom are discussed later in this chapter.

THE DOCTOR-PATIENT (CLIENT) RELATIONSHIP

The subject of enhancing communication between doctor and patient is not a new one. During the days when patients went to one doctor for all their ills this was not as much of a problem as it is currently in the age of superspecialization and fragmentation of medical care. It is also developing that the necessary improved communication be on a different level, an equal one. Previously, instructions to physicians were confined to advice to "listen" to the patient, accept and understand his or her feelings, not to judge, and try to read body language.[15] If today's patients are to become partners in their own health care, many more aspects must be addressed.

During the course of an illness and its traditional treatment, most patients experience feelings of loss of control, powerlessness, and a lack of predictability.[16] These are all common occurrences in the traditional active-passive physician-patient relationship. Such a relationship is appropriate for some medical situations (emergencies, trauma, surgery) but not all. The situation in which two parties are mutually involved in the effective management of a health problem is an "adult-adult" communication. Schain[17] says "this type of interaction should reinforce the qualities of individuality, autonomy, and personal dignity for the patient as well as preserve a high level of regard for the skills, opinions, and expertise of the physician." Of course, a relationship of this nature is dependent upon the patient acquiring an adequate amount of relevant knowledge. There are many opinions on how this should be done, and each situation will be different. Questions to be considered by the physician include what information to dispense at what time and in what manner.

In addition to direct verbal dispensing of information, the physician might maintain in the waiting room a bulletin board for health education articles and a patient library with literature on specific diseases, as well as a health encyclopedia and appropriate books on self-care.[18] In the consulting room, anatomy models and illustrations of diseases along with a PDR for patient use might be made available.

Obviously, this kind of mutual participation would not be appropriate for all patients, but it can be used with many more than it is currently allowed with most resources being made available for use at the patient's discretion. Cues should be taken from the attitude projected by the patient. Schain classifies patients as either "Monitors" (information seekers) or "Blunters" (information avoiders). "Monitors" will often have acquired much information on their own and actively request more, while "Blunters" will leave all decisions up to the doctor.

In the past, physicians often classify patients with "Monitor" characteristics as demanding[19] and praise what they call the "good patient" who is conforming, dependent, and ingratiating. Glogow[20] feels, however, that faster recovery may occur for the "bad patient" who is "characterized as aggressive, bold, and defiant, has a driving desire to recover and does so more quickly"; and that perhaps the labels of "good" and "bad" should be reversed if illness outcome is used as the criterion.

A patient who is involved significantly in the management of an illness may be less likely to hold the physician responsible when the desired outcomes are not achieved. Ross Egger,[21] a family physician in Daleville, Indiana, says that his patients are involved in their care to the degree that if they wanted to sue him, they would also have to sue themselves: "Once a patient becomes involved in his illness, he shares the responsibility for his treatment and the outcome."

Communication is usually considered something that comes naturally and doesn't require any special skill. This is not the case, however, as all of its elements must be understood if it is to be successful. For example, communication is a circular process and requires feedback in order to be complete. Because patients are usually under stress when they are receiving information about their illness, it has been recommended that the doctor use the three-step plan used by good speakers who want their audience to remember the message.[22] They tell the listeners what they are going to tell them; then they tell them; finally, they tell them what they have told them. Other techniques for communicating information can be learned.

Beyond eliciting feedback from the patient, the physician can initiate a mutually written listing of important problems. This has been found to correlate highly with patient satisfaction. Patient awareness that a doctor attempted to negotiate differences between them has been found to correlate more positively than with symptom relief.[23]

Since so much of the success of patient self-responsibility depends on its adoption by physicians, much more research needs to be conducted on the attitudes of physicians and other health care providers toward teaching self-care techniques to patients and on provider behavior, that is, what the provider actually does about encouraging consumer-initiated treatment.[24]

GIVING THE PATIENTS THEIR MEDICAL RECORDS

In 1973, an article appeared in the *New England Journal of Medicine* by Budd Shenkin and David Warner[25] on the subject of giving copies of complete medical records (physician and hospital) to patients. This article was widely discussed and became quite well known for its radical thesis. At this writing, the feeling in the general medical community has changed little if at all and the subject of complete disclosure to patients of all relevant facts including physician qualifications still strikes terror in the heart of conservative medical practitioners. However, with this greater exposure of heretofore unpublicized information, there would certainly be a more definite incentive to practice high-quality medicine. Many other advantages would result. The record would serve to educate the patient as well as to provide a complete available history of all medical procedures conducted and drugs administered. The "whole-person" could always be "seen at a glance" by physicians consulted later on who read the record.

A study of record sharing with patients conducted at the University of Vermont noted that "97 of 100 randomly chosen patients felt less worried about their own health after reviewing their records."[26] Positive results were also noted in areas of compliance with medication requirements and life-style change. These patients went beyond reading their record and actually had the opportunity to "audit" the care received. The patient actively agreed or disagreed with the history as written, and reviewed and evaluated the plans for clarity.

It was noted that patients were somewhat reluctant to do this auditing on their own and appeared to be reluctant to question the physician's judgment and understanding. Physicians, on the other hand, found the experience to be highly positive and eventually were able to share records with many more patients than they had originally estimated. The doctors "discovered that honesty between physician and patient leads to better communication, which, in turn, helps the patient to deal more effectively with his problem." They also noted great improvement in their own performances as a result of the performance-based audit and found that as patients showed greater understanding of health problems, they were "more comfortable about giving them increased responsibility for self-management of chronic health problems."

Similar positive results were found at the University of Massachusetts Health Service where a Personal Life Health Plan was utilized.[27] This record contained, in addition to what can be found in a medical record, a past health history, a family health history, tables of individualized risks of morbidity (a health hazard appraisal—see Chapter 3), and a health maintenance plan. All of this material was held by the patient and results showed a high degree of usage of it by the patient.

CHRONIC DISEASE AND THE NEW HEALTH CARE PARTNERSHIP—CONTRACTING FOR HEALTH

Long-term treatments are usual today in which informed patient participation is essential for effective control. Some health professionals take the management of a chronic disease one step further and set up a written contract to be signed by the patient, physician, and other involved health workers. It provides a concrete form for the establishment of goals. This technique of patient participation has been popularized by Donnell Etzwiler[30] who has used it extensively in his Diabetes Education Center in Minneapolis. A mutually signed contract immediately creates a situation whereby the patient experiences a sense of control.[31] The contract basically defines the responsibilities and tasks of both parties in the management of an individual's health problem. It can be made formal or informal as desired. It can also be open-ended and renegotiable by either party at any time.[32] Expectations by the physician may be raised or lowered as necessary.

In many of these contracts, a form of reward is chosen by the patient if the desired behavior is carried out. In one study (hypertension) the patients were encouraged to choose tangible rewards over and above praise. A frequently chosen reward (in addition to books, money, magazines) was more time with the health provider.[33]

Contracts have also been found to be useful with persons who do not yet have a chronic disease but who are at high risk. The Well Aware About Health project discussed in Chapter 20 of this book describes a health improvement plan contract which identifies at least one negative behavior, sets goals for changing that behavior, and lists educational sessions the participant will attend. Additionally, as many of the chronic diseases are life-style induced, the patient needs to become involved in health maintenance well before the appearance of any symptoms.

The diseases which lend themselves to individual attempts at prevention as well as patient participation in their treatment include cancer, heart disease, diabetes, arthritis, obesity, alcoholism, respiratory diseases, renal disease, hypertension, and mental illness.

Hypertension was one of the first of the chronic diseases to lend itself to active participation by the patient. Studies have shown that patients who are active in their treatment are more likely to have their blood pressures under control, to understand their
treatment plan, and to follow through on recommendations.[28] Some hypertension
health workers, in defining critical patient behaviors in high blood pressure control, go
even further and view the patient as the decision maker and problem solver, with the
professional functioning as advisor and guide. In a study conducted for the National
Heart, Lung, and Blood Institute,[29] patients were rated on knowledge, attitude, and
skill for critical behaviors such as making the decision to control blood pressure, taking
medication as prescribed, and resolving problems that block achieving blood pressure
control. In making the decision to control blood pressure, the patient demonstrates
that he or she is ultimately in charge.

A similar contract was utilized with health professionals who had high-risk life-style
behaviors.[34] Subsequent to an administered health hazard appraisal, the participants
signed formal contracts (drawn up by an attorney) with the Utah Public Health Association. The individual wrote into the contract those self-determined changes deemed
necessary to reduce his or her risk for disease. A self-determined penalty in case of failure was also written in. The most frequently contracted for changes were for exercise
programs and weight reduction. Others were increased wearing of seat belts, eliminating
junk foods, breast self-examination, and more sleep. Of the 75 participants, 21 were
100 per cent successful and 56 (or 75 per cent) accomplished 50 per cent or more of
their contracted changes.

MENTAL HEALTH AND INCREASED SELF-RESPONSIBILITY

by Raymond A. Faber, M.D.

The treatment contract as well as all of the principles of patient sharing of responsibility, is particularly applicable to the fields of psychiatry and psychology.

For those health professionals who are mental health workers (psychiatrists, psychologists, nurses, social workers, and other counselors) the patient-provider partnership
provides particular opportunities to optimize maintaining and achieving a high level
of mental health. Utilizing a "customer" approach, the patient and clinician can mutually set appropriate goals and then negotiate how best to reach these goals.[35-37]

A written treatment contract has been proposed by Rosen[38] and endorsed by
others[39] as an effective means of involving psychiatry patients in their own care. The
contract contains five sections: treatment goals, time parameters, specific treatment
methods and personnel, the patient's role, and signing of the contract by all involved
parties. In negotiating the treatment goals the nature of the therapeutic relationship
becomes more equal as the patient gets the opportunity to make choices regarding
treatments offered. Goals need to be stated very specifically and clearly. The negotiation of such a contract can in itself be very therapeutic. By taking on more of a
consumer role, the patient gains a sense of mastery, which all too often is list in the
forced dependency of traditional treatment approaches which often result in demorali-
zation and helplessness.

As a prelude to a contract, an interesting concept has been described wherein patients
are first educated about their conditions in a hospital classroom setting.[40]

When suicide is a risk, a verbal contract can help monitor its seriousness.[41] The patient is asked to state and mean, "I will not kill myself." This is qualified with the sec-

ond aspect of their contract, "until." Immediate plans can then be made according to the patient's ability to make the contract for a given time period.

The patient who threatens suicide and accosts the therapist with "and what are you going to do about it" must be helped to assume responsibility for his or her actions which cannot be abrogated to a therapist or anyone else.[42]

In the field of behavior therapy patient-provider contracts are a standard tool. Such contracts allow for the identification of very specific problems. Successful use of contracts has been reported in treating obesity, smoking, obsessive-compulsive disorders, and marital discord.

In dealing with obesity, smoking, or obsessive-compulsive disorders, quantification of the problem and treatment goals are easily accomplished (such as number of cigarettes smoked or number of rituals performed in a time period).[43] Being able to monitor their problems often is a cause for patient optimism, as they are then able to "rise above" the problem by writing it down. In abiding by a contract, patients learn self-discipline, achieve their specific goals, and contingency rewards, and gain new self-awareness that they are not helpless victims.

Marital discord is a somewhat more complex issue. Here the clinician is a third party who monitors a contract between the couple, and change comes about by reinforcing targeted behaviors.[44]

No single aspect of mental health care demands more patient responsibility than psychotherapy. In fact, the patient may do a more substantial part of the "work" involved than the therapist. One of the major strategies in psychotherapy is for the patient to accept responsibility for his or her behavior and subsequent predicament. This may be easy in terms of earnest verbalization, but too often the patient pays only lip service to being responsible and it is a major obstacle to truly understand and accept his or her role in personal problems.

Collaboration and cooperation are critical elements in successful psychotherapy.[45] In no way can a therapist impose truth on the patient without the patient's shaping that truth, and only when the patient is so inclined. This phenomenon of resistance is only too well known and universal. It is only when the patient realizes his or her role in the initiation and maintenance of symptoms, that he or she can in turn do something to alleviate the dilemma. The patient's hope for cure comes with the realization that he or she is not a passive victim but the latent healer of his or her illness.

Patient participation in medication treatment decisions can help minimize the dose of medication to which patients are exposed, thus allowing for optimal outcome with minimal risk. It has been demonstrated that patients used less Valium when they could get it on demand than when they were assigned a fixed dosage regimen.[46] This suggests that when patients are active participants in their treatment and hence taking less medication, they may be at lower risk for abusing and becoming dependent on such medication. Additionally, the daily timing of doses may be left up to patients receiving antidepressants. If daytime anxiety is especially troublesome, several daily doses may be optimal, whereas if insomnia is a major difficulty, a single nightime dose may work best.

PROGRAMS EMPHASIZING INDIVIDUAL PARTICIPATION IN HEALTH

The first and best known of the medical self-care courses was started in Virginia in 1970.[47] The Course for Activated Patients taught patients how to handle common illnesses and injuries, how to use the health care system appropriately (consumerism), to increase their knowledge about health problems and health promotion, and to accept more responsibility for their own and their families self-care. The classes included not only didactic lectures but also demonstrations, experiments, role playing and field trips, and other active involvement. It was discovered during these courses that many skills previously in the domain only of the health professional were able to be learned by lay persons. Persons learned, for example, to monitor vital signs (blood pressure, pulse, temperature, respiration rate) and to describe and record them, and what appropriate actions and treatments were then advisable.

These courses proved so popular that many health professionals in other parts of the country started similar programs and there are now hundreds in most states in the United States and Canada.

The Health Activation Network located in Vienna, Virginia, and a product of the original courses, offers periodic meetings designed to teach persons to start their own courses and acts as a clearinghouse for self-care classes nationwide.

An example of a project set up to deal with a particular health problem is the Cold Self-Care Center, developed at the University of Massachusetts Student HMO at Amherst.[48]

In non-HMO settings colds often never reach professional attention but in prepaid situations, there is frequent use of professional resources for these self-limiting illnesses. Therefore, much motivation exists in an HMO for a method for efficient and effective (nonprofessional, if possible) care of minor, uncomplicated colds. The Center at the University of Massachusetts promotes active decision making by consumers, emphasizes the self-limited nature of the illness, and teaches the limitations of cold medications. The consumers are helped to decide whether they have just a common cold or need professional care; if self-care is feasible, they are taught how to exercise it. After 2 years of implementation of this project, it was determined that a saving in patient visits had occurred of over 2,500 per year. A consumer survey determined that 20 per cent of users referred themselves for professional care for their next cold. It was thus inferred that the Cold Self-Care Center clarified the criteria for seeking professional care and increased confidence in self-care.

Among self-care teaching programs described in the literature, some are concerned with a particular malady (diabetic, hypertension, arthritis, preventive gynecology, self-medication for asthmatics, gonorrhea self-screening, kidney disease, throat-culture), and others are comprehensive as is the Course for Activated Patients in Virginia. Some of the activities which have been taught in classes are insulin injection, urine testing, breast self-examination, cervical self-examination, taking blood pressures, taking throat cultures, ear wax irrigation, kidney dialysis, physical therapy for arthritis, hyposentization injections, first aid for common injuries, and emergency care.[49]

Increased responsibility is also a learnable and valuable tool for children as well as adults, as was demonstrated by a project conducted at the UCLA elementary school with first-, third-, and sixth-graders, to study the behavior of children who are involved with their own health care.[50] Sick children who referred themselves to the school nurse were given a report of their health exam and were then asked to select one of several treatment plans. It was found that they usually made the most appropriate choice of treatments. Each was then allowed to choose the immediate steps to be taken (going home, lying down, returning to class). Most of these choices were also appropriate. This study demonstrates that children also have the ability to participate in their own care.

In another study, which emphasized teaching self-help medical skills to children, a survey before and after was taken of the children asking them to choose the person most responsible for maintaining their health: "mother, doctor, teacher, or myself." Before the study only 21 chose "myself," but at the conclusion of the study, the figure had increased to 85 per cent.[51]

In many public and private schools health education is assuming a new position of importance and is no longer taught as an afterthought by gym teachers.[52] The new curricula often utilize the school nurse or doctor as a teacher and use the actual illness experiences of children as learning opportunities. Children are capable of learning a great many of the same skills that adults learn in their self-care courses. An example of an excellent health education program was conducted at the Mary Hooker School in Hartford, Connecticut.[53] This program incorporates the existing medical and dental clinic services provided for the children. The children actually participate in their own care and as "helping paraprofessionals" in the care of fellow students. With the aid of staff doctors, the children learn how to read throat cultures and recognize symptoms of many disorders that require a clinic visit. In the dental program, children hand instruments to the dentists and help prepare fillings. In these programs children react quite positively to being included in the previously forbidden world of doctors and are eager to learn things about which they have always been curious. Home programs include teaching children how to use the instruments in the "Black Bag" and even provide stethoscopes for them.

Some physicians hold adult self-care classes for their own patients in their offices. Dr. Walt Stoll of Lexington, Kentucky, teaches his students 300 "protocols" that tell them all they need to know about many illnesses and injuries. He provides each client with a 30-page booklet which spells out doctor's and client's responsibilities and includes information on how his clients can most effectively use him as a tool in their own health care. It includes a complete listing of free emergency phone numbers, information on appointments, phone calls, insurance, and other office procedures. It also includes a self-care guide to the dozen problems most frequently seen in Dr. Stoll's practice.

Dr. Keith Sehnert incorporated much of the subject matter from his Activated Patient Course in one of the first self care books entitled *How to Be Your Own Doctor (Sometimes)*.[54] He advocated that patients acquire a black bag of their own and become familiar with the contents. Many similar books by physicians and other health professionals then followed.[55-59]

The Southwest Medical Plan, an HMO in San Antonio, Texas, dispenses free of charge to all members a copy of the self-care book *Take Care of Yourself*[60] by Donald H. Vickery and James F. Fries when these members attend an orientation session.

A study reported by Dr. Steven Moore, an internist in Seattle, Washington, found that when groups of patients were given self-care books to study and seminars on self-care, their physician visits dropped significantly. The most significant findings were for the visits for coughs, colds, and sore throats, down 15 per cent.[61]

The area of patient self-medication has received special attention both as a means of improving regimen compliance and because of its controversial nature. On March 31, 1980, a symposium in Washington, D.C., was held by 12 authorities in the field of self-medication.[62] Speakers included physicians, economists, pharmacists, consumers, and representatives of the drug industry and the Food and Drug Administration. It was generally acknowledged that certainly self-medication is not a new phenomenon, but what is new is a professional acknowledgment that it does exist and it has always been an important way in which individuals have tried to improve their health. Over-the-counter (OTC) agents do provide definitive medical care in many instances. In fact, it was held that the status of many prescription drugs could be changed so that consumers could obtain them on their own. Examples mentioned were typical acne antibiotic solutions and tar products for control of psoriasis. What is needed is more education and more information on OTC drug labels (such as complete lists of ingredients, information about possible side effects, contraindications). Education should, of course, include the point that there may not be a medication for every unpleasantness. What is also needed is a return to the previously held theories of training pharmacists to aid persons in self-care. Pharmacists can give consumers advice about OTC products. They can also funtion in a triage manner, that is, advising when an OTC product might not provide relief and the person should see a physician, or whether, perhaps, no drug is required at all.

In the area of prescription drugs and appropriate compliance, it has long been shown that patients' inappropriate use of medications has caused higher hospitalization rates and increased visits to physicians. In a study conducted at United Hospitals, St. Paul, Minnesota, "inpatients self-administered their medication under the supervision of hospital staff members so that they could be familiar with their medications after they left the hospital."[63] Education and positive reinforcement was also given. A follow-up study after discharge showed that the program had substantially improved patient compliance with medication regimens. An approach such as this is more realistic than including patients in the standard "Here, swallow this!" routine and then expecting instant home compliance with what might be, for the patient, a complicated regimen.

An approach such as this is even more important with the largest group of self-medicators: the elderly. Many individuals in this group have one or more chronic illnesses that require several medications; and many also have failing memories, hearing, and sight which make learning and implementing appropriate self-medication difficult. Education is particularly important for these patients and an example of an excellent program in this area is being conducted at Augustana Hospital in Chicago.[64] The program consists mainly of organizing the seniors into groups to provide information to combat the most common and potentially dangerous self-medication habits (overusing OTC drugs, taking medicines irregularly, sharing medicines with friends, saving old medicines, doubling dosages for faster relief).

Programs for teaching persons to take more responsibility for their own health are proliferating in widely scattered areas of the health care system. While many are in already established traditional care such as HMOS, some have been set up purely for the purpose of promoting health.

The Common Health Club in Santa Rosa, California was established through an initial grant from the Department of Health, Education and Welfare (DHEW) but is now self-sufficient. It is a nonprofit program with 4,000 members and provides low-cost screening tests and general health education. It sees itself as complementary to the physician-centered health care system which provides diagnosis and treatment. The club is not itself affiliated directly with any medical group, hospital, or other health organization. Its emphasis is on self-responsibility and positive life-style changes and toward these goals includes multiphasic testing, blood tests, x-rays, EKGs, fitness tests, stress reduction classes, transactional analysis classes, a common health problems class, a home physical examination class, and a health hazard appraisal. Consumer skills are also taught to aid in making efficient use of the health care delivery system.

Some HSAs are taking quite an active role in health promotion (see Chapter 19). The Western Massachusetts HSA in West Springfield, Massachusetts, has even established a regional health promotion center to provide consumer services. Lifeways serves health and nonhealth service agencies, schools, and government with the goal of promoting the general well-being in the region. Some of their projects include an alcohol abuse prevention program, an auto safety media campaign, stress workshops, health education for schools, and health information workshops and seminars.

Among HMOs the Arizona Health Plan in Phoenix, Arizona, is a good example of a "health surveillance program" which is designed to keep people healthy from the point at which they first join. Their classes (24 in all) include holistic health, assertiveness training, heart risk factors, relaxation skills, contraception, understanding depression, and many classes dealing with individual diseases. Evaluation of all members includes a risk appraisal questionnaire which is followed up by counseling with a trained nurse practitioner. Enrollment is then scheduled for the relevant courses. The goal of this method, which is designed for the well patient, is to retain the participation of those who are well and avoid the costly shift of membership toward those who have chronic illnesses.

Organizations set up by consumers for promoting individual self-health responsibility are very much in evidence at this writing. The Health Research Group in Washington, D.C., formed out of a collaboration between Ralph Nader and Dr. Sidney Wolfe, its current director, is well known for its many victories for consumers by playing the role of watchdog for health issues. One of their current efforts concerns an attempt to make public PSRO ratings for doctors so that consumers could see which doctors and hospitals provide the best care. Some of their publications include *A Guide for Compiling a Directory of Physicians, Getting Yours: A Consumer's Guide to Obtaining Your Medical Records*, and *Trimming the Fat Off Health Care Costs: A Consumer's Guide to Taking Over Health Planning*.

Other consumer organizations are the Consumer Coalition for Health (Washington, D.C.), a clearinghouse for information on how consumers can analyze their local health institutions and implement new programs; The National Women's Health Network (Washington, D.C.), active in many women-consumer issues; the Center for Medical Consumers and Health Care Information (New York City), which sponsors a library and newsletter and helps consumers make informed health care decisions by providing them with an accurate, independent source of health information; and the coalition for the Medical Rights of Women (San Francisco), which is working to improve medical care for women through grassroots action.

An example of a consumer group on a local level is the Consumers' Health Group in Evanston, Illinois. Among the goals of its 1,000 members are to assist individuals to devise and use their own resources for maintaining health and to encourage and support a knowledgeable public. Among their activities are the compiling of a Directory of Evanston Primary Care Physicians, a senior citizens health maintenance program which aims to make the older person a working partner in the maintenance of his or her health, a series of workshops (nutrition, home health care, hearing problems), and a school health project (similar to and suggested by the "Know Your Body" program discussed in Chapter 13).

INDIVIDUAL RESPONSIBILITY FOR HEALTH AND THE FUTURE

The concepts discussed here are not new, but general acceptance and implementation of them is far from widespread at this point. Attitudes cannot be changed overnight and it would be unrealistic to expect habit and beliefs that took 50 years to become established to be easily changed. Indeed, many professionals will not be moved at all, such as the doctor who recently wrote that the personal encounter between physician and patient is necessarily marked by authoritarianism, paternalism, and domination, and that these are essential to good medical care.[65] Some physicians, however, do see the inevitability of patient responsibility for health though they don't necessarily welcome it; a headline in the December 1980 issue of *Clinical Psychiatry News* read "Physicians' Biggest Competition Predicted to Come from Patients."[66] Then there are the physicians and health professionals, such as the contributors to this text and most of those cited in this chapter, who feel that patients should be equal participants in their care and should be educated to take better care of themselves.

Beyond the greater individual desire to influence one's own health, a major motivating factor will be one of economic self-defense on the part of government and business. This year employers will spend $63 billion on health insurance for workers and their dependents; 5 years ago they spent only $15 billion.[67] Lower cost alternatives are going to be eagerly sought out and government and business will become deeply involved with health promotion.

A government-developed health insurance plan should contain self-care incentives, to ensure that costs do not go even higher, and provide funds for consumer classes on basic health care and the home treatment of chronic illnesses.[68] More and better health education is crucial, as most people are unaware of the natural history of common disease and its treatment. Public schools are ideal locations for introducing high-quality self-care programs as children are one of the groups most in need of self-care education. Other foci for increased self-care training should be the elderly and women.

The near future should see a much greater role for nurses in the areas of self-care and health promotion as they begin to move out of the hospitals and assume roles independent from physicians. There will be increased numbers of nurse practitioners whose focus is often on wellness rather than disease and who can do some of the work doctors have done in the past. They will be doing much of the necessary lay education. Professional education of nurses, and physicians as well, will be broadened to introduce curricula early in their training that emphasize aspects of the patient-professional relationship.

An enormous amount of research is needed on the effectiveness of all new efforts in teaching consumers to share responsibility. We are entering a new era and must tread slowly until the most efficacious methods emerge from the many being attempted. Consumer satisfaction, consumer effectiveness and competency in illness situations, and containment of health care costs are crucial outcomes to evaluate.[69] Techniques are needed to ensure that lay persons maintain skills at high levels of effectiveness over long periods of time.

One danger that should be kept in mind as consumers receive health education is that their increased activity may be dominated and controlled by professionals rather than increasingly responsible individuals having a cooperative relationship with the professional structure and thus modifying the basic dependency relationship that they are working to overcome. This and other dangers accompanying the fledgling movement make the road ahead uncertain as we attempt to achieve a better balance between traditional health priorities and individual needs.

REFERENCES

1. Levin, Lowell, "Self-Care: An Emerging Component of the Health Care System." *Hospitals and Health Services Administration* (Winter 1978), pp. 17–25.

2. Ardell, Donald B., *High Level Wellness: An Alternative to Doctors, Drugs, and Disease*. Emmaus, Pa: Rodale Press, 1977.
3. Marieskind, Helen, "The Women's Health Movement." *International Journal of Health Sciences* 5 (1975), pp. 218–223.
4. Illich, Ivan, *Medical Nemesis*. New York: Random House, 1976.
5. Carlson, Rick J., *The End of Medicine*. New York: John Wiley & Sons, 1975.
6. Schwartz, Jerome L., "Motivating for Health—The Self-Care Concept." *Society of Prospective Medicine Proceedings*, 1977.
7. Rothstern, William G., *American Physicians in the Nineteenth Century*. Baltimore: Johns Hopkins University Press, 1972.
8. Thomas, Samuel, *New Guide to Health*. Boston: E. G. House, 1832.
9. Alcott, William A., *The Home Book of Life and Health*. Boston: Phillips, Sampson and Co., 1856.
10. Levin, Lowell, Katz, Alfred, and Holst, Eric, *Self-Care: Lay Initiatives in Health*. New York: Prodist, 1976.
11. Levin, Lowell, "The Layperson as the Primary Health Care Practitioner." *Public Health Reports* 91 (1976), pp. 206–210.
12. Fleming, G. and Anderson, R., *Health Beliefs of the U.S. Population: Implications of Self-Care*. Chicago: Center for Health Administration Studies, 1976.
13. Pratt, Lois, "Changes in Health Care Ideology in Relation to Self-Care by Families." *Health Education Monographs* 5 (Summer 1977), pp. 121–135.
14. Milio, Nancy, "Self-Care in Urban Settings." *Health Education Monographs* 5 (Summer 1977), pp. 136–144.
15. Bogdonoff, M.D. et al., "The Doctor—Patient Relationship." *Journal of the American Medical Association* 192 (April 5, 1965), pp. 131–134.
16. Schain, Wendy S., "Patient's Rights in Decision Making: The Case for Personalism Versus Paternalism in Health Care." *Cancer* 46 (1980), pp. 1035–1041.
17. Ibid.
18. Currie, Bruce and Renner, John, "Patient Education: Developing a Health Care Partnership." *Postgraduate Medicine* 65 (1979), pp. 177–182.
19. Groves, James E., "Taking Care of the Hateful Patient." *New England Journal of Medicine* 298 (1978), pp. 883–887.
20. Glogow, E. "The 'Bad Patient' Gets Better Quicker." *Social Policy* 4 (1973), pp. 72–76.
21. Egger, Ross L., "I Make My Patients Be Their Own Doctors." *Medical Economics* 55 (1978), pp. 83–85.
22. Benarde, Melvin and Mayerson, Evelyn, "Patient-Physician Negotiation." *Journal of the American Medical Association* 239 (1978), pp. 1413–1415.
23. Starfield, Barbara et al. "Patient-Doctor Agreement About Problems Needing Follow-Up Visit." *Journal of the American Medical Association* 242 (1979), pp. 344–346.
24. U.S. Department of Health, Education, and Welfare, *Consumer Self-Care in Health*. Pub. No. (HRA) 77-3181. Washington, D.C.: Department of Health, Education and Welfare, 1977.
25. Shenkin, Budd and Warner, David, " Giving the Patient His Medical Record: A Proposal to Improve the System." *New England Journal of Medicine* 288 (1973), pp. 688–692.
26. Bronson, David L., Rubin, Alas S., and Rufo, Henry M., "Patient Education Through Record Sharing." *QRB* 4 (1978), pp. 2–4.
27. Giglio, R. et al., "Encouraging Behavior Changes by Use of Client-Held Health Records." *Medical Care* 16 (1978), pp. 757–764.
28. Schulman, Beryl A., "Active Patient Orientation and Outcomes in Hypertensive Treatment." *Medical Care* 17 (1979), pp. 267–280.
29. Deeds, Sigrid A. et al., "Patient Behavior for Blood Pressure Control." *Journal of the American Medical Association* 241 (1979), pp. 2534–2537.

30. Etzwiler, Donnell D., "Why Not Put Your Patients Under Contract." *Prism, the American Medical Association* (January 1974), pp. 1–3.
31. Steckel, Susan and Swain, Mary Ann, "Contracting with Patients to Improve Compliance." *Hospitals, Journal of the American Nursing Association* 51 (1977), pp. 81–84.
32. Currie and Renner, *Postgraduate Medicine*.
33. Steckel and Swain, *Hospitals, Journal of the American Nursing Association.*
34. Warner, H. Lynn, "Health Hazard Appraisal—An Instrument for Change." *Proceedings of the Thirteenth Meeting of the Society of Prospective Medicine.* Bethesda, Md.: Health and Education Resources, 1978.
35. Lazare, A., Eisenthal, S., and Wasserman, L., "The Customer Approach to Patienthood." *Archives of General Psychiatry* 32 (1975), pp. 553–558.
36. Lazare, A., Eisenthal, S., and Frank, A., "A Negotiated Approach to the Clinical Encounter." In *Outpatient Psychiatry*, A. Lazare, ed. Baltimore: Williams and Wilkins, 1979, pp. 157–171.
37. Hefferin, E., "Health Goal Setting." *Military Medicine* (1979), pp. 814–822.
38. Rosen, B., "Written Treatment Contracts." *British Journal of Psychiatry* 133 (1978), pp. 410–415.
39. Editorial, "Sign Here for Treatment." *Lancet* (February 3, 1979), p. 252.
40. Osmond, H., Mullaly, R., and Bisbee, C., "The Medical Model and the Responsible Patient." *Hospital and Community Psychiatry* 29 (1978), pp. 522–524.
41. Drye, R., Goulding, R., and Goulding, M. "No Suicide Decisions: Patient Monitoring of Suicide Risk." *American Journal of Psychiatry* 130 (1973), pp. 171–174.
42. Murphy, G. and Guze, S., "Setting Limits: The Management of the Manipulative Patient." *American Journal of Psychotherapy* 12 (1960), pp. 30–47.
43. Skuja, A., "A Self-Control and Contingency Contracting Weight Reduction Program." *Psychological Reports* 38 (1976), pp. 1267–1270.
44. Weiss, R., Birchler, G., and Vincent, J., "Contractual Models for Negotiation Training in Marital Dyads." *Journal of Marriage and Family* 36 (1974), pp. 321–330.
45. Bonime, W., "Dynamics and Psychotherapy of Depression." In *Current Psychiatric Therapies*, Vol. 2, J. Masserman, ed. New York: Grune and Stratton, 1962.
46. Winstead, D. et al., "Diazepam on Demand." *Archives of General Psychiatry* 30 (1974), pp. 349–351.
47. Sehnert, Keith, "Medical Self-Care: An Old Remedy Recurs." *Virginia Medical* (1978), p. 8.
48. Estabrook, Barbara, "Consumer Impact of a Cold Self-Care Center in a Prepaid Ambulatory Care Setting." *Medical Care* 17 (1979), 1139–1145.
49. Green, Lawrence et al., "Research and Demonstration Issues in Self-Care: Measuring the Decline of Medicocentrisim." *Consumer Self-Care in Health.* DHEW No. HRA-3181. Washington, D.C.: Department of Health, Education and Welfare, 1977.
50. Lewis, Mary Ann, "Child-Initiated Care." *American Journal of Nursing* 74 (April 1974), pp. 652–655.
51. Sehnert, Keith, "On Teaching Self-Care to Children." *Medical Self-Care* 2 (Spring 1977), pp. 8–9.
52. Ferguson, Tom, "Teaching Medicine to Kids." *Teacher,* November-December 1979. 1979.
53. Clark, Matt, "Doctoring Yourself." *Newsweek* 93 (1979), p. 89.
54. Sehnert, Keith, *How To Be Your Own Dr. (Sometimes).* New York: Grosset and Dunlap, 1975.
55. Galton, Lawrence, *The Complete Book of Symptoms and What They Can Mean.* New York: Simon and Shuster, 1978.
56. Belsky, Marvin and Gross, Leonard, *How to Choose and Use Your Doctor.* New York: Arbor House, 1975.

57. Levin, Arthur, *Talk Back to Your Doctor*. New York: Doubleday, 1975.

58. Freese, Arthur, *Managing Your Doctor*. Briarcliff Manor, N.Y.: Scarborough House, 1975.

59. Gots, Ronald and Kaufman, Arthur, *The People's Hospital Book*. New York: Crown Publishers, 1978.

60. Vickery, Donald M. and Fries, James F., *Take Care of Yourself*. Reading, Mass.: Addison-Wesley, 1976.

61. "Doctor Says Self-Care Can Save Money." *Health Care Week* 2 (December 18, 1978), p. 8.

62. *Self-Medication: The New Era . . . A Symposium*. Washington, D.C.: The Proprietary Association, 1980.

63. D'Altroy, Lawrence H. et al., "Patient Drug Self-Administration Improves Regimen Compliance." *Hospitals, Journal of the American Hospital Association* 52 (1978), pp. 131–136.

64. Plant, Janet, "Educating the Elderly in Safe Medication Use." *Hospitals, Journal of the American Hospital Association* 51 (1977), pp. 81–87.

65. Ingelfinger, Franz J., "Arrogance." *New England Journal of Medicine* 303 (December 1980), pp. 1507–1511.

66. "Physicians' Biggest Competition Predicted to Come from Patients." *Clinical Psychiatry News* 8 (December 1980), p. 5.

67. Ibid.

68. Stokes, Bruce, "Self-Care: A Nation's Best Health Insurance." *Science* 205 (August 1979), p. 2.

69. U.S. Department of Health, Education, and Welfare. *Consumer Self-Care in Health.*

Index